Microbiology for Veterinary Technicians

TRACY H. VEMULAPALLI, DVM, MS, DACLAM
Clinical Assistant Professor of Laboratory Animal Medicine
Department of Comparative Pathobiology
College of Veterinary Medicine
Purdue University
West Lafayette, IN

G. KENITRA HAMMAC, DVM, PhD, DACVM
Clinical Assistant Professor of Veterinary Diagnostic Microbiology
Department of Comparative Pathobiology
College of Veterinary Medicine
Purdue University
West Lafayette, IN

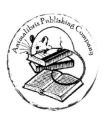

Notices:

This book contains information obtained from
authentic and highly regarded sources. Every
effort has been made to identify copyright
holders and their permission for the use of any
copyrighted materials. Reprinted materials are
quoted courtesy of or with permission, and the
source of the material is indicated. Open
access/public domain images are marked as such.
Reasonable efforts have been made to publish
reliable information, but the authors and the
publisher cannot assume responsibility for the
validity of all materials or for the consequences
of their use.

Knowledge and best practices in the field of
veterinary medicine and microbiology are
constantly evolving. As new knowledge surfaces,
the classification of organisms as well as the
diagnostics used to identify them may change.

ISBN-10: 0692560475
ISBN-13: 978-0692560471

Published by Animalibris Publishing Company
295 Zinnia Street
West Lafayette, IN 47906

Printed in the United States of America

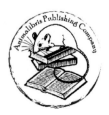

Tracy H Vemulapalli is a veterinarian on
faculty at the College of Veterinary Medicine at
Purdue University where she is a Clinical
Assistant Professor of Laboratory Animal
Medicine. She has a Master's Degree in
Molecular Bacteriology and has been a
diplomate of the American College of
Laboratory Medicine since 2009. She has
experience in small animal private practice, food
safety, and infectious disease research, including
Animal Biosafety Level 3 (ABSL3) work.

G Kenitra Hammac is a veterinarian on faculty
at the College of Veterinary Medicine at Purdue
University where she is a Clinical Assistant
Professor of Microbiology. She heads the
Indiana Animal Disease Diagnostic Laboratory's
Microbiology Section. A diplomate of the
American College of Veterinary Microbiology
since 2014, she has extensive experience in
diagnostic microbiology as well as several years
of experience in small animal private practice.

DEDICATION

To my family, for all their love and support. To my Master's degree and laboratory animal residency advisors, Drs. Nammalwar Sriranganathan and Jerry Davis for their valuable mentorship over the years. To my students, who challenge me every day; I learn as much from you as I hope you do from me. And to my grandmother, Hazel Hearne, who encouraged me to keep writing.

Tracy H. Vemulapalli

To my husband, whose keen sense of adventure and opportunity propelled me into an exciting career in infectious disease. To my children who remind me daily of the joy of learning. To the veterinary technicians who taught me the real world of veterinary practice when I was a young, naive DVM.

G. Kenitra Hammac

Preface

The genesis of this textbook came three years ago when I was asked to become the instructor of record for an undergraduate microbiology class taught at Purdue University's College of Veterinary Medicine that is geared towards the veterinary technician. The administration at the college was looking for someone to restructure the course to meet the changing demands of the veterinary technician and technologist. There was a short timeline to get the class structured and ready for that first semester. Excited at this new challenge, I immediately set about gathering materials for the laboratories and lectures. It was then that I ran into the first major stumbling block – which textbook to use? As I looked and looked it soon became clear to me that far from having to peruse many texts and whittle them down to a single best choice, there were *no* current microbiology textbooks written for veterinary technicians. In fact, the one and only textbook I was able to find was written more than twenty years ago and was no longer in print; I managed to get a copy from a used bookstore. Needless to say, I was flummoxed. Daily, members of the veterinary team are confronted with infectious diseases. Each year, we are confronted with new pathogens that threaten the health and welfare of our patients. And it's my job as an educator to ensure that my students are ready for that challenge. As a veterinarian, I have the utmost respect for the incredible expertise that a licensed veterinary technician or technologist can bring to the veterinary team. Yet they need access to good sources of material from which to learn and consult. Thus, it was clear that the creation of a microbiology textbook for veterinary technicians was more than just a little overdue.

In this book, we have strived to provide pertinent, up-to-date information regarding many different aspects of microbiology. Part I is designed to give the veterinary technician a foundation of basic microbiological structure and function, the role of the immune system in microbial diseases, as well as discussing therapeutics commonly in use today. Parts II and III cover the most common bacterial and fungal agents, respectively, encountered in veterinary medicine today. In Part IV of this book, we discuss diagnostics available to the veterinary technician. While we endeavored to include the latest tests available, newer diagnostic tests are constantly being developed. Such is the speed of medical discovery. In addition, this book mentions specific manufacturers of tests, especially if they are commonly used in clinical practice (e.g., SNAP® tests, IDEXX). Information regarding the relative accuracy and precision of such tests is given if this information is published within the peer-reviewed scientific literature. It should be stated that such information is not an endorsement of the products by the authors of this book, nor do the authors have any financial interests in these products.

Throughout the book, special attention was paid to facets of the veterinary technician's role as a member of the veterinary team. Veterinary technicians are often asked to take a history from the owner of an animal prior to the veterinarian performing the physical exam. Thus, included in this textbook are discussions on aspects of history-taking related to particular diseases and pathogens (e.g., timing of spontaneous abortions in pregnant animals can sometimes help rule-out certain diseases). Another common task the technician is asked to perform is delivering the discharge instructions and relaying educational information to clients (i.e., client education). Common points to discuss with clients regarding important issues such as biosecurity, zoonotic potential, and prognosis of various infectious diseases are laid out in each chapter. Lastly, there is an important aspect that directly affects the health and welfare of each and every member of the veterinary team – zoonotic diseases. Therefore, important safety precautions for pathogens with the potential to infect humans are discussed.

A note about image credits: all photos and illustrations obtained from outside sources have been given appropriate credit within the figure legend. All other (uncredited) images (e.g., photos, charts, and illustrations) are the work of the authors and they solely retain the copyright to them. However, for those interested in reproducing our images, prior written permission may be obtained.

Finally, on behalf of Kenitra and myself, I would like to express our thanks for all the contributors and reviewers of this book. We are grateful for the support and patience of all those involved in this project, especially when short turnaround times were needed. We also wish to thank all of the veterinary technician students we have had the privilege in getting to know as they pursue their degrees in veterinary technology. The feedback they gave us, both on the class and on their "wish list" for what to include in a textbook, was invaluable. We hope that veterinary technician students (past, present, and future) find this book useful both as a textbook and as a frequently consulted reference.

Tracy H Vemulapalli
West Lafayette, IN
December 1, 2015

ACKNOWLEDGMENTS

This work would not have been possible without the important contributions of numerous colleagues, friends, and family. First, we owe a huge debt to the many scientists and veterinary professionals who let us include their color images in this book. Microbiology is in no small part a *visual* science and the inclusion of these wonderful images will help veterinary technicians understand the importance and complexity of microbes and the diseases they cause. Thank you so much for your generosity.

In creating a brand new textbook, it takes a significant amount of time to map out the proposed scope of the book. We gratefully acknowledge the help and advice of our colleagues, but most especially to Dr. Mohamed Seleem, DVM, PhD who really helped in fine-tuning the scope of this book to our unique audience: veterinary technician and technology students. Throughout the process, this book has undergone numerous revisions and edits with the goal of making it a most useful and easy-to-understand textbook. Many thanks to Julie Roarhig and Josh Clark (instructors in our veterinary technician program) who tirelessly reviewed the manuscript for readability, content errors, and general editing. Josh, you are now officially a member of the "That/Which Police."

Special thanks to Manuel (Manny) Benitez for providing the laboratory support that allowed us to take such beautiful microbiology photos. You are the master of "streaking for isolation"! We owe you one!

A big thanks to our families for putting up with us for the more than two years that we spent from concept to completion on this book. Finally, an apology to our children who accidentally saw a larger-than-life-sized photo of caseous necrosis on our computer monitor. We hope you'll forgive us someday.

Contents

Part I:

Fundamentals of Veterinary Microbiology

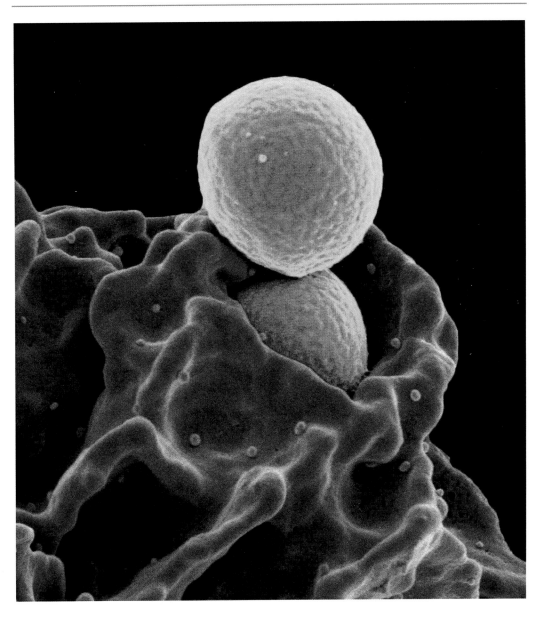

Photo (previous page):

MRSA, ingestion by neutrophil. Colorized SEM. Courtesy of the National Institute of Allergy and Infectious Diseases (NIAID). NIH Image Bank, Washington, DC, 2009.

Chapter 1:

An Introduction to Microbiology

"Science knows no country, because knowledge belongs to humanity, and is the torch which illuminates the world."

— *Louis Pasteur, 1876*

What is Microbiology?

Simply put, **microbiology** is the "branch of biology that deals with microorganisms and their effects on other living organisms."[1] These tiny organisms include bacteria, viruses, some fungi, and some parasitic organisms.

Why is Microbiology so Important?

Microbiology plays many useful roles in our lives. Life on earth was made possible because of bacteria (e.g., global geochemical cycles, creation of an ozone layer by adding molecular oxygen).The term **microbes** refers to microscopic organisms. Talk to people about microbes and most will think of germs and the diseases they cause. In reality, most microbes do not cause harm at all.

Many microbes, contrary to harming us, actually protect us from disease. For example, the human gastrointestinal tract contains well over 100 trillion microbes. If you could remove these bacteria from the gut, they would weigh almost 2 kg! These bacteria live in a peaceful, mutually beneficial relationship with their hosts (i.e., us). What do we get out of it? The bacteria eat and metabolize the food that we eat and break it down into usable molecules that are carried into our bloodstream and then into the cells that need the energy from those molecules. We get our food broken down more easily and the bacteria get a free meal. It's a "win-win" situation!

In addition, bacteria are used in the food industry (Figure

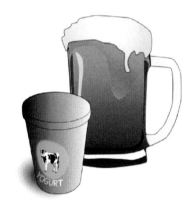

Figure 1.1: **Microbes play a significant role in our day-to-day activities.** Bacteria, through a process called fermentation, are used to create a variety of different food products such as yogurt and beer.

---

[1] Stedman, Thomas Lathrop. The American Heritage Stedman's Medical Dictionary. 2nd ed. Boston: Houghton Mifflin, 2004. Print.

1.1). They act as bioconversion "machines" in processes like fermentation and nitrogen capture. Fermentation of milk by the bacterium *Lactobacillus acidophilus* creates yogurt. Other products that require fermentation include such foods as beer and sauerkraut. Bacteria are also involved in nitrogen capture and utilization. For example, soybeans interact with nitrogen-fixing soil bacteria called rhizobia. The rhizobia give the soybeans nitrogen while the soybeans provide much needed carbohydrates as a source of energy for the rhizobia.

A Short History of Microbiology

Many scientists and non-scientists alike have made significant contributions to the field of microbiology. It is impossible in a few short paragraphs to do their contributions justice. Here are the contributions from just a few of the key individuals that helped propel the discipline forward and increase our understanding of the microscopic world.

Anton van Leeuwenhoek (1632-1723)

Born in 1632, Anton van Leeuwenhoek thought he would follow his father's merchant footsteps and become a cloth seller in his native Holland. However, in his spare time, the ever curious Leeuwenhoek became a self-taught scientist. While others of his era gazed at things far bigger than themselves – the stars, planets, and the celestial heavens – Leeuwenhoek was fascinated by what could not be seen. Not yet, anyway. His biggest and most memorable contribution to the field was the invention of the light microscope. It was well known that glass could be ground into the shape of a lens and that things would appear much larger than they really were when viewed through these lenses. Grinding his own glass to make the most precise lenses necessary, he spent countless hours perfecting this new apparatus. One day after a heavy rainstorm, he placed a drop of rain water on the end of a very finely pointed glass straw. He viewed the tiny raindrop using one of his new lenses and observed the teeming life within. As the single-celled organisms contained within the raindrop darted to and fro under his gaze, he recorded all that he saw, naming the creatures "**animalcules**" to distinguish them from inanimate molecules. He began to look at everything he could get a hold of and scrutinized them using his immaculately constructed lenses. Leeuwenhoek meticulously recorded everything he observed. Modern microscopy was born.

Louis Pasteur (1822-1895)

Almost two hundred years after Leeuwenhoek's discovery of tiny animalcules, a French chemist by the name of Louis Pasteur was using his skills to strengthen acceptance of **germ theory**, the idea that microorganisms are the cause of diseases. This professor of chemistry went on to prove that some bacteria could survive, indeed even depended upon living, in an environment completely devoid of oxygen. Today, we call these bacteria **anaerobes**. He identified the parasite that was infecting silkworms and devastating the silk industry and developed methods to ensure only disease-free silkworms were used in breeding, thus saving the industry. He created the process of super-heating and then cooling liquids, such as milk, to render them free from bacteria in a process we now call **pasteurization**. Pasteur also created the first vaccines for anthrax, rabies, and chicken cholera.

We might not have life-saving vaccines were it not for a happy little accident in Pasteur's laboratory. Pasteur had already hit upon the idea that giving a person or animal "a little" of a disease, like *Bacillus anthracis*, might protect one from dying from the actual disease (i.e., anthrax). The problem was in deciding the dose. Not enough bacteria in the inoculation and the individual would not develop immunity to the natural disease. Too much and the individual wouldn't need protecting – they'd need an undertaker. This was hardly the kind of risks most people were willing to take.

Pasteur began to tinker with how to make vaccination safer. He chose to experiment on a vaccine to protect chickens from a deadly disease known as fowl cholera. The initial results, as you might imagine, were rather hit-or-miss. Then one day, during one experiment, Pasteur gave a set of unvaccinated chickens a "little" dose of cholera. When Pasteur entered the laboratory the next day, he was shocked to find that not one of the chickens had gotten sick or died. In fact, they were happily strutting about completely unfazed. Thinking that they'd used a bad batch of culture, Pasteur again dosed the chickens with a proven live fatal dose of cholera bacteria. Again, the chickens lived. An investigation revealed that the original cholera culture was an old one and that the cholera bacteria had been weakened by age. This first dose protected the chickens from the second otherwise fatal dose. This was the way to make vaccines safer! They must be weakened to a point that they could not cause the death of the animal but the animal would mount an immune response to them. Vaccines can be made from weakened or killed bacteria or viruses. This was the beginning of the creation of the "modified-live" and "killed" vaccines that we use to this day.

Joseph Lister (1827-1912)

Those in the medical field owe a huge debt of gratitude to English surgeon Joseph Lister, the father of aseptic technique. In his clinical practice, Dr. Lister noticed that open bony fractures often resulted in copious amounts of pus being produced. He surmised that the cause of the suppuration (i.e., pus formation) was due to the "decomposition" of the tissues. If he could only prevent this decomposition, perhaps his patients might stand a better chance of surviving the surgery and making a better long-term recovery. To do this, he had to find a way to destroy any of the "septic" germs that were introduced into the wound at the time of the accident or in the time that had elapsed before the patient was brought to the surgery table. Indeed, it was these same germs that were responsible for much of the decomposition of the tissues.

His solution: carbolic acid. Gauze sponges soaked in a dilute solution of carbolic acid were applied to the open fracture site to kill any bacteria present. Patients treated with this "antiseptic" solution survived and thrived as compared to those patients who did not receive Lister's care. He published his findings in 1867, just two years after the American Civil War ended. Lister quickly broadened usage of antiseptics to include swabbing the intact skin to cleanse it in preparation for surgery. In an era before the use of latex surgical gloves, he insisted that anyone performing or assisting in surgery should "purify" their skin using carbolic acid. Perhaps some of his patients still weren't enamored with the idea of going through surgery – who is? But at least they knew they'd now stand a good chance of surviving it!

Robert Koch (1843-1910)

Someone charting Robert Koch's early medical career would never have guessed this young doctor's eventual impact on microbiology. After graduating from the University of Gottingen in Germany, he spent his internship doctoring the insane in an asylum in Hamburg. Shortly thereafter, after he became a village doctor, his wife gave him a microscope as a gift so that he could develop a hobby. Koch was not satisfied with the state of medicine during this time. For all of Pasteur's (and numerous others') elegant experiments on the presence of microbes and the refutation of spontaneous generation, little was known about the link between microbes and disease. Luckily for science – and us – Koch was a stickler for good scientific method. It was not sufficient to prove something once. It must hold true again and again and under a myriad of different conditions.

Koch's biggest and most lasting contribution to microbiology started with a disease that left veterinarians and physicians alike stumped – anthrax. At the time of Koch's work, anthrax (Chapter 8) was killing whole herds of animals in a most horrific fashion. They became ill with the disease, and death followed soon afterward. This was no peaceful way to die; animals literally bled out of every orifice of their body. When Koch set to investigating anthrax, he noticed that he could isolate some unusual looking long rod-shaped bacteria from the tissues of animals ill with or that had died from anthrax. But were these *particular* rod-shaped bacteria to blame? After all, our bodies are filled with bacteria. At the same time, he could never find any of these rod-shaped bacteria in healthy animals. What he did next is what sets him apart from his scientific predecessors. He decided that he had to get some of these bacteria from the ill/dead animals, grow the bacteria in pure culture, and then give it to an animal known to be free of these odd little rod-shaped bacteria. If the healthy animal developed the disease it must be because of the bacteria he'd grown in pure culture. In every species of animal he tried – and he tried quite a few – the animals developed and died from anthrax. From these experiments Koch developed a series of five postulates. In order to prove that a microbe is responsible for the disease condition seen in the animal or person, all of Koch's Postulates must be fulfilled (see "The Key to Causation: Koch's Postulates").

The Key to Causation: Koch's Postulates
Microorganisms must be:
1. Present in every person/animal with the disease
2. Absent in healthy individuals
3. Capable of being isolated and grown in pure culture
4. Capable of causing the same disease when inoculated into a healthy host
5. Re-isolated from the experimentally infected host

When Do Koch's Postulates Fail Us?
There are times where scientists cannot fulfill all of the postulates set forth by Koch. The biggest obstacle is often in isolating the organism and growing it in a pure culture. Some microbes are incredibly picky about where and how they wish to live. Some microbes require a life spent inside living cells and, thus, depend on cell-based culture systems. While both cell-free and cell-based culture procedures have improved since Koch's death in 1910, there are still some organisms (e.g., certain intracellular bacteria, prions) that cannot be grown in culture. These, therefore, fail to fulfill all of Koch's postulates even though they may indeed be the cause of a given disease.

The Five Kingdoms
Scientific classification is a hierarchical system of grouping organisms by similar structure and function. Over the years, many classification systems have been developed – most famously by Swedish biologist Carl Linnaeus. Using the modern system of classification, all life on the planet Earth can be grouped into one of the five main kingdoms. Each kingdom is made up of many phyla. Each phylum is split into many classes. For our purposes, the lowest and most specific taxonomic nomenclature is at the species level. However, even species can be further divided into subspecies and varieties. The often cited mnemonic "King Philip Came Over For Good Spaghetti" can be used to help students remember the taxonomic hierarchy (Figure 1.2).

The five kingdoms are: Monera, Protista, Fungi, Plantae, and Animalia. Bacteria and fungi, both covered in this textbook, are classified under the kingdoms Monera and Fungi, respectively. Each kingdom has several features which distinguish them from one another. Examples of these distinguishing features may be seen in Table 1.1.

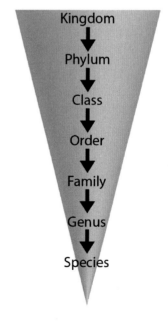

Eukaryotes versus Prokaryotes
The simplest division between organisms is whether or not they can

Figure 1.2: Scientific classification of organisms.

be classified as prokaryotes or eukaryotes. Prokaryotes are unicellular organisms and are found within the kingdom Monera. Eukaryotes may be unicellular or multicellular and may be found in the other four kingdoms of life. The differences between prokaryotes and eukaryotes lie mainly in their cellular organization and are summarized in Table 1.2.

Table 1.1: The five kingdoms

	Monera	Protista	Fungi	Plantae	Animalia
Cell type	Prokaryote	Eukaryote	Eukaryote	Eukaryote	Eukaryote
Organization	Unicellular	Unicellular	Uni- or Multicellular	Multicellular	Multicellular
Cell wall	Yes*	Variable	Yes	Yes	No
Nutrition	Absorption or photosynthesis	Ingestion or absorption	Absorption	Absorption or photosynthesis	Ingestion
Reproduction	Asexual	Mostly asexual	Both asexual & sexual	Both asexual & sexual	Mostly sexual
Example	Bacteria	Amoeba	Fungi	Plants	Humans

*Some exceptions exist, e.g., mycoplasmas do not have a cell wall.

Table 1.2: Key differences between prokaryotic and eukaryotic cells

Structural Characteristic	Eukaryotic Cell	Prokaryotic Cell
Nucleus surrounded by nuclear membrane	Present	Absent
Number of Chromosomes	More than one	One[†]
Cell type	Usually multicellular	Unicellular
Selected Organelles: Lysosomes	Present	Absent
Microtubules	Present	Absent
Cytoskeleton	Present	May be absent
Endoplasmic Reticulum	Present	Absent
Mitochondria	Present	Absent
Golgi Apparatus	Present	Absent
Cell size	10-100 µm	1-10 µm

[†]A few bacteria are known to carry two chromosomes, but they are the exception to the rule.

Further Reading

Lister, Baron Joseph. "The Classic: On the Antiseptic Principle in the Practice of Surgery." *Clinical Orthopaedics and Related Research*® 468 8 (2010): 2012-16.

Chapter 2:

Tools of the Trade – Microscopy

"The microscope or the telescope, which of the two has the grander view?"

— *Victor Hugo, Les Miserables, 1862*

Introduction

In order to become proficient at microbiology, members of the veterinary team must become proficient users of the tools of the trade. Of the many tools used, the microscope is one of the most valuable. In this chapter we will discuss the types of microscopes available, when to use them, and their relative merits. Additionally, we will learn the different methods by which we can estimate the size of an organism we are viewing through the microscope. This is a vital skill that will help us when attempting to identify microorganisms by sight.

Before we discuss the different types of microscopes, there are several properties that apply to all microscopes. One of the most important features of a microscope is its ability to distinguish between two closely positioned objects. **Resolution** is defined as the shortest distance between two points on a specimen that can be distinguished visually by the observer. The term **magnification** indicates how enlarged an object appears (i.e., the **image size**) when compared to the actual size of the object being observed. The specifications of resolution and magnification are very important to consider when choosing which microscope type is required to best visualize a particular sample.

Types of Microscopes

Light Microscopy

The most common instrument found in today's microbiology laboratory is the **light microscope**. The light microscope is also referred to as a light field microscope, to differentiate it from the dark field microscope (discussed next). As its name suggests, in light microscopy it is the transmission of light through the specimen that allows us to visualize the specimen. Some of the light that traverses through the specimen is absorbed by it, and therefore the specimen appears darker than the surrounding brightly illuminated field. This provides some contrast allowing us to visualize the specimen. However, a dye, or stain, is often required to enhance visualization of the specimen. Stains are discussed later in this chapter. The resolution limit of most light microscopes is approximately 0.2-1 micrometer (μm). Units of measurement used in microscopy are reviewed in Table 2.1.

Table 2.1: Common units of measure used in microbiology

Unit	Prefix	Absolute measurement (m)
meter (m)		1
centimeter (cm)	*centi* = one hundredth	0.01 (10^{-2})
millimeter (mm)	*milli* = one thousandth	0.001 (10^{-3})
micrometer (μm)	*micro* = one millionth	0.000001 (10^{-6})
nanometer (nm)	*nano* = one billionth	0.000000001 (10^{-9})
Angstrom (Å)		0.0000000001 (10^{-10})

Dark Field Microscopy

In dark field microscopy, unstained specimens are illuminated against a black background. Dark field microscopy is particularly useful in microbiology for visualizing extremely thin spiral-shaped bacteria known as spirochetes (see Chapter 16). Spirochetes are so thin and threadlike that they cannot be easily visualized using light microscopy even when stained with a cytological dye for better contrast. Depending upon the quality of the microscope, the resolution limits of dark field microscopy are typically around 0.2 μm. Dark field microscopes are usually only found in reference microbiology laboratories.

Electron Microscopy

As stated above, the resolution limit of most light microscopes is approximately 0.2-1 micrometer (μm). This is just about the size of most bacteria. In order to see smaller structures, such as viruses, requires the use of electron microscopy. Electron microscopy allows for the visualization of objects that are as small as or smaller than 1 nanometer (nm), which is equal to 1 millionth of a millimeter! An electron microscope creates an image of the sample by first bombarding it with electrons. The scatter of these electrons are then collected and recorded as an image.

There are two types of electron microscopes: the **scanning electron microscope** (SEM) and the **transmission electron microscope** (TEM). A scanning electron microscope is used to visualize the surface of structures. Transmission electron microscopes are used to visualize the internal structures of an object, such as the organelles of a eukaryotic cell. Given the highly technical nature of these microscopes, there use is limited to research institutions and some reference laboratories.

Using the Light Microscope Effectively in Microbiology

In the rest of this chapter we will discuss how to most effectively use the light microscope, the most common type of microscope used in veterinary medicine, to aid us in our study of microbiology.

A good quality binocular microscope, with adjustable ocular lenses, is vital to both clinical and research microbiology laboratories. The microscope should have at least three objective lenses: 10x, 40x (high dry), and 100x (oil immersion) objectives. The one that is of the most utility for visualizing bacteria will be the 100x objective. Because bacteria are very small, it is important that the sample is well lit. Therefore, the veterinary technician should be well acquainted with the proper setup and adjustment of the microscope (e.g., adjustment of the sub-stage condenser, iris diaphragm, and diffuser). Refer to the user's manual of your microscope to ensure proper setup before attempting to visualize specimens.

Magnification

As mentioned above, magnification indicates how enlarged an object appears (i.e., the image size) when compared to the actual size of the object being observed. The total magnification of an object is the product of the magnification number of the ocular and the objective lenses. Most light microscopes have 10x ocular lenses.

> **Example:** When viewing a bacterium at the high dry objective (40x) any objects will be magnified 400 times.
>
> Ocular × Objective = Total magnification
>
> (10) × (40) = 400

Estimating Size Using a Light Microscope

When trying to identify bacteria, it is useful to be able to estimate their size. This can help in the ultimate diagnosis of the bacteria responsible for the animal's infection. There are several methods the veterinary technician can use to estimate the size of the bacteria when examining glass slides. Some light microscopes have a built-in ocular ruler, called a **reticle** (Figure 2.1). The reticle must be calibrated using a calibrated **stage micrometer slide**. Objects in the microscope field of view will appear larger or smaller depending upon the objective lens used. Therefore, the object is measured using the micrometer and a conversion factor is used to determine the actual size of the object being observed.

If an ocular reticule is not available, a veterinary technician can use a "biological micrometer" to determine the size of the bacteria viewed on the glass slide. This technique requires the comparison of the size of the bacterium to a reference cell. The two most common reference cells used are the red blood cell (RBC) (Figure 2.2) and the neutrophil. In the dog, the size of a healthy RBC is approximately 7 µm in diameter, while the neutrophil is 12 µm on average.

Table 2.2 lists the average RBC diameter of the common species seen in veterinary medical practice.

Table 2.2: Average size of the erythrocytes of common veterinary species

Species (Adult)	RBC size (µm)
Dog	7.0
Cat	5.8
Rabbit	6.4
Horse	5.5
Cow	5.8
Pig	6.0

Stains Used in Light Microscopy

In order to most effectively visualize a specimen, it is often necessary to apply a dye, or **cytological stain**, to it. Numerous stains are available. We will discuss the most common stains used in veterinary microbiology laboratories. Some stains merely provide enough contrast to aid in visualization while others stains aid in the differentiation of one cell type or structure from another.

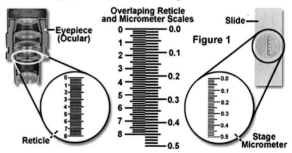

Eyepiece Reticles and Stage Micrometers

Figure 2.1: Comparison of an eyepiece reticle and a stage micrometer. Photo used with permission by Nikon, Inc.

Cytologic Stains

There are numerous stains available to the veterinary technician to aid in the visualization of cytological specimen preparations. Stains commonly used to visualize bacterial cells include: Gram, Acid Fast, India ink, Methylene Blue, and Giemsa stains. To visualize fungi and yeast, typical stains used include: Lactophenol cotton blue, India ink, Gomori Methenamine Silver (GMS) and Periodic acid-Schiff (PAS).

Specifics as to determining when to use and how to apply each of these cytological stains will be covered in Chapter 22.

Tissue Stains

Veterinarians often send tissues to a pathology laboratory for histologic examination. For example, they might send a small piece of a "lump" found on the skin of the dog. *What is causing the mass? Inflammation? Infection? Cancer?* When the sample is processed for histopathology, a stain is applied to allow better visualization and contrast of the histological structures of the specimen, just as in cytology. The most common stain is Hematoxylin and Eosin (H&E) stain. While this stain is quite good at visualizing mammalian histologic tissue structures such as epithelial skin cells and the adnexa, it is not a good stain for visualizing bacteria or fungi. Special stains such as the Brown and Brenn, a tissue Gram stain, are needed. Histologic specimens are best examined by a board-certified veterinary pathologist.

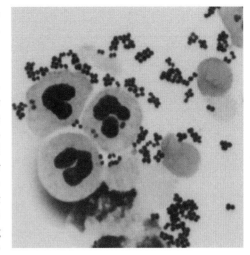

Figure 2.2: **Using a patient's blood cells as an internal micrometer for measuring the size of bacteria present in a sample.** The diameters of neutrophils (~12 μm) and red blood cells (~7 μm) can be used to estimate the size of bacteria if they are simultaneously present in a sample. Using this method, you could line up about 12 of the bacteria end-to-end across the diameter of the neutrophil. Therefore, the bacterial cocci in this sample are estimated to be approximately 1/12th the diameter of the neutrophil, or approximately 1 μm in diameter. Photo courtesy of Dr.Craig Thompson, Purdue University.

For Further Reading

JoVE Science Education Database. General Laboratory Techniques. Introduction to Light Microscopy. JoVE, Cambridge, MA, (2015). Web. http://www.jove.com/science-education/5041/introduction-to-light-microscopy

Stockham, Steven L., and Michael A. Scott. *Fundamentals of Veterinary Clinical Pathology.* 1st ed. Ames: Iowa State Press, 2002.

Weiss, Douglas J., and Jane K. Wardrop. *Schalm's Veterinary Hematology.* 6th ed. United States: Wiley, John & Sons, Incorporated, 2010.

Chapter 3:

An Introduction to Bacteria

"If you don't like bacteria, you're on the wrong planet. This is the planet of bacteria."

— *Craig Venter (geneticist, first to sequence the human genome), 2007*

Introduction

In chapter 1, we discussed the differences between prokaryotic and eukaryotic cells. In this chapter we will expand on the structural characteristics of bacterial cells and how they differ from eukaryotic cells.

Bacterial Cell Structures

Bacterial DNA

Deoxyribonucleic acid (DNA) contains the genetic sequences encoding all of the structural and functional components of a cell (Figure 3.1). Bacteria generally only have one **chromosome** (DNA), although there are a few exceptions (e.g., *Brucella suis*). Bacteria may also carry additional DNA in the form of plasmids. A **plasmid** is a circular double-stranded piece of DNA. Plasmids are self-replicating. That is, plasmids have all of the required "machinery" for making additional copies of themselves and do not have to rely on the host's (in this case, the bacterium's) replication mechanism. Plasmid DNA often encodes useful, but not entirely necessary, genes. If the plasmid were to be lost from the bacterium, the bacterium could still survive. Many plasmids contain genes encoding for antibiotic resistance. Antibiotic resistance is an ever-growing concern in veterinary medicine and will be covered in subsequent chapters.

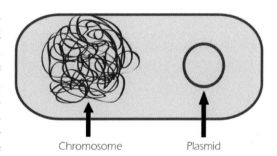

Figure 3.1: **Bacterial chromosome and plasmid.** The chromosome is a highly folded circular, double-stranded piece of DNA. The genes that are necessary to sustain life are contained in the chromosome. The majority of bacterial species carry only one chromosome per cell. In contrast, a single bacterium may carry from 1-20 plasmids. Like chromosomes, plasmids are made up of circular, double-stranded DNA. Helpful, but not absolutely necessary genes, are often found on plasmids (e.g., antimicrobial resistance genes).

The Cytoplasm

The cytoplasm is not just the location where the bacterial DNA sloshes about. In fact, it is a very congested and busy place. The bulk of the cytoplasm is made up of water. However, within the watery matrix many other essential components are found. These include:

- Enzymes
- Dissolved oxygen (not all bacteria)
- Essential nutrients
- Building blocks of life – proteins, carbohydrates, lipids
- Nucleic acids – DNA, RNA
- Ribosomes
- Waste products

The Cell Wall

The cell wall is responsible for holding all of the constituents of the cytoplasm contained within. It also acts as a protective barrier for the bacterium. The cell wall consists of many different layers. Associated with the cell wall, the **cell membrane** consists of a double layer of phospholipid sheets. Interspersed within the cell membrane are various structural proteins, some of which aid in the transport of nutrients across the cell membranes and into the bacterial cell. **Peptidoglycan** is a structural polymer consisting of polysaccharide and peptide chains. The two most common components of the peptidoglycan layer are teichoic acid and lipoteichoic acid.

The actual number and type of these layers within the cell wall differs between different bacterial species. These differences can be seen most dramatically by the way in which the cells take up a common cell stain, the **Gram stain**. The so-called "gram-negative" bacteria have walls that consist of a layer of peptidoglycan sandwiched in between the inner and outer cell membranes. Gram-positive bacteria cell walls contain only a single (inner) cell membrane and an outer layer of peptidoglycan. The layers can be seen in Figure 3.2.

A third category of bacteria that relies on its response to staining, the acid-fast bacteria, will be discussed in a subsequent chapter. More information as to how the cell wall structure relates to its Gram stain characteristics can be found in Chapter 22.

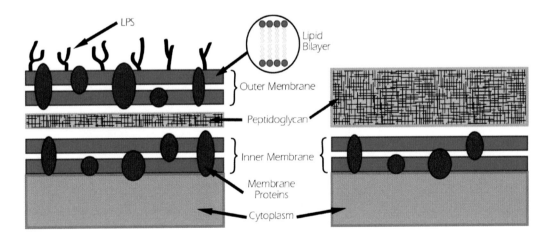

Figure 3.2: Bacterial cell wall of gram-negative (left) and gram-positive (right) bacteria. Both types of bacteria contain cytoplasm, an inner membrane, and a peptidoglycan layer. However, the amount of peptidoglycan in gram-positive bacteria greatly exceeds that of gram-negative bacteria. Gram-negative bacteria carry the additional structures of an outer membrane and lipopolysaccharide (LPS). For specifics on each of these structures and their relevance, see body text.

Capsule

Some bacteria are capable of producing a **capsule**. The capsule is an outer protective layer made up of polysaccharides. Some capsules also contain various lipids and proteins. Many bacterial capsules are **antiphagocytic**, meaning that macrophages and other immune cells that would normally engulf (eat) the bacterium cannot do so. Also, encapsulated bacteria tend to be harder to kill when using disinfectants, such as bleach or quaternary ammonia compounds (e.g., Pine-Sol® cleaner).

Lipopolysaccharide (LPS)

Lipopolysaccharide, or LPS, is a unique feature of gram-negative organisms found in the phospholipid layer of the outer membrane of gram-negative bacteria. Lipopolysaccharide is made up of three subunits: lipid A, core oligosaccharide and O-antigen (Figure 3.3). We know from biochemistry that, by themselves, saccharides (sugars) are not very antigenic. However, the lipid A phospholipid (also called: **endotoxin**) can produce a process called **endotoxic shock** in people and animals. Endotoxic shock is characterized by a hyperactive immune system that creates severe, generalized inflammation.

The amount of LPS present on a bacterium's surface influences their appearance on artificial growth media like agar. Bacteria producing large amounts of LPS will appear "smooth" while bacteria producing little to no LPS are deemed to have a "rough" appearance (Figure 3.4).

Bacterial Cell Morphology

Bacteria come in all shapes and sizes. Along with a bacterium's Gram stain characteristic, cell shape can be very helpful when trying to identify which genus and species of bacteria are responsible for a given infection. When bacterial cells reproduce by asexual division, the divisions between the cells can give rise to several different cell arrangements. These arrangements include chains, tetrads, and clusters. The term **pleomorphic** is used to describe bacterial genera that can assume more than one shape type depending upon

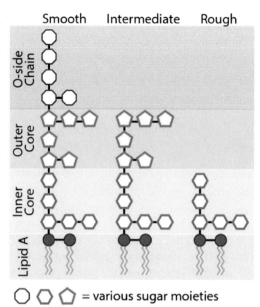

○ ⬡ ⬠ = various sugar moieties

Figure 3.3: The structure of lipopolysaccharide (LPS). LPS is made up of several subunits including lipid A, core polysaccharides, and the oligosaccharide (O) side chain. Lipid A is a lipid which anchors the LPS to the outer membrane of gram-negative cells. Various sugar molecules make up the core and O-side chain of LPS.

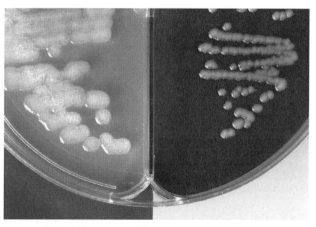

Figure 3.4: Smooth and rough forms of *Bacillus anthracis*. Colonies on the left (bicarbonate agar) are producing copious LPS resulting in smooth colonies. The colonies on the right (blood agar) aren't, thus resulting in the rough colony phenotype. The rough colonies look "drier" and more "pixilated" than the glistening smooth colonies. Courtesy of the Public Health Image Library, PHIL #1165, Centers for Disease Control and Prevention, Atlanta, 1980.

the environmental conditions the organism is found under. Figure 3.5 summarizes the typical shapes and arrangements of bacterial cells.

Flagella

Some bacteria are equipped with structures that help them move (i.e., motile bacteria). **Flagella** consist of three or more thread-like proteins, called flagellins, that are twisted upon each other like a rope. The ropelike flagella can then spiral and twist (e.g., like the propeller on a motor boat) and both power and steer the bacterium to its destination. The location and number of the flagella helps determine the type and direction of motility the bacterium is capable of executing (Figure 3.6). **Monotrichous** bacteria possess a single polar flagellum. **Amphitrichous** bacterium contain two flagella, one on each pole (end) of the bacterium. **Peritrichous** and **lophotrichous** bacteria contain multiple flagella. Flagella associated with lophotrichous bacteria are localized to one pole of the bacterium, where as peritrichous flagella are interspersed over the bacterium's entire surface.

Pili and Fimbriae

Pili are long, thick hair-like structures made of polymerized protein molecules, called pilin. They arise from the bacterial cytoskeleton and traverse the cell wall and capsule (if present) and may be visualized protruding from the cell surface. Pili are most often found on gram-negative bacteria. Functionallly, pili attach the bacterium to different surfaces. This is important for two reasons. One, attachment is the first step to colonizing a surface. In the case of **pathogenic** (i.e., disease-causing) bacteria, this may be followed by invasion into the cell. Second, pili are important for sexual reproduction of some species of bacteria. This specialized pilus is termed the **sex pilus**. Sexual reproduction (or "conjugation") and the role of the sex pilus will be discussed later in this chapter. **Fimbriae** are tiny, bristle-like structures distributed evenly over the entire surface of the bacterial cell (Figure 3.7). Like pili, they aid bacteria in adhering to surfaces. Unlike flagella, neither pili nor fibriae are used in motility.

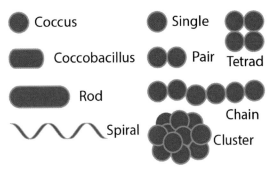

Figure 3.5: Common bacterial shapes and cellular arrangements. Cocci (sing.: coccus) are bacteria that are spherical. Elongated bacteria are referred to as rods, or alternately as bacilli (sing: bacillus). A bacterium that is an extremely short, rounded rod is classified as coccobacillus. Threadlike bacteria that assume a spiral shape are called spiral organisms. When examining bacteria in the microscope, bacteria may assume many cellular arrangements including singles, pairs, tetrads, chains, and clusters.

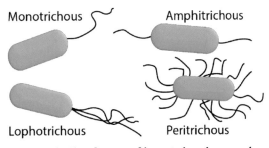

Figure 3.6: Classification of bacteria based on number and location of flagella present. For an explanation of each term, see the body text.

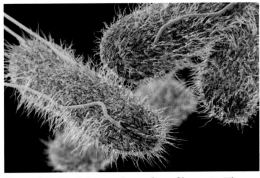

Figure 3.7: Fimbriae on the surface of bacteria. The surface of the bacteria seen here, *Salmonella* serotype Typhi, are covered with numerous thin, wispy fimbriae. The thicker, rope like structures are flagella. Courtesy of the Public Health Image Library, PHIL #16877, Centers for Disease Control and Prevention, Atlanta, 2013.

Factors Affecting the Survival and Growth of Bacteria

Nutrition

Bacteria are very busy microbes. They attach and colonize surfaces. They reproduce faster than rabbits – some at a doubling rate of 20 minutes! They may even cause disease. All of this furious activity requires energy in the form of food. So what's on the dinner plate of a typical bacterium?

The primary food source for bacteria is carbohydrates. Carbohydrates provide a carbon source from which new chemical compounds are made, such as amino acids and sugar molecules. They also provide energy. Glucose is the most common "carb" source for bacteria.

Other sources of nutrition include proteins, water, and minerals. Proteins provide a ready source of nitrogen which can be broken down into amino acids and then rebuilt into new and different proteins based on the bacterium's needs. Other elemental needs are in the form of phosphorus, sulfur, iron, and calcium.

Temperature: The Story of the Three Little Bacteria

Some of us love the summer and hate those long frigid winters. Others can't wait for the first snowfall and droop miserably in the long, hot muggy summers. Each of us has a unique preference for a certain temperature. Bacteria are no different.

Each species of bacteria has a temperature range that is necessary for ideal growth. If those same bacteria find themselves outside of their optimal temperature range, their growth rate suffers. If they find themselves well outside of their ideal range, the bacteria may not be able to survive. **Psychrophiles** are those bacteria that love the cold; they grow best at anywhere from 0-30°C. **Thermophiles** (Figure 3.8) like it hot! Their preferred temperature range is between 40-80°C. Some thermophiles may even survive the process of pasteurization. And finally, just like Baby Bear in the story "Goldilocks and the Three Bears," **mesophiles** find the intermediate temperature range between 20-40°C *just* right." In fact, some mesophiles have a very tight temperature range in which to grow optimally; this is usually at or just below normal body temperature, between 35-37°C.

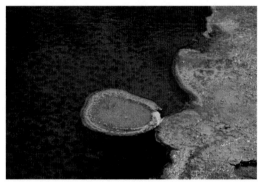

Figure 3.8: **Thermophiles can live in some pretty steamy places.** Here is a bacterial mat (orange) floating atop the sulfurous waters of one of the many hot springs near "Old Faithful", Yellowstone National Park, Wyoming.

Bacterial Respiration

While bacteria don't contain lungs, they do need to respire, that is, exchange gasses in order to provide energy in the form of electrons for their cellular processes. We can classify bacteria by the primary gas and the amount of that gas they use for respiration (Table 3.1).

Table 3.1: Terms used to describe gas requirements for respiration.

Term	Gas Requirement for Respiration
Aerobic	Grow only in the presence of free oxygen
Anaerobic	Grow only in the absence of oxygen
Facultative Anaerobic	Grow in the absence/presence of free oxygen, BUT must obtain oxygen from oxygen-containing compounds (e.g., inorganic sulfates)
Microaerophilic	Grow best in oxygen levels *less than in air*
Capnophilic	Require 3-10% carbon dioxide in the environment to initiate growth

Preferred Living Location

Some bacteria, like *Brucella* species, can readily live and survive within mammalian cells. These are called **intracellular pathogens**. Those that can live either in or outside of mammalian cells, such as *Corynebacterium pseudotuberculosis*, are called **facultative intracellular pathogens**. A few species (e.g., *Lawsonia intracellularis, Anaplasma marginale*) are **obligate intracellular pathogens**; they must live inside cells and do not survive for long if not within a cell.

Bacterial Reproduction

Binary Fission

Bacteria reproduce by a process of asexual reproduction called **binary fission** (Figure 3.9). In binary fission, the original cell undergoing asexual reproduction is denoted the **parent cell**. The parent cell begins the process of binary fission by making a duplicate copy of its chromosomal DNA. Once the duplication process is complete and there are two copies of the chromosomal DNA, each copy binds itself to a spot on the plasma membrane. In addition to the duplication of DNA, each new cell will need all of the other components (e.g., ribosomes, vacuoles, enzymes) that were in the original parent cell. The cell duplicates these components along with the plasma membrane as the cell wall continues to grow and expand. As the duplication process comes to completion, the cell membrane begins to invaginate or "pinch" in the middle. At this time the duplicated contents of the parent cell separate with one set going toward one side of the cell and the other set going into the opposite side. The attachment of each set of chromosomal DNA to the plasma membrane facilitates their separation into opposite sides. The invagination proceeds and the bacterium continues to make a new cell wall in the form of a **cross-wall**. Once the new cell wall is complete, the two cells separate. Binary fission results in the formation of two **daughter cells**. These daughter cells (i.e., progeny) are genetically identical to the parent cell and are often referred to as genetic **clones**.

The process of binary fission of an individual parent bacterium and its daughter cells is often referred to as **clonal expansion** (Figure 3.10). This means that one parent leads to two identical daughter cells. These two daughter cells each create two more identical daughter cells (i.e., four identical cells total at this point). This process continues to

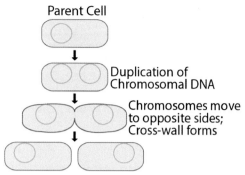

Parent Cell

Duplication of Chromosomal DNA

Chromosomes move to opposite sides; Cross-wall forms

Daughter Cells

Figure 3.9: Asexual reproduction of microbes often occurs via a process called binary fission. The parent cell first creates a duplicate copy of its chromosomal DNA. As the cytoplasm expands, each copy of the chromosomal DNA moves to opposite sides of the enlarged cell. An invagination, called a cross-wall, begins to move toward the center of the cell. Once the two sides touch, the two cells pinch off and two daughter cells are formed.

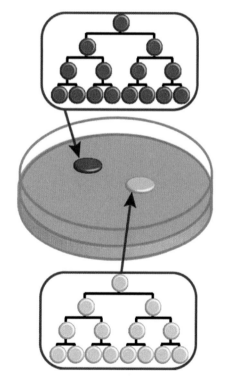

Figure 3.10 Clonal expansion of a parent cell leading to the creation of a colony. If the original cell is resistant to penicillin (orange colonies), then all daughter cells will be resistant to penicillin. If the original cell is susceptible to penicillin (yellow colonies), all progeny will be susceptible as well. Clonal expansion results in the visible appearance of a colony on the agar plate.

repeat itself, creating greater and greater numbers of daughter cells from the one original parent cell. The time from parent cell to the creation of two daughter cells is known as the **generation time** of the bacterium. The generation time can also be thought of as the time it takes to double the population of bacteria in a given space.

Bacterial Colonies

In the laboratory, we can inoculate a single bacterium onto an agar plate. An agar plate is both a solid surface for the bacterium to attach to and a source of nutrients. The bacterium uses these nutrients to provide the necessary energy and building blocks for clonal expansion. The dividing bacteria lay on the agar surface one beside the other in an ever-increasing circle of growth. It takes many cycles of binary fission to create enough daughter cells for a person to see them with the naked eye. The small circular patch of clonally expanded bacteria is known as a **colony**.

Clinical Correlation: Generation Time

Generation time can greatly influence the day-to-day operations of veterinary clinical practice.

For example: *Staphylococcus aureus*, a bacterial species of the skin, has a generation time of approximately 30 minutes.

- How long will it take for the bacteria to accumulate on a given surface, such as the plastic of the intravenous catheter?
- How long before the bacteria accumulates in the body?

Questions like these can influence decisions like when to change out IV catheters, how often to sanitize examination tables, and more.

Because each colony is the progeny of one parent cell, all cells in the CFU carry the identical DNA. This means that if the original parent cell carries a gene making the bacterium resistant to a particular antibiotic (e.g., penicillin), all the resulting daughter cells in every generation created after the parent cell will be resistant to that same antibiotic (Figure 3.10).

Strains and Isolates

Common terms that may be used to describe bacteria are bacterial strain and bacterial isolate. An **isolate** is a pure culture derived from a single colony that arose from a single organism or, in this case, bacterium. A **strain** is a group of isolates that are indistinguishable from each other yet can be differentiated from a completely different group of isolates.

Bacterial Growth Cycle

Bacteria replication and colony growth do not occur in a completely linear fashion. The bacterial growth cycle can be broken down into four parts (Figure 3.11). First, when a group of bacterial cells

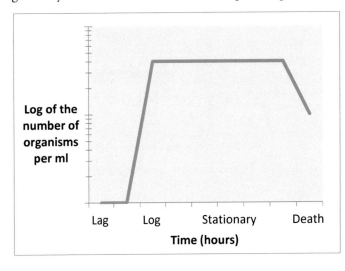

Log of the number of organisms per ml

Lag   Log   Stationary   Death

Time (hours)

Figure 3.11: The bacterial growth curve. The growth curve can be broken down into four distinct phases. In the *lag phase*, the bacteria must adjust to their new environment, thus binary fission is minimal. Once sufficient resources have been obtained at the new location, the bacteria can undergo binary fission. This is called the *log phase* and is the period of maximum growth. During the *stationary phase*, the number of replicating bacteria equals those that are dying, thus the total number of organisms appears static. During the *death phase*, waning nutrients and toxic increases in waste products lead to dying organisms outnumbering living, replicating organisms.

find themselves in a new environment, they must take time to adjust to the different parameters within that environment (e.g., available oxygen, type of nutrients present). This adjustment period is called the **lag phase**. During this phase, most of the bacteria within the group or colony are not actively dividing. Once the bacterial cells have adjusted to their environment, they can put forth most of their energy into dividing at regular intervals. Thus, the **logarithmic (log) phase** is the period of maximum growth rate. During the **stationary phase**, there begins to be an exhaustion of available nutrients accompanied by the accumulation of toxic waste products produced by the bacteria themselves. With this shift in available nutrients, bacterial cells begin to die. In the stationary phase, the growth rate equals the death rate. The last phase of the growth cycle, the **death phase**, occurs when the death rate significantly outpaces the growth rate due to a severe depletion of available nutrients along with a significant increase in toxic waste products.

Escaping Death: Sporulation

Early explorers came to the New World in search of the mystical Fountain of Youth as a way to cheat death. While there is no fountain of youth, some bacteria have found a unique way to (at least temporarily) avoid destruction, thus enabling them to survive and flourish in better times.

The armor needed to weather such tough environmental conditions as extreme heat, cold, drying, and damage from chemicals comes in the formation of thick-walled **endospores**. A few genera (e.g., *Bacillus* and *Clostridium*) are capable of forming endospores. Once the bacterium senses that an environmental condition is present, the bacterium begins to package all of the important contents within the cytoplasm needed for survival in the endospore. The endospore survives in this inactive state, while the **vegetative** (i.e., actively growing and developing) portion of the bacterium dies. The location of the endospore within a bacterial cell differs amongst the different spore-forming bacteria (Figure 3.12). Once more favorable growing conditions return, the endospore sporulates and releases the vegetative form of the bacterium.

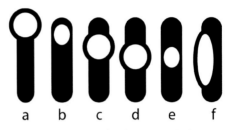

a   b   c   d   e   f

Figure 3.12: **Types of endospores.** The location of the endospore (white) residing inside the vegetative cell (black) varies in location. This largely depends upon the particular species of bacteria. Terminal endospores (a,b) are located on one or the other pole of the vegetative cell. Central endospores (d,e) are located in the middle. Subterminal spores are those that are located between these first two extremes (c). Lateral endospores are pushed to one side (f).

Bacterial Cell Niches

A bird's wings allow it access to the tree tops and the skies above. A fish's gills make it uniquely suitable to life underwater. Overtime, bacteria have developed favorite places (or **niches**) to which they are well suited. Some bacteria can access a wide variety of niches, while others can only occupy a very narrow niche. Bacteria that cause disease in animals tends to come from two different sources: those that live in or on individuals and those that may be found in the environment.

Client Education:
King of the Endospores

Endospores of *Bacillus anthracis*, the bacterium that causes anthrax in both cattle and humans, are especially hearty. Its spores have been known to survive *over one-hundred years in the soil!*

This makes the clean-up of infected pastures extremely difficult and unrealistic.

Microbes Associated with a Host

Microbes either found on or in an individual animal (including humans) may include **normal microflora**, opportunistic microbes, or pathogens.

Normal Microflora

These bacteria live on or within the body of normal, healthy individuals. They are also referred to as **commensals**. Normal microflora do not cause the host any harm. In fact, normal microflora have essential functions that benefit the host. For example, the normal microflora of the gastrointestinal system aids in the breakdown of food as well as the synthesis of key vitamins such as vitamin B. The removal of commensals can open up niches in or on the body that may be filled by harmful bacteria and result in disease. Actions that can cause the elimination of commensals include using the wrong antibiotic or an antibiotic at too high a dose.

Pathogens

A **pathogen** is a microorganism that causes disease. There are two major types of pathogens. **Obligate pathogens** (also called **primary** or **"frank" pathogens**) almost always cause disease when contracted by an individual. The second type of pathogen is the opportunistic pathogen (discussed below).

Opportunists

An **opportunistic pathogen** is a microorganism that does not normally cause disease in healthy, immunocompetent animals or people. However, these microorganisms can cause disease under certain conditions. For example, when the host is immunocompromised (e.g., patient undergoing cancer chemotherapy) its immune cells cannot adequately eliminate the opportunistic pathogen; this pathogen is able to multiply within the body and cause disease. Sources of opportunistic infections may include both environmental microbes and commensal organisms.

Zoonoses and Anthroponoses

Infectious microorganisms can be transmitted within animal species, between animal species, and between animals and humans. **Zoonoses** are diseases humans can acquire from animals or animal-origin products. For example, the fungus causing ringworm, *Microsporum canis*, can be transmitted to people by touching the lesion on an infected cat.

Disease transmission is not unidirectional. Human diseases that are transmittable to animals are called **anthroponoses**. In the wild, monkeys do not suffer from the measles. However, humans are the natural host for the measles virus. Transmission of the measles virus from an infected human results in serious disease in the affected monkeys.

Zoonoses and anthroponoses are not limited to transmission via live animals. Animal products may also carry diseases with them. Several cases of transmission of anthrax have occurred in people obtaining improperly cured leather products (e.g., drums made from cow hide) from places such as Africa where the causative agent, *Bacillus anthracis*, is not uncommon. The people became ill after touching, inhaling, or accidentally ingesting the infective endospores that were present in the leather.

Client Education: Zoonoses

Microbes causing zoonotic diseases are further classified as either frank or opportunistic zoonotic pathogens. In people with compromised immune systems (e.g., infants, elderly, cancer chemotherapy patients), an agent that wouldn't normally cause disease may cause a serious opportunistic infection in these individuals.

Do not assume that your client, their family, or their friends are 100% healthy. Always explain to them the risks of zoonoses.

Rules of Bacterial Nomenclature

When writing the names of bacterial species, it is important to use proper bacterial nomenclature. The bacterial genus is always capitalized and the species is written using all lowercase letters. The genus and species are both italicized. When italics are not possible (e.g., you are writing out the name by hand), the genus and species may be underlined. If the bacterial species also has a subspecies, the letters "ssp." (i.e., not italicized) are added and then the name of the subspecies (i.e., italicized) follows. When referring to the condition or disease that the bacterial species causes, the word is not capitalized nor is it italicized. Table 3.2 shows examples of proper bacterial nomenclature.

Table 3.2: Examples illustrating the rules of bacterial nomenclature

Rule	Example
Genus species	*Streptococcus equi* (typed) <u>Streptococcus equi</u> (hand-written)
Genus abbreviation*	*S. equi*
Genus species & subspecies	*Streptococcus equi* ssp. *equi*
Condition or disease	streptococcal infections
When referred to as a group	streptococci

*Note: the abbreviation may only be used if genus has previously been defined.

Further Reading

Rothschild, Lynn J., and Rocco L. Mancinelli. "Life in Extreme Environments." *Nature* 409 6823 (2001): 1092-101.

Sneath, Peter. "Bacterial Nomenclature." *Bergey's Manual of Systematic Bacteriology: Volume One: The Archaea and the Deeply Branching and Phototrophic Bacteria*. Eds. Boone, David, Richard Castenholz and George Garrity. 2nd ed. United States: Springer-Verlag New York Inc., 2001.

Zimmer, Carl. "A Weakness in Bacteria's Fortress." *Scientific American* 312 1 (2014): 40-45.

Chapter 4:

Sterilization, Sanitation and Disinfection

"I trust I may be enabled in the treatment of patients always to act with a single eye to their good."

– Joseph Lister, 1857

Introduction

As a part of the veterinary team, it is of vital importance that the veterinary technician have a thorough understanding of the key concepts related to aseptic technique, sterilization, sanitation, and disinfection. Our patients' lives quite *literally* depend upon it. A number of terms are used when describing sterilization, sanitation, and disinfection. They are summarized in Table 4.1.

Table 4.1: Terms related to sterilization and disinfection

Term	Definition
Sterilization	The killing or removal of all microorganisms in a material or on an object.
Disinfection	The reduction of the number of pathogenic microorganisms to the point where they pose no danger of disease.
Antiseptic	A chemical agent that can safely be used externally on living tissue to destroy microorganisms or to inhibit their growth.
Disinfectant	A chemical agent used on inanimate objects to destroy microorganisms.
Sanitizer	A chemical agent typically used on food-handling equipment and eating utensils to reduce bacterial numbers so as to meet public health standards. Sanitization may simply refer to thorough washing with only soap or detergent.
Bacteriostatic agent	An agent that inhibits the growth of bacteria
Germicide	An agent capable of killing microbes rapidly; some such agents effectively kill certain microorganisms but only inhibit the growth of others.
Bactericidal agent	An agent that kills vegetative (actively growing) bacteria. Most such agents do not kill spores.
Fungicide	An agent that kills fungi
Sporicide	An agent that kills bacterial endospores or fungal spores

Reducing the Likelihood of Infection

As a part of the veterinary team, there are several ways for the veterinary technician to reduce the likelihood of transmitting infection to a patient. These include proper hand washing and the use of aseptic technique, proper sanitation, and disinfection.

Proper Hand Washing

The single most effective method available to prevent the transmission of infectious organisms is proper hand washing. Good technique ensures that all surfaces of the hands, fingers, and nails are adequately scrubbed during hand washing. The skin underneath the fingernails is the space most commonly missed or inadequately cleansed when washing hands (Figure 4.1). Surgical scrub brushes often come with a nail "pick" to aid in cleaning the dirt underneath fingernails (Figure 4.2). Contact time is also important. Hand washing prior to handling veterinary patients should take a minimum of twenty seconds. Pre-surgical hand scrubbing requires at least ten minutes of contact time.

Aseptic Technique

For procedures performed under sterile conditions, members of the veterinary team use aseptic technique. Aseptic technique involves practices and procedures performed under controlled conditions with the goal of minimizing contamination and decreasing the likelihood of transmitting an infection to a patient. To ensure uniformity and compliance with these practices and procedures, it is a good idea for the veterinary team to develop a set of **standard operating procedures** (SOPs). For surgery, these SOPs might include a set way to prepare the patient for surgery by first shaving and then cleansing the surgical site using the same method for each patient. Other SOPs might include:

- Proper hand washing technique
- Donning and doffing the surgical gown and gloves
- Proper handling of sterile equipment and instruments

Sterilization

Sterilization is the killing or removal of all microorganisms in a material or on an object. There are no "degrees" of sterility; an object is either sterile or not sterile. **Sterility** means that

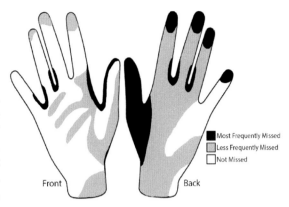

Figure 4.1: Sites frequently missed when handwashing. When handwashing, particular attention should be paid to areas such as the webs of the fingers, the thumb, and around and under nailbeds. These are the sites most frequently missed when handwashing.

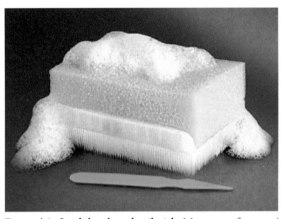

Figure 4.2: Scrub brush and nail pick. Many manufactures of surgical scrubs produce prepackaged surgical hand scrub brushes and nail picks. It is important to use the nail pick to thoroughly clean under the nails as this is one of the most frequently missed areas in handwashing. See also: Figure 4.1, above. Courtesy and © Becton, Dickinson and Company. Reprinted with permission.

Remember this: Antibiotics and Aseptic Technique

While the veterinarian may need to prescribe antibiotics to a patient based on the disease the animal is suffering from, remember that antibiotics are no substitute for aseptic technique. Put yourself in the animals "shoes" and remember…

Someday YOU may be the patient!

there are no living organisms in or on a material. A number of physical methods may be used to achieve sterilization. These include:

- Heat
- Radiation
- Filtration
- Sonication

Heat

Heat is a preferred agent and most widely used method of microbial control for all materials not damaged by high temperature. It rapidly penetrates thick materials not easily penetrated by chemical agents. It can be divided into moist and dry heat.

Moist heat, because of its penetrating properties, is a widely used physical sterilization method. Boiling water destroys vegetative cells of most bacteria and fungi and inactivates some viruses, but it is not effective in killing all kinds of spores. However, if water is heated under pressure, its boiling point is elevated, so temperatures above 100°C can be reached. This is normally accomplished by using an **autoclave**. Complete sterilization can be achieved after 15 minutes in an autoclave at a pressure of 15 psi (i.e., pounds per square inch) and 121°C. In this procedure it is the increased temperature, and not the increased pressure, that kills microorganisms. (Steam at 134 °C can achieve in 3 minutes the same sterility that hot air at 160°C takes two hours to achieve)

To prepare items for autoclaving, all containers should be unsealed and articles should be wrapped in materials that allow steam penetration. Large packages of dressings and large flasks of media require extra time for heat to penetrate them. Likewise, packing many articles close together in an autoclave lengthens the processing time to as much as 60 minutes to ensure sterility. It is more efficient and safer to run two separate, uncrowded loads than one crowded load. Several methods are available to ensure that autoclaving achieves sterility.

Autoclave indicator tape consists of yellow or white indicator stripes and pressure-sensitive adhesive. When the steam sterilization is completed, the color of the indicator strips will turn from yellow or white to dark brown or black. The complete color change occurs in 15 to 20 minutes at 121°C. These tapes are not fully reliable because they do not indicate how long appropriate conditions were maintained. Sometimes they change color within a few minutes at the high temperature.

Biological indicators are another method for ensuring sterility. The Centers for Disease Control and Prevention (CDC) recommends weekly autoclaving of a culture containing heat-resistant endospores, such as those of *Geobacillus stearothermophilus*, to check autoclave performance. Endospore strips are commercially available to make this task easy (Figure 4.3).

Dry (oven) heat penetrates substances more slowly than moist (i.e., steam) heat. It is usually used to sterilize metal objects and glassware and is the only suitable means of sterilizing oils and powders. Objects are sterilized by dry heat when subjected to 171°C for 1 hour, 160°C for 2 hours or longer, or 121°C for 10-16 hours or longer –

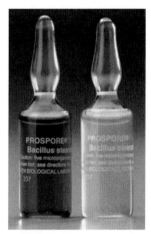

Figure 4.3: Biological indicators containing *Geobacillus stearothermophilus.* Obtaining a negative culture after an autoclave run is the only direct way to truly validate that an autoclave is achieving the time, temperature, and pressure necessary to achieve sterility of the objects placed within. The indicator is placed at the center of a load and allowed to go through the entire autoclave cycle. The vial contains a pH indicator that turns from purple (negative for growth) to yellow (positive for growth) when growth of the spores is detected. Thus, an autoclave would "pass" this test only if the vial remained purple (no growth) after the autoclave run finished. Courtesy of Lab Alley at Labsupplyoutlaws.com, Cleveland.

depending on the volume of the load. An open flame is a form of dry heat used to sterilize inoculating loops and the mouths of culture tubes (See Chapter 22).

Radiation

Four general types of radiation—ultraviolet light, ionizing radiation, microwave radiation and strong visible light (under certain circumstances)—can be used to control microorganisms.

Ultraviolet (UV) light (Non-ionizing) consists of light of wavelengths between 40 and 390 nanometers (nm), but wavelengths in the 200-nm range are most effective in killing microorganisms by damaging DNA and proteins. Ultraviolet light is absorbed by the purine and pyrimidine bases of nucleic acids. Such absorption can permanently destroy these important molecules. Ultraviolet light is especially effective for inactivating viruses. However, it kills far fewer bacteria than one might expect because of DNA repair mechanisms. Once DNA is repaired, new molecules of RNA and protein can be synthesized to replace the damaged molecules. Ultraviolet light is of limited use because it does not penetrate glass, cloth, paper, or most other materials, and it does not go around corners or under lab benches. It does penetrate air, effectively reducing the number of airborne microorganisms and killing them on surfaces in operating rooms and rooms that will contain caged animals.

X-rays, which have wavelengths of 0.1 to 40 nm, and gamma rays, which have even shorter wavelengths, are both forms of **ionizing radiation**. Ionizing radiation damages DNA and produces peroxides, which act as powerful oxidizing agents in cells. This radiation can also kill or cause mutations in human cells if it reaches them. It is used to sterilize plastic laboratory and medical equipment as well as pharmaceutical products.

Filtration

Filtration is the passage of a material through a filter, or straining device. Sterilization by filtration is used mostly for liquids and requires filters with exceedingly small pores. Membrane filters, thin disks with pores that prevent the passage of anything larger than the pore size, are widely used today. They are usually made of nitrocellulose and have the great advantage that they can be purchased pre-sterilized and discarded after use.

Sonication

Ultrasonic vibration, also termed **sonication**, is a mechanical method of microbial control used to remove microbes from the surface of instruments and teeth. Ultrasonic vibration utilizes high frequency sound waves to generate "shock waves" that are conducted through living structures or liquids. The force exerted by these shock waves leads to the rupture of microbial membranes and their removal from surfaces. Ultrasonic vibration is used to clean surgical instruments, dental instruments, teeth, pacemakers, hearing aids, test tubes and small electronics.

Sanitation

Even the best autoclaves and disinfectants (discussed below) will fail to eliminate or reduce, respectively, the amount of microbes on a surface or in an object if there is too much organic material present. Therefore it is important to use proper sanitation procedures prior to autoclaving or applying the disinfectant. First, every surface of the object to be autoclaved or disinfected must be cleaned to remove any **organic material** (e.g., dirt, blood, pus) that may be present. This typically involves the use of soap and water. Once the surface has completely dried, the object or surface may be either autoclaved or disinfected, as appropriate.

Disinfection Methods

Disinfection is the act of reducing the number of pathogenic organisms on objects or in materials so that they pose no threat of disease. Agents called **disinfectants** are typically applied to inanimate objects, and agents called **antiseptics** are applied to living tissue. Although most disinfectants are too harsh for use on delicate skin tissue, a few agents are suitable as both disinfectants and antiseptics (e.g., isopropyl alcohol).

Chemical Agents for Control Of Microbial Growth

The **potency**, or effectiveness, of a chemical antimicrobial agent is affected by the number of micro-organisms present, time, temperature, pH, and concentration. The death rate of organisms is affected by the length of time the organisms are exposed to the antimicrobial agent, as was explained earlier for heat. Thus, adequate time should always be allowed for an agent to kill the maximum number of organisms. The death rate of organisms subjected to a chemical agent is accelerated by increasing the temperature. Increasing temperature doubles the rate of chemical reactions and thereby increases the potency of the chemical agent. Acidic or alkaline pH can increase or decrease the agent's potency. A pH that increases the degree of ionization of a chemical agent often increases its ability to penetrate a cell. Such a pH can also alter the contents of the cell itself. Finally, increasing concentration may increase the effects of most antimicrobial chemical agents, with the exception of 100% ethanol. High concentrations may be **bactericidal** (i.e., kills the bacteria), whereas lower concentrations may be **bacteriostatic** (e.g., growth inhibiting). Manufacturers of disinfectants have validated their brand of disinfectant; therefore, it is very important to follow the label recommendations on how strong or dilute to make a disinfectant solution. Some disinfectants come at a "ready-to-use" concentration and thus should not be further diluted; they should simply be used "as is".

The time needed to properly disinfect a given surface is dependent upon the particular disinfectant used and which microbial agent(s) you are trying to kill or inactivate. For example, SporKlenz®, a disinfectant containing the active ingredients hydrogen peroxide and peracetic acid, is rated to inactivate *Staphylococcus aureus* at 20°C with a minimum contact time of 10 minutes. Note that not all organisms will be listed on a given label. If the organism you are looking for is not listed, use the guidelines for an organism with similar hardiness. For example, SporKlenz® does not list a specific contact time for Canine Parvovirus. Since Mouse Parvovirus is similar and is listed, you may use that contact time.

Chemical antimicrobial agents kill microorganisms by participating in one or more chemical reactions that damage cell components. Agents can be grouped by whether they affect proteins, membranes, or other cell components.

Reactions That Affect Proteins:

Much of a cell is made of protein, and all its enzymes are proteins. Alteration of protein structure is called **denaturation**. In denaturation, hydrogen and disulfide bonds are disrupted, and the functional shape of the protein molecule is destroyed. Any agent that denatures proteins prevents them from carrying out their normal functions. When treated for a short time with mild heat or with some dilute acids, alkalis, or other agents, proteins are temporarily denatured. After the agent is removed, some proteins can regain their normal structure. However, most antimicrobial agents are used in a strong enough concentration over a sufficient length of time to denature proteins permanently. Permanent denaturation of a microorganism's proteins kills the organism. Denaturation is bactericidal if it permanently alters the protein so that the protein's normal state cannot be restored. Denaturation is bacteriostatic if it temporarily alters the protein, and the normal structure can be recovered.

Reactions That Affect Membranes:

Membranes contain proteins and so can be altered by all the preceding reactions. Membranes also contain lipid and thus can be disrupted by substances that dissolve lipids. Surfactants are soluble compounds that reduce surface tension, just as soaps and detergents break up grease particles in dishwashing water. Surfactants include alcohols, detergents, and quaternary ammonium compounds, such as benzalkonium chloride, which dissolve lipids. Phenols, which are alcohols, dissolve lipids and also denature proteins. Detergent solutions, also called wetting agents, are often used with other chemical agents to help the agent penetrate fatty substances. Although detergent solutions themselves usually do not kill microorganisms, they do help get rid of lipids and other organic materials so that antimicrobial agents can reach the target organisms.

Reactions That Affect Other Cell Components:

Other cell components affected by chemical agents include nucleic acids and energy-producing systems. Alkylating agents can replace hydrogen on amino or alcohol groups in nucleic acids. Certain dyes, such as crystal violet, interfere with cell wall formation. Some substances, such as lactic acid and propionic acid (i.e., end products of fermentation), inhibit fermentation and thus prevent energy production in certain bacteria, molds, and some other organisms.

Assessing the Success of Disinfection: Techniques for a Clinical Setting

It is important for all members of the veterinary team to be confident in the methods of sanitation and disinfection used in the clinical, hospital, and laboratory settings. It is not enough to rotely follow cleaning and disinfecting SOPs. *We must prove that those procedures worked at achieving good sanitation.* Otherwise, we find ourselves working under a sense of false security – and our patients will suffer because of it.

Replicate Organism Detection and Counting (RODAC) plates

Replicate Organism Detection and Counting (**RODAC**) plates are solid agar microbial media plates used for the detection and enumeration of aerobic (i.e., oxygen-loving) bacteria present on a surface (e.g., surgery table). RODAC plates are most often used to assess the efficacy of a sanitation program such as within a clinic, hospital, or laboratory. More details on the methods for using RODAC plates are discussed in the laboratory methods chapter (Chapter 22) of this book.

ATPase Bioluminescence

ATPase bioluminescence is another methodology for assessing the success of a sanitation program. All prokaryotic and eukaryotic cells use the molecule adenosine triphosphate (ATP) for energy. This system can detect how much ATP is present on a surface. Thus, this test is a good test for detecting organic material. It does not detect whether or not there are live cells or organisms present. It is used to determine how clean a surface is. *Therefore, it cannot tell us if microorganisms are present;* for that, you need to use something like a RODAC plate (see above). Testing requires a kit that includes the ATPase swabs and a luminometer. The swabs are used to wipe a portion the surface that was recently cleaned (e.g. 4" x 4" section of countertop). The swab has a chemical on it that contains ATPase, an enzyme capable of breaking down ATP. When the ATP breaks down, there is a release of luminescence (i.e., glow) that the luminometer can detect. The greater the glow, the greater the amount of ATP, and thus the greater organic material, present on the surface.

Biofilms

Bacteria have developed many ways to access areas that they can then successfully inhabit and reproduce. Perhaps one of the most challenging environments is a liquid one. The flowing nature of rivers, streams, and water pipes makes it hard for bacteria to stay stationary and grow. However, some bacteria are more than up to the challenge. These bacteria can stay affixed to the stones in the river or the sides

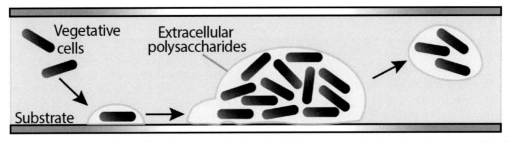

Figure 4.4: Anatomy of a biofilm. Vegetative cells (purple rods) flowing in a liquid medium (e.g., water, blood) come into contact with a substrate (e.g., water pipes, endothelial cells, IV catheter) and adhere to the surface substrate. Once they adhere, the bacteria produce copious amounts of extracellular polysaccharides (yellow). These polysaccharides are largely impervious to fluid pressure and even antimicrobials. At times, the sheer force of the flowing water or blood becomes too intense, causing a portion of the biofilm to break off. This piece flows free and attaches on a downstream substrate or lodges (in the case of the bloodstream) in distant sites such as body organs.

of the water pipes with the help of biofilms. A **biofilm** is a grouping of bacteria with a distinct architectural structure (Figure 4.4). Briefly, a biofilm is made up of two main parts: a core of bacteria and an outer layer of extracellular polysaccharides. The bacteria produce these extracellular polysaccharides and cover themselves with it. As sugars, the polysaccharides are very sticky and help in the attachment of the biofilm to surfaces like the inside of water pipes. Like capsules, these polysaccharides are antiphagocytic (see Capsule, Chapter 3). They are also relatively resistant to antibiotics.

While biofilms may seem to be nothing more than a simple blob of bacteria and sticky polysaccharide, this community of bacteria is actually quite intelligent. It may seem strange to use the term "intelligent" for organisms without a brain. However, they actively communicate to each other in a process called "quorum sensing". **Quorum sensing** involves the regulation of gene expression within the population of bacteria in response to the density of the cell population. In biofilms, this is used to coordinate the production of proteins and other materials needed to keep the population at its optimal level. For example, a population too large is in danger of being dislodged from the surface it is stuck to and swept downstream. Too small a population is in danger of being easily killed by host defenses. Bacteria populations can also use quorum sensing to determine how to best respond to external threats such as decreased available nutrients and avoidance of toxic compounds. Seems a pretty "smart" way to survive, doesn't it?

Biofilms in Veterinary Medicine

Intravenous (IV) catheters have a structure not unlike that of a tiny water pipe. The small lumen of the catheter is a prime spot for the formation of biofilms. They are especially susceptible to colonization by skin commensals such as *Staphylococcus aureus*, among others. These biofilms are subject to the forces of blood pressure. The constant pulsating of the blood can cause a small portion of the biofilm to break off and rush down the bloodstream. These packets of bacteria can then access other distance parts of the body, such as the liver or kidneys.

The formation of biofilms within the catheter lumen is one reason that IV catheters should be replaced on a regular basis (e.g., once every three days) in those patients that require long-term fluid therapy. Some catheters are coated with substances (e.g., Teflon®) in an effort to slow down the generation of biofilms. However, to date, no coatings have completely prevented the formation of biofilms.

In addition to IV catheters, biofilms can form on other medical devices, such as urinary catheters and orthopedic implants. Consequently, it is imperative that aseptic technique is used when placing medical devices.

As noted above, all water pipes carry biofilms. Regardless of how well the water treatment at the municipal treatment facility worked, it is impossible to eliminate the biofilms from the miles of piping to buildings, such as a private homes or veterinary hospitals. The presence of these biofilms is rarely a problem for most of our healthy patients. But what about debilitated, immunocompromised patients? These patients may become ill with bacteria that a healthy individual could successfully fight off. For this reason, members of the

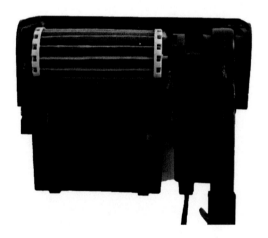

Figure 4.5: An aquarium filter as a beneficial biofilm. Many hobbyist aquarium filtration systems contain some sort of "biofiltration" system. Briefly, biofiltration systems serve two purposes: to remove large waste products (e.g., feces) and detoxify the water by removing dissolved nitrogenous waste products such as ammonia. The conversion of toxic ammonia to less toxic nitrates is performed via nitrogen-fixing bacteria. These bacteria need a substrate upon which to grow, adequate water flow, and oxygenation of that water. The corrugated water wheel shown here fulfills all of those requirements. Water is sucked up from the tank and flows over the water wheel causing it to turn thus aerating the water.

veterinary team should engage in regular discussions about what water source (e.g., tap water, autoclaved water, and IV fluids) will be used to deliver oral or parenteral fluid therapy in these patients.

Removing Biofilms

Methods to reduce the amount of biofilms present on surfaces are available. Ultrasonic cleaners use ultrasonic waves to break apart and disperse biofilms off of objects such as surgical instruments. Even manual scrubbing of surgical instruments can help to reduce the amount of biofilm present. However, care should be taken when hand washing instruments not to cause pitting of the surface of the instruments. Using bleach at a concentration of higher than 1:10 (i.e., 1 part full-strength bleach to 10 parts water) or soaking instruments in bleach for a prolonged period can pit stainless steel. These small pits and crevices are ideal places for future biofilms to attach.

Beneficial Biofilms

Not all biofilms are damaging to our patients. An example of beneficial biofilms can be found in our aquatic patients. Aquariums use biological filters (Figure 4.5) laden with biofilms to maintain water quality. Fish produce nitrogen waste in the form of ammonia-containing compounds. Ammonia in high quantities is toxic to fish. However, nitrogen-fixing bacteria such as *Nitrosomonas* and *Nitrobacter* species colonize the biological filters and help detoxify the water by degrading ammonia into the less toxic substances of nitrites and nitrates, respectively. Nitrates can then be eliminated through periodic water changes. Disrupting or eliminating these beneficial biofilms can cause dangerously high ammonia levels in the water and can hurt or even kill the fish.

Further Reading

Bordi, Christophe, and Sophie de Bentzmann. "Hacking into Bacterial Biofilms: A New Therapeutic Challenge." *Annals of Intensive Care* 1 1 (2011): 19.

Ednie, Douglas, Ronald Wilson, and Max Lang. "Comparison of Two Sanitation Monitoring Methods in an Animal Research Facility." *American Association for Laboratory Animal Science* 37 6 (1998): 71-74.

Lemmen, Sebastian W., et al. "Comparison of Two Sampling Methods for the Detection of Gram-Positive and Gram-Negative Bacteria in the Environment: Moistened Swabs versus RODAC Plates." *International Journal of Hygiene and Environmental Health* 203 3 (2001): 245-48.

Nakamura, R. K., et al. "Hand Hygiene Practices of Veterinary Support Staff in Small Animal Private Practice." *Journal of Small Animal Practice* 53 3 (2012): 155-60.

Chapter 5:

Microbial Pathogenesis & Immunity

Introduction

Whether or not exposure to a microbe leads to disease depends on three interrelated factors. If any one of these factors is out of balance, disease can develop. This is known as the **host-agent-environment triad** (Figure 5.1). The host is more susceptible to pathogens if its immune system is not functioning properly or if it is already engaged in a fight with another pathogen (e.g., virus). If the latter is the case, the host may not be able to fight off this second invader (e.g., pathogenic bacteria) and worsening disease may result. A microbe (i.e., agent) can overwhelm even the heartiest and healthiest of hosts if they are present in very large numbers. Finally, the environment can play a role in an animal's susceptibility to disease. For example, in 2005, when dogs and other animals were abandoned during the emergency evacuation of New Orleans in the wake of Hurricane Katrina, the animals faced rising waters from the breached levee system. This water was not clean and served as a breeding ground for many different pathogens. In addition, many animals could not stay dry and this caused the skin to lose its ability to act as a barrier to infection. Added to that was the immunosuppressive effects of stress from the forced separation from their human companions. It is no wonder that many animals suffered, and some died, from infectious diseases.

Bacterial Pathogens: Basic Classifications

Bacteria are classified into groups based on their disease-causing ability. Commensal microorganisms, also simply referred to as **commensals**, are those microorganisms which normally reside in a host without causing any infection or disease. These microorganisms are also referred to as **normal microflora**. In fact, commensals contribute in many ways to the maintenance of host health. A **pathogen** is a microorganism capable of causing disease in its host. One that always causes disease in a given host is called a **primary (frank) pathogen**. Some microbes only cause disease under certain circumstances. For instance, a microbe may be incapable of causing disease in an otherwise healthy animal. However, if the animal becomes immunosuppressed for any reason (e.g., concurrent infection, immune disorder, or the animal is undergoing

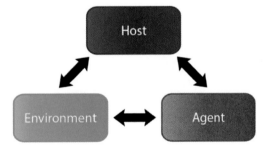

Figure 5.1: The host-environment-agent triad. With germs all around us, why aren't we perpetually ill? If a host's immune system is strong, the microbe (agent) is weak, and the environment is clean, individuals infected with microbes can fight them off without ever feeling anything other than wonderful. But should any one of these parameters be out-of-balance, such as a decrease in host immune defenses or a particularly strong microbe, an individual can quickly find themselves becoming ill.

chemotherapy), the same microbe can now cause disease. A microbe capable of causing disease only in these limited circumstances is called an **opportunistic pathogen**. An opportunistic pathogen may also cause disease when it is introduced into a site of the body where it does not normally reside or have access. Such is the case for *Staphylococcus aureus*, a normal inhabitant of the skin. While *Staphylococcus* causes no damage when on intact skin, it can cause a variety of problems should it become introduced into the host's bloodstream via a cut or open wound. It is important to realize that the same microbe may be considered part of the normal microflora in one animal species (or body location), yet it may act as an opportunistic or primary pathogen in another species (or location). Many dogs and cats carry *Pasteurella multocida* in their normal oral microflora. When a dog or cat bites a person, the introduction of the *Pasteurella* into the bite wound via their sharp teeth can cause an infection and inflammation in the form of large abscesses.

Pathogenesis and Infectious Disease

A pathogen moves through several different stages along its way to successfully propagating itself in a host (Figure 5.2). The establishment, development, and progression of disease caused by an infectious agent is known as the agent's **pathogenesis**.

Resumé of a Successful Pathogen

There are several steps that a microorganism must undertake if it is to become a successful pathogen. These steps are:

1. **Entry** of the pathogen into the body
2. **Attachment** of the pathogen to some tissue(s) within the body (e.g., intestinal epithelium)
3. **Multiplication** of the pathogen within the host
4. **Invasion** or spread of the pathogen within the host
5. **Evasion** of host immune defenses
6. **Damage** to host tissue(s)

The secret of a truly successful pathogen is the ability to damage the host just enough that it can access the niche(s) it needs to in order to survive, but not so much that it causes the immediate death of the animal. A pathogen that causes death too quickly may do so before it has a chance to multiply and infect other hosts. Without new hosts, a pathogen would quickly cease to exist. The time period between the exposure of the host to the pathogen and the first clinical signs is known as the **incubation period** (Figure 5.2). Even though the patient isn't showing clinical signs, they *may still be infectious during this period*. The next step in the pathogenesis of disease is the **prodromal period**. This period consists of early, usually non-specific, signs of a disease that occur *just before* the characteristic signs of the disease appear. The illness proceeds and can be followed by one of three outcomes. In individuals with a healthy immune system, a complete resolution of clinical signs and

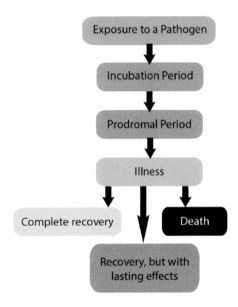

Figure 5.2: Steps involved in microbial infections and possible outcomes. Infections begin with an initial exposure to the pathogen. During the incubation period, affected individuals are asymptomatic but still capable of transmitting the infection to others. Non-specific signs of illness (e.g., ADR = "ain't doing right") occur during the prodromal period followed by signs of overt, recognizable illness. Finally, infection may result in complete recovery, recovery with deficits, or death. This depends on the ability of the host to mount a successful immune response.

return to health follow. Sometimes the pathogen causes enough damage that a complete recovery is not possible and the individual must cope with lingering health issues (e.g., kidney insufficiency or decreased mobility due to damage to muscle and bone). Those individuals which either get a very large dose of the infectious agent or whose immune system is suppressed eventually succumb to the disease resulting in the death of that individual.

Virulence and Virulence Factors

A **virulent** microbe is one that is highly pathogenic. Pathogenic microorganisms have the ability to cause disease because they possess arsenals of virulence factors. **Virulence factors** are attributes that enable pathogens to attach to the host, escape destruction by the immune system, or cause disease. A single bacterial species may contain both virulent and **avirulent** (i.e., non-pathogenic) strains. For example, *Escherichia coli* (*E. coli*) is part of the normal microflora of the intestinal tract. However, toxigenic *E. coli* (i.e., toxin-producing strains of *E. coli*) cause scours (diarrhea) in calves.

Remember this: Flu-like Symptoms

"Flu-like" symptoms are an excellent example of what can happen during the prodromal period. These symptoms are very non-specific and can occur prior to many diseases. They include:

- Fever (with or without chills)
- Headache
- Myalgia (muscle pains)
- Weakness/feeling tired

This is why, during the prodromal period, it is almost impossible to predict which pathogen is actually causing the disease!

Attachment Factors

Two key attachment factors that bacteria possess are pili and adhesins. Recall from Chapter 3 that **pili** are bacterial structures that enable a bacterium to attach to either the cell surface of the host or, in the case of the sex pilus, to another bacterium. **Adhesins** (also known as "ligands") are special molecules on the surface of pathogens enabling the recognition and binding to particular host cell receptors. The specificity of the adhesins to specific host receptors is one reason why some pathogens will preferentially colonize one area of the body over another (e.g., skin versus intestinal tract).

Escape

Bacteria possess many different structures that aid in their escape from capture and destruction by the immune system. In the last chapter, we saw how flagella are used to propel bacteria toward a food source. However, a bacterium can also use its flagella to move away from host immune cells like macrophages and neutrophils that would otherwise phagocytose (i.e., "eat") the bacterium. Another virulence factor, leucocidin, is a toxin produced by and exported out of some bacteria. This toxin can kill the host's white blood cells allowing the bacterium's escape from the host's immune system. Some bacteria are able to make a capsule which physically protects the bacteria from components of the immune system. Like leucocidin, having a capsule aids the bacteria in escaping phagocytosis.

Causing Disease

As stated in the previous section, a successful pathogen is one that causes just enough damage to the host to keep the bacterium alive and multiplying, but not so much that the host dies quickly. *Helicobacter pylori*, the bacterium that causes stomach ulcers, has found a way to survive in a very unforgiving environment, the stomach. The stomach uses hydrochloric acid to break down the food we eat. The high level of acid drives the pH down to about 2.0. This is extremely caustic. (If you've ever tried the experiment of leaving a baby tooth overnight in soda pop – which has about the same pH – you know exactly how destructive stomach acid can be. *Hint:* It wasn't the tooth fairy that made the tooth completely disappear!) *Helicobacter* has developed a way of effectively hiding from the acid by tunneling through the mucin layer to where the pH is not quite so caustic (Figure 5.3). However, it is

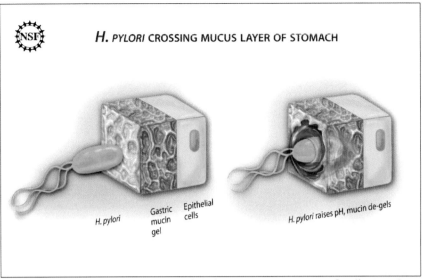

H. PYLORI CROSSING MUCUS LAYER OF STOMACH

H. pylori   Gastric   Epithelial
              mucin   cells
              gel

H. pylori raises pH, mucin de-gels

Figure 5.3: *Helicobacter pylori* **escapes a hostile environment using its flagella.** In order to escape the life-threating stomach acid (pH ≈ 2.0), *H. pylori* first raises the pH of the stomach mucin layer. Then, using its flagella it tunnels into the softened mucin which then re-seals over the bacterium providing much needed protection from the caustic hydrochloric acid. Courtesy of the NSF Multimedia Gallery, National Science Foundation, Arlington, Virginia, 2010

this same tunneling action which allows it to eventually cause stomach ulcers.

Toxins are poisonous substances found in various pathogens. They generally fall into one of two categories. **Endotoxins** are part of the cell wall structure of gram-negative bacteria (e.g., LPS). Endotoxins can cause serious, adverse physiologic effects like fever and shock. **Exotoxins** are poisonous proteins secreted by a variety of pathogens. Examples of exotoxins include: neurotoxins, enterotoxins, exfoliative toxins, erythrogenic toxins, and leucocidins.

Throughout the book, we'll see how other bacteria and fungi cause diseases in our veterinary patients.

Who Will Save Us? The Immune System to the Rescue!

The immune system is composed of three interrelated components: host tissue barriers, the "innate" immune response, and the "adaptive" immune response. These three act like layers of protection surrounding the host.

The First Line of Defense: Host Barriers

We're literally crawling with bacteria on our skin! You could shower three times a day and they'd still be there. Many are normal microflora, while others are not. So why don't these bacteria cause disease?

The Skin

The so-called "first line of defense" consists of host tissue barriers like the skin. Intact skin is like the castle of the Middle Ages whose stone walls protected the citizenry within (Figure 5.4). Intact skin provides many different defense properties that work quite well at resisting the attack of most microbial pathogens. For one, the skin is relatively dry. Bacteria need a certain amount of moisture to survive. Keratin, one of the key materials making up the epidermis, provides waterproofing to the skin keeping it dry. The skin also has a low basal pH making it relatively inhospitable to most bacteria. In addition, skin cells contain antibacterial substances such as lysozyme and antimicrobial peptides. **Lysozyme** destroys bacteria through its ability to disrupt the polysaccharides in the cell wall. **Antimicrobial peptides**, such as defensins and cathelicidins, are produced by the skin cells. These peptides form a kind of chemical shield against pathogens on the surface of the skin. Finally, removal of bacteria from the external surface of the skin occurs when the skin cells slough.

Mucin

Mucin is a group of mucoproteins found in various substances of the body such as saliva, gastric juices, and other mucous secretions. Mucin is released from the apical membrane of epithelial cells and forms a protective barrier which limits the exposure to commensal bacteria and prevents adhesion of pathogenic organisms. It also protects the epithelial layer from harmful products produced by bacteria, such as toxins and **reactive oxygen species** (ROS). If the epithelium were a castle (Figure 5.4), then mucin acts as the protective "moat" in front of the castle.

Secretory Immunoglobulin A (IgA)

A third component of the body's first line of defense comes in the form of secretory immunoglobin A (IgA). The body produces different types (called isotypes) of immunoglobulins (commonly referred to as antibodies), such as IgA, IgE, IgG, and IgM. B-lymphocytes secrete IgA which is then transported to the mucosal surfaces of the body. IgA molecules prevent microbial pathogens and toxins from traversing the epithelium by a series of actions that result in the entrapment and clearance of these entities from the body. (To continue the castle analogy, you can think of IgA as if the moat were stocked with alligators!) Some bacteria have developed ways to bind and destroy IgA, thus getting past this valuable defense mechanism.

The Second Line: The Innate Immune Response

The bodies of animals and humans alike possess many redundancies. If one system fails, the other tries to compensate. The immune system is no exception. The innate immune system serves as a second, non-specific, line of defense. It is composed of many factors, including phagocytes, extracellular killing mechanisms, the inflammatory response, and the complement system. Effective killing and elimination of pathogens via the innate immune system requires the coordination of all of these factors. Such coordination is accomplished in part through **cytokines**, signaling molecules that can stimulate or inhibit different functions of different cells of the immune system. The basic steps involved are: marking pathogens as foreign, ingestion of the pathogens, and destruction of the pathogens.

Marking Pathogens as Foreign: The Complement System

The **complement system** consists of a large number of plasma proteins that possess the ability to attach and break down pathogen cell walls, attract phagocytes, and stimulate inflammation. The first step in the complement cascade can involve complement proteins binding directly to microbes or to microbes coated with antibodies (see Humoral Immunity, below). As more and more complement proteins interact, they stimulate inflammation and recruit inflammatory cells to the scene, including phagocytes (see Ingestion of Pathogens, below). The endpoint of the complement cascade is the formation of the **membrane attack complex (MAC)**, a protein tube which creates a pore in the bacterial plasma membrane and induces cell lysis. This is a bit like the childhood prank

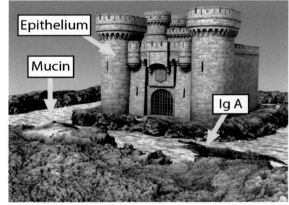

Figure 5.4: The skin as a formidable fortress. The epithelium (castle) constitutes a formidable barrier blocking the entry of pathogens. However, it is not acting alone. In many places, a layer of mucin (moat) coats the epithelial cells. In addition, IgA is freely floating in the mucin layer (alligators). This means that pathogens have to successfully cross the mucin moat while dodging IgA alligators before they even get to the epithelium. And they better have some serious tools by which to damage and enter the solidly built epithelial cells.

of pushing a pencil low into a Styrofoam cup full of a beverage and then quickly removing it (and laughing at the unfortunate kid whose drink is now soaking the school lunch table). In this case, the MAC "pencil" is hollow and doesn't need to be removed to do its damage. The cytoplasm of the pathogen rushes out of the MAC, thus effectively killing the cell.

The inflammatory response generated by complement produces multiple effects which enhance the body's ability to combat pathogens. Increasing local blood flow, activation of phagocytes, and increasing capillary permeability all allow for the localization of phagocytic cells to the area where the infection is occurring. The inflammatory response activates local clotting in an attempt to wall off the region and prevent spread of the pathogen. Inflammation also results in an increased local temperature which both inhibits the activities of the pathogen while increasing the activity and productivity of the immune system. If an infection becomes systemic, the hypothalamus reacts by increasing the body's temperature (i.e., fever). Fever has a stimulatory effect on immune cells and an inhibitory effect on pathogens.

Ingestion of Pathogens:
The Professional Phagocytes

One of the most important cell types in the innate immune system is the group known as **phagocytes.** These cells are professional "eating machines." Neutrophils, macrophages, and monocytes are all capable of engulfing and removing pathogens and debris from the body (Figure 5.5). During infection and injury, damaged host cells and pathogens each emit a chemical trail of bread crumbs in the form of **chemoattractants.** An example of a chemoattractant is the C5a peptide of the complement system. Phagocytes are attracted to and follow these chemoattractants and begin their attack.

First, the phagocyte attaches to the microbe and engulfs it by wrapping its plasma membrane around the microbe, creating a **phagosome**. The phagosome fuses with the cell's **lysosome**, a vesicle containing numerous hydrolytic enzymes capable of breaking down proteins, lipids, nucleic acid, and polysaccharides. The digestible parts of the microbe are recycled for use as nutrients and

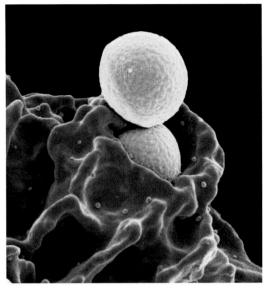

Figure 5.5: **A neutrophil (purple) phagocytosing Methicillin-Resistant** *Staphylococcus aureus* **(MRSA, yellow).** Colorized SEM. Courtesy of the National Institute of Allergy and Infectious Disease and the Public Health Image Library, PHIL #18168, Centers for Disease Control and Prevention, Atlanta, 2009.

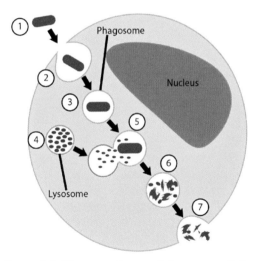

Figure 5.6: **The macrophage and the process of phagocytosis.** (1) The microbe emits chemoattractants that signal to the macrophage that foreign material is in the vicinity. The macrophage moves to and attaches to the microbe whereupon, (2) the microbe is ingested and (3) a phagosome is formed. (4) A lysosome moves within the cytoplasm toward the phagosome. (5) Fusion of the phagosome with a lysosome follows creating the phagolysosome. (6) The microbe is quickly digested leaving only indigestible material. (7) The indigestible material is discharged into the extracellular environment.

energy by the phagocyte; any indigestible material is released back into the body.

The most common phagocytes involved in pathogen destruction are **neutrophils** and **macrophages**. The first phagocytes "on scene" at the site of pathogen infiltration are the neutrophils. Macrophages arrive slightly later to kill any pathogens (e.g., bacteria) that the neutrophils failed to kill in an effective "one-two knockout punch". Additionally, macrophages initiate tissue repair by removing dead, dying, or damaged cells in the area.

The Common Denominator

What do phagocytes and the complement system have in common? They have the ability to detect small differences in the molecules located on the outer surfaces of pathogens and thereby identify these organisms as foreign or "non-self". This ability, however, is limited to a relatively small number of molecules, called **pathogen-associated molecular patterns** (or PAMPs). For bacteria, many of these PAMPs are associated with cell structures such as the peptidoglycan or lipoteichoic acids within the cell wall. Host cells possess specific receptors that recognize the common molecular patterns of PAMPs. These pattern recognition receptors allow innate protection against a wide array of bacterial invaders. A more specific, tailored approach to the elimination of the multitude of potential microbial invaders requires the ability to recognize an even larger set of foreign cell components. The adaptive immune system brings this ability to the table.

The Adaptive Immune Response: "The Buck Stops Here!"

A pathogen lucky enough to make it past the first two lines of defense, will find that it still must contend with the body's formidable adaptive immune response. The adaptive immune response possesses not only the ability to recognize microbes but can also kill them and store vital information about the pathogen and how to best eliminate it if a reinfection occurs in a process called "memory". The adaptive immune response can be divided into two parts: humoral immunity and cell-mediated immunity (CMI). The humoral response is required for protection against extracellular bacterial, fungal, and parasitic infections. The elimination of viruses from the host, as well as some intracellular bacteria and parasites (e.g., intracellular protozoa like *Toxoplasma*), requires CMI.

Humoral Immunity

In the humoral response, antibodies mark pathogens for removal by complement or macrophages. Two types of lymphocytes are very important in this process: B-lymphocytes (B cells) and T-lymphocytes (T cells). **B-lymphocytes** originate from the bone marrow; **T-lymphocytes** originate from the thymus. B cells take up exogenous antigen and present it to a subtype of T cells (helper T cells), which in turn activate B cells. This process is highly specific because, unlike in the innate immune system, adaptive immunity targets only those microbes that activates it. For example, each B-lymphocyte is able to recognize only a single antigen. When the B-lymphocyte ingests and processes its matching antigen (e.g., a particular cell wall component of a particular bacterium), it displays the antigen on its surface in a structure known as the major histocompatibility complex II (MHC-II). Helper T cells (also called CD4+ or Th cells) recognize the displayed antigen and produce chemical messages called **cytokines** that activate the B-lymphocyte causing it to start replicating, which is called clonal expansion. Some of these activated B-lymphocytes increase in size and begin producing antibodies that are specific to the antigen; these cells are called **plasma cells**. The cytokines also cause a subset of the B-lymphocytes to become **memory cells**. Memory B-lymphocytes are long-lived cells that are capable of quickly transforming into plasma cells should they meet the same antigen much (sometimes years!) later. The antibodies produced by plasma cells coat the pathogen. This antibody coating is attractive to macrophages thus destruction by phagocytosis is enhanced. The antibody-coated pathogens are also less likely to attach to host cells and cause infection. Additionally, antibody coated pathogens are better targets for killing by the complement system, thus eliminating them from the body. Antibodies that are specific to toxins can bind with them and prevent them from causing damage to the host cells (think about anti-snake venom!),

Antibodies are, however, incapable of marking intracellular pathogens, which reside (hide!) within host cells. This requires a different approach in the form of CMI.

Cell-mediated Immunity (CMI)

Intracellular pathogens avoid many of the host innate and humoral immune defenses by hiding within host cells, mostly in macrophages. CMI is a process whereby these pathogens are processed and presented in a form that the immune system will then recognize as foreign. Most nucleated cells are capable of processing and presenting endogenous antigens (i.e., antigens coming from cell cytoplasm) on their cell surface via MHC-I molecules. Cytotoxic T cells (also called CD8+ T cells) bind MHC class I molecules, recognize the antigen and proliferate to become killer T cells; some of the proliferating cells become long-living memory cytotoxic T cells. Cytotoxic T cells can recognize and kill host cells that are infected by the intracellular pathogens. Cytotoxic T cells kill their target cells by releasing granules containing two groups of proteins called perforins and granzymes onto the target cell surface. Perforins make a hole in the target cell membrane through which granzymes enter and cause cell death. Helper T cells (CD4+ T cells) are also very important for CMI; cytokines produced by these cells help activation of cytotoxic T cell and macrophages. Note that the helper T cells of CMI produce a different set of cytokines than those involved in humoral immunity. Activated macrophages can kill intracellular pathogens by secreting cytolytic enzymes and nitrous oxide.

Mechanisms by Which Pathogens Escape the Immune Response

It should be no surprise that while our immune system works hard to protect us from infectious diseases, pathogens develop ways of working around the immune system. Individual pathogens may possess a single or several different strategies. These can include antigenic variation, camouflage, and the ability to destroy antibodies. The human immunodeficiency virus (i.e., HIV, the causative agent of AIDS) evades the immune system by changing its surface antigens thereby constantly avoiding the antibody and CMI response of the immune system. Some pathogens, like *Staphylococcus aureus*, are able to conceal their foreign nature inside the host by coating themselves with proteins belonging to the host (e.g., fibrin). Upon interacting with the fibrin-coated pathogen, the host immune cells erroneously identify the pathogen as self. Finally, pathogens like the bacterium *Haemophilus influenza* can destroy the host's antibodies via an enzyme called IgA protease.

Immunology-based Diagnostic Tests

When someone mentions performing a serology test, they are referring to tests that look for evidence of specific antibodies in a patient's blood. For example, if you want to know if a horse is infected with West Nile Virus (WNV), one way to test is to look for WNV-specific antibodies in the horse's serum. Techniques for determining if antibody is present vary in their detection methods and include: radioactivity, fluorescence, color change, precipitation, and agglutination. Serology tests include enzyme linked immunosorbent assays (ELISA), indirect fluorescent antibody tests (IFA), and precipitation and agglutination tests, to name a few. Common examples include the microscopic agglutination test (MAT) for *Leptospira* and the Coggins tests for equine infectious anemia (EIA). For further details on test methods, refer to chapter 41 of Veterinary Immunology (see Further Readings, below).

Diseases of the Immune System

Despite the checks and balances in the immune system, immunological diseases do occur. Such diseases can generally be categorized as either autoimmune diseases or immunodeficiencies. The immune system is designed to spring to action only when there is a danger to host health posed by invading microorganisms. A healthy immune system can differentiate self-antigens from non-self-antigens, and react to only non-self antigens, but not to self-antigens; the system is tolerant to self. **Autoimmune diseases** occur when the immune system loses this tolerance and reacts (attacks!) self-antigens. Two examples are myasthenia gravis in which the body makes antibodies (known as auto-antibodies) against the acetylcholine receptors at neuromuscular junctions resulting in muscle weakness, and pemphigus foliaceous in which the body makes autoantibodies against cellular connections in the skin, resulting in vesicular (blister-causing) skin disease. **Immunodeficiencies** occur when a component of the immune system is lacking. For example, cyclic neutropenia occurs in gray collies making them more susceptible to diseases. In bovine leukocyte adhesion deficiency, neutrophils are unable to attach to endothelial cells of blood vessels and therefore cannot emigrate from blood vessels and move toward the site of infection. Severe combined immunodeficiency (SCID) in foals results in no functional T or B cells due to a missing enzyme required for the formation of antigen receptors.

Further Reading

Colville, Thomas P., and Joanna M. Bassert. "Chapter 9: Blood, Lymph, and Immunity." *Clinical Anatomy and Physiology for Veterinary Technicians*. 2nd ed. St. Louis, Mo.: Mosby Elsevier, 2008.

Tizard, Ian R. "Chapter 41: Immunological Diagnostic Techniques. *Veterinary Immunology*. 9th ed. St. Louis, Mo.: Elsevier/Saunders, 2013. Print.

Chapter 6:

Antimicrobial Drugs & Drug Resistance

Introduction

In the news, we hear about them on an increasingly frequent basis. A new "superbug" appears in hospitals and doctors' offices and there are few if any drugs to kill it. The media clamors for the medical community to develop a "magic bullet" – a super drug to kill a superbug. But what causes the development of these superbugs? What drugs currently exist to cure our veterinary patients of microbial pathogens? How do microbes develop resistance to them?

An **antimicrobial drug** is one that kills a microorganism or inhibits its growth. **Antibiotics** and **antifungals**, which target bacteria and fungi respectively, are both considered antimicrobials. Antimicrobial drugs have been around less than one hundred years. In 1928, Alexander Fleming discovered a fungus contaminating one of his petri dishes he had used to grow bacteria on. This, however, was no ordinary fungus. It killed the bacteria nearest to it on the petri dish. The mold was *Penicillium notatum* and the substance it produced would be harvested and come to be known as penicillin. Few people paid attention to his discovery when he published his findings a year later. However, penicillin would make an effective debut in World War II as a treatment for combat-related infections; the US produced over 400 million units by the end of the war. It wouldn't be until after World War II that production would skyrocket and society would realize the true potential of the power of antibiotics.

This chapter will focus on antibiotics. Antifungals will be briefly discussed in chapters 19-21.

Antimicrobial Drugs

Selective Toxicity

The Middle Age alchemist, Paracelsus, understood that all things must be done in moderation. The most effective medicine becomes poisonous if taken at too high a dose. With antimicrobial drugs a concept developed known as **selective toxicity**. A drug that has selective toxicity causes more harm to the pathogen than to the host. The basis for selective toxicity comes from the ability of the antimicrobial drug to recognize structures or processes of the pathogen, *but not the host*. In the case of some antibiotics, they are able to target the bacterial cell wall which has a vastly different structure than animal cells. This enables them to penetrate and disrupt the bacteria's cell wall without causing

You tell 'em, Paracelsus!

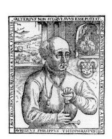

"Solely the dose determines that a thing is not a poison."

Paracelsus (1493-1541)

damage to the host's cells.

Selective toxicity can be indirectly measured by calculating a drug's **therapeutic index**. A drug's therapeutic index is calculated using the formula below:

$$Therapeutic\ Index = \frac{Maximum\ Tolerated\ Dose}{Minimum\ Therapeutic\ Dose}$$

A drug that has a therapeutic index of 8 is more effective and less toxic to the patient than a drug with an index of 1. Whenever possible, a drug with the highest therapeutic index should be chosen. However, there are some situations where the benefits justify the risk of using a drug with a low therapeutic index. For example, a patient's risk of dying from an extremely aggressive form of cancer outweighs the risk of toxicity inherent in some chemotherapy drugs.

Spectrum of Activity

The range of microorganisms an antimicrobial drug can kill or inhibit is known as its **spectrum of activity** (Figure 6.1). **Broad spectrum** antimicrobials target a wide range of pathogens. **Empirical treatment** is the practice of choosing an antimicrobial based on a practitioner's "best guess" as to the identity of the pathogen. Often this happens when treating a serious infection where it would be inadvisable to wait for the identification of the pathogen prior to beginning treatment. Drug selection may also be made without identifying the pathogen during the first-occurrence of the pathogen, e.g., "routine" infections of the ears or urinary tract. Broad spectrum antimicrobials make a good empiric choice in such situations. However, they are not without risk. Because their target range is wide, broad spectrum antimicrobials may also affect the body's normal microflora. Remember that loss of normal microflora can give the opportunity for other microbes – some pathogenic – to colonize the body.

On the other hand, **narrow spectrum** antimicrobials target a more limited range of microbes. To be most effective, this requires the correct identification of the pathogen. The benefit is that narrow spectrum antimicrobials are less disruptive to the body's normal microflora.

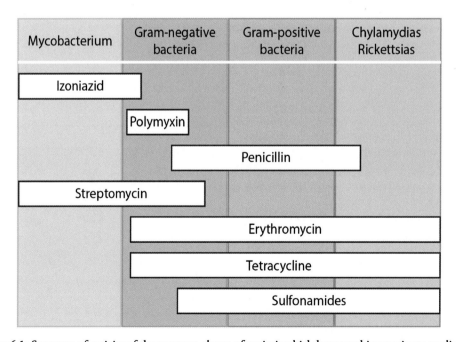

Figure 6.1: Spectrum of activity of the common classes of antimicrobial drugs used in veterinary medicine.

To Kill or Not to Kill...

Antimicrobials act against pathogens in one of two ways. **Bacteriostatic** drugs inhibit the growth of the pathogen allowing the host immune response time to eliminate the pathogen. These drugs are suitable for minor infections. They are not a good choice in severe infections or when the host's immune system is suppressed (e.g., FIV-infected cats, or dogs receiving chemotherapy). **Bactericidal** drugs actually kill the pathogen directly. Removal of the pathogen occurs through the phagocytic activities of cells like macrophages. Some antibiotics can be both bacteriostatic and bactericidal, depending on the dose, duration of exposure, and the state of the invading bacteria. Examples of bacteriostatic and bactericidal drugs are given in Table 6.1.

Table 6.1: Examples of bacteriostatic and bactericidal antimicrobials used in veterinary medicine.

Bacteriostatic	Bactericidal
Chloramphenicol	Aminoglycosides
Clindamycin	Beta-lactams
Erythromycin	Metronidazole
Sulfonamides	Rifampin
Trimethoprim	Quinolones
Tetracyclines	Vancomycin
	Trimethoprim-sulfa

Remember this:
Bactericidal and Bacteriostatic Drugs Don't Mix!

Bacteriostatic drugs often slow down the growth of the bacteria it targets. This is antagonistic to the actions of most bactericidal drugs. This is the reason that we don't prescribe a bacteriostatic drug in combination with a bactericidal drug.

Mechanisms of Action

Antimicrobial drugs use a variety of ways to eliminate pathogens. These can be classified into five groups based on their mechanism of action. These mechanisms include:
- Inhibition of cell wall synthesis
- Disruption of plasma membrane function
- Inhibition of protein synthesis
- Inhibition of nucleic acid synthesis
- Inhibition of enzyme activity

Inhibition of Cell Wall Synthesis

β-lactam antibiotics, such as penicillins and cephalosporins, kill bacteria by blocking the formation of cross-linkages that stabilize peptidoglycan. This inhibits division and destabilizes the cell wall, leading to rupture of the bacterium. This action is specifically targeted to prokaryotic cells as eukaryotic cells lack a cell wall (i.e., no peptidoglycan).Other antibiotics that interfere with peptidoglycan formation include vancomycin and bacitracin. Drugs that interfere with cell wall synthesis are bactericidal.

Disruption of Plasma Membrane Function

Like the cell wall, the integrity of the plasma membrane is key to the survival of bacteria. Some antibiotics act by targeting the phospholipids within the membrane. Polymyxins are cationic detergents that interfere with the cell membrane, resulting in increased permeability and loss of the cytoplasm and cell contents. Because the structure of the plasma membrane of bacteria and eukaryotic cells are extremely similar, the use of these types of antibiotics is typically limited to topical use. Polymyxin B is often one of the main active ingredients in the so-called "triple antibiotic" ointment found over-the-counter in most drug stores. The polymyxins selectively target gram-negative bacteria; the specificity is due to the presence of certain phospholipids in the cell membrane and the fact that gram-negative bacteria have an exposed cell membrane, unlike gram-positive bacteria whose cell membrane is covered by a thick layer of peptidoglycan. Drugs that target the cell membrane are bactericidal.

Inhibition of Protein Synthesis

Protein synthesis occurs during translation of mRNA. In order to translate the mRNA, ribosomes are needed. By their very nature, ribosomes are proteins themselves. They consist of two protein subunits that fit together to make a larger protein. These subunits are referred to by their relative size, which is calculated in something called Svedberg units. The "S" of a 70S ribosome, for example, stands for 70 Svedberg units. We will use the Svedberg units to readily differentiate between the different subunits of prokaryotic and eukaryotic ribosomes; their exact measurements are not important for us here.

Let us now briefly review the process of protein synthesis. First, mRNA is transcribed from the host DNA. In our case, the host could be either a eukaryote (e.g., dog or horse) or a prokaryote (e.g., bacteria or fungus). Here, let us follow the process of prokaryotic translation as an example. Once the bacterial host DNA has been transcribed into mRNA, the mRNA is transferred to a ribosome that is floating in the bacterial cytoplasm. The mRNA lays atop the smaller ribosomal subunit whereupon the larger subunit comes down on top of the mRNA, thus surrounding it. Once closed around the mRNA, the ribosome begins reading the genetic code of the mRNA and simultaneously produces the corresponding protein.

Two types of ribosomes are produced: a 70S and an 80S ribosome for bacteria and animals, respectively. Bacterial 70S ribosomes contain a 30S and 50S subunit, whereas animal cytoplasmic 80S ribosomes contain 40S and 60S subunits. Antibiotics that inhibit bacterial protein synthesis target the 30S or the 50S subunits, and thus they are fairly specific for bacteria. However, eukaryotes also contain 70S ribosomes within their mitochondria that may also be targeted by antibiotics. It is thought that this non-specific targeting of the 30S subunit of 70S ribosomes is the reason behind the occasional toxicity to the kidneys (i.e., nephrotoxicity) and ears (i.e., ototoxicity) of animals while using antibiotics such as gentamicin, an aminoglycoside. With these antibiotics, care must be taken to thoroughly check the animal's health records and establish if they have a prior history of damage to these organs. Also, the veterinarian should decide whether the current illness or condition is likely to increase the likelihood of damage to these organs. If so, it is best to steer clear of these types of antibiotics. For example, if it is determined that pre-existing kidney damage exists or the animal is very dehydrated, it is best to avoid the use of aminoglycosides so as to avoid worsening existing kidney damage.

Examples of drugs able to inhibit protein synthesis include: tetracycline, gentamicin, chloramphenicol, and amikacin. Drugs that interfere with protein synthesis are bacteriostatic.

Inhibition of Nucleic Acid Synthesis

Nucleic acid synthesis is an important task for bacterial cells. Without DNA replication, bacteria cannot copy genomic DNA and produce daughter cells. Without RNA transcription, DNA cannot be read and produce messenger RNA which will later be translated to form proteins necessary for the bacterial cell's day-to-day operations. Fluoroquinolones (e.g., enrofloxacin and ciprofloxacin) inhibit DNA gyrase, an enzyme essential in bacterial DNA replication. Because bacterial RNA polymerase is structurally different from animal RNA polymerase, drugs like rifampin can block RNA transcription. Drugs that interfere with nucleic acid synthesis are bactericidal.

Inhibition of Enzyme Activity

Bacteria produce numerous enzymes to help carry out the myriad of chemical reactions required for cell growth, maintenance, and replication. Drugs that target essential enzymatic reactions by binding to the enzymes active site can disable the essential pathway and slow the bacteria down, making it an easier target for phagocytes. For example, synthesis of folic acid (i.e., vitamin B) is very important for many bacteria. Many sulfa drugs, such as sulfamethoxazole-trimethoprim, inhibit different enzymes along the folic acid synthesis pathway (Figure 6.2). Individually, they are bacteriostatic, but together, because they are targeting two points in the pathway, they are bactericidal (Table 6.1).

Combination Therapies

While most infections may respond to a single antimicrobial, other more serious infections may require prescribing multiple antimicrobials to effectively eliminate the infection. Combining antibiotics can have two main outcomes. **Synergism** occurs when the administration of two drugs together exerts an additive effect (i.e., a better outcome than if each antibiotic were given singly). Streptomycin and penicillin act synergistically. Penicillin damages the bacterial cell wall allowing for better penetration by streptomycin. Some drugs come already formulated as combination drugs. Sulfamethoxazole-trimethoprim is one such drug combination. **Antagonism** occurs if drugs that are used in combination are less effective than when each is used alone. An example of an antagonistic combination of antibiotics is tetracycline and penicillin. Tetracyclines inhibit bacterial cell growth through their ability to inhibit protein synthesis. Penicillin, however, requires normal bacterial cell growth in order to be effective. Combinations of antibiotics should be chosen so as to maximize synergism and avoid antagonism.

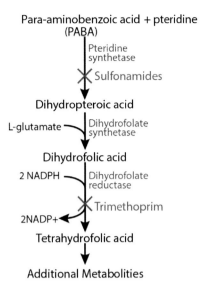

Figure 6.2: Inhibition of the folic acid synthesis pathway. Both sulfa drugs and trimethoprim (red X's) can block various portions of the folic acid synthesis pathway leading to a decrease in available folic acid. Folic acid, vitamin B, is essential for bacterial cell function.

Client Compliance

As a veterinary technician, you may be asked to go over with the owner the medications prescribed to the pet or livestock animal. During this time, you should inform the owner about the importance of client compliance. Research has shown that low doses of bactericidal antibiotics can mutate the bacterial genome. These mutations may play a critical role in the emergence of resistance to one or multiple classes of antibiotics. Forgetting to give the medication, skipping doses, or not giving the right dose can all cause the concentration of the drug within the body to fall to these low, subtherapeutic levels. Likewise, a client may be tempted to stop administering antibiotics to their pet before the prescription is finished because the client thinks the pet is better and doesn't need to take the rest of the medication. It is our duty to explain that while it is very good that the pet appears to feel better, some microbes may yet remain. It is vital to the ultimate health of the animal to kill these remaining bacteria, lest the bacteria mutate and become resistant to many (or all) antibiotics used to treat the infection.

Antibiotics and Viral infections

It is important for clients to understand that as helpful and even lifesaving as antibiotics can be, they are not useful for all types of infections. For example, antibiotics are not effective in treating viral infections. In fact, the use of an antibiotic in this instance may potentially harm the patient as many broad-spectrum antibiotics are capable of killing off some of the normal microflora. The loss of normal microflora may allow the virus to access more sites and cause a more severe infection. Discussing the merits and limitations of antibiotic use in our veterinary patients will help clients to understand how and when it is best to prescribe antibiotics for their animals.

There is one very specific exception to the "rule" discussed in the previous paragraph. Sometimes a virus does not exist as the sole infection. Instead, the virus causes the initial damage and opens up an area of the body that bacteria can successfully colonize. These bacteria are responsible for what are called "secondary" infections; most often, they occur secondary to a viral infection. For example, people can be infected by various cold viruses (e.g., rhinoviruses) that can cause damage to not only the nasal epithelium but also the back of the throat. *Streptococcus pyogenes*, a bacterium, can take advantage of the damaged pharyngeal epithelium and colonize these tissues which leads to a disease may of us may have intimate experience with – "Strep" throat! At this point, when the physician diagnoses Strep throat, he or she will prescribe antibiotics – not against the rhinovirus, but against the secondary invader, *Streptococcus pyogenes*. In clinical practice, the veterinarian may suspect that microbes (i.e., particularly bacteria) may be taking advantage of the damage done by a viral infection and will prescribe antibiotics to kill the bacteria before they can weaken the patient even further. A common example of microbial synergism in veterinary medicine is bovine respiratory ("shipping") disease which begins with a viral infection, followed by bacteria infecting the respiratory tract and causing most of the pathology.

Antibiotic Resistance

Antibiotic resistance is a significant problem affecting both human and veterinary medicine today. The discovery and approval of new antibiotics is currently at an all-time low. Therefore, it is critical for the health and welfare of both humans and animals that we use antibiotics appropriately.

Methods of Resistance

Just as antibiotics have several different methods of action, there are different methods bacteria can use to develop resistance. Bacteria are constantly being bombarded by threats to their survival. Heat, cold, ultraviolet (UV) radiation, caustic chemicals, and antibiotics are but a few. In any population of bacteria, there are at least a few possessing traits or characteristics that allow them to survive a given threat. Such a trait makes the bacterium more "fit" for survival. For example, a bacterium that produces more capsule than its "brothers and sisters" may better survive in the presence of a threat, such as high stomach acid production. This bacterium not only survives the threat, but reproduces, passing that trait – in this case, enhanced capsule production – to all of its progeny. The more often the bacteria encounter the same threat or "pressure," the more often the susceptible bacteria without the trait die and the bacteria that are able to resist the threat live and produce more progeny. This **selective pressure** leads to a shift in the population of bacteria where the majority of individual bacterium are able to survive the threat. In the case of antibiotics, this means that an antibiotic that initially could kill almost all of the bacteria within a population will no longer be effective. There are several mechanisms by which a bacterium can gain a fitness advantage over other bacteria in the population, and below some of the major categories of mechanisms are listed.

- Altered target
- Enzyme degradation
- Efflux

Altered Target

As described earlier, antibiotics employ specific mechanisms of action directed at particular targets. Bacteria possessing an altered target will be resistant to antibiotics that can no longer bind to their intended target and exert their effect. A high profile example of this is the altered penicillin binding protein (PBP) produced by the methicillin resistant staphylococci such as methicillin resistant *Staphylococcus aureus* (MRSA) and *S. pseudintermedius* (MRSP). Another example of an altered target is fluoroquinolone resistance. Bacteria resistant to fluoroquinolones possess DNA gyrases that are mutated and thus no longer contain the active site that fluoroquinolones bind to, thereby making the bacteria impervious to the antibiotic.

Enzyme degradation

Some bacteria possess enzymes capable of degrading particular antimicrobials, rendering the antimicrobial ineffective against the bacterium. For example, bacteria that possess the enzyme β-lactamase are able to cleave the β-lactam ring (Figure 6.3) of penicillin through a process of hydrolysis, thus rendering it non-functional. As early as 1940, just a few years after penicillin was introduced onto the market, reports of *E. coli* resistant to the drug were being reported. Later, it was discovered that when penicillin was coupled with clavulanic acid, the clavulanic acid blocked the action of the β-lactamase enzyme and protected the activity of penicillin.

Extended spectrum β-lactamases (i.e., bacteria containing a modification of the β-lactamase enzyme) confer resistance to third generation cephalosporins as well; however, these bacteria are still inhibited by clavulanic acid. Trade names of this drug combination include Augmentin®, used in human medicine, and the veterinary product Clavamox® (Pfizer).

Efflux

Certain bacteria possess channels within their cell wall that are capable of actively exporting antimicrobials and other compounds out of the cell. In this scenario, the antimicrobial enters the bacterium through a channel or porin, called an efflux pump (Figure 6.4). The efflux pump promptly pumps the antimicrobial back out into the extracellular environment thus preventing the lethal intracellular accumulation of the drug inside the cell. Gram-negative bacteria and mycobacteria are two groups of bacteria that possess efflux pumps. This is a common mechanism of resistance against tetracyclines.

DNA mutations and genetic transfer

Every time a bacteria divides, it must first make a copy of its DNA so that it can pass one copy of its genetic material to each of its two daughter cells in a process called DNA replication. DNA replication does not always result in a perfect copy. Accidental substitutions of base pairs, small deletions, and small insertions may occur. These mutations may be lethal to the bacterium and thus the mutation is removed from the population. However, many small mutations are not lethal. In fact, a mutation in the bacterial DNA may result in the production of an altered gene product which is advantageous to the bacterium.

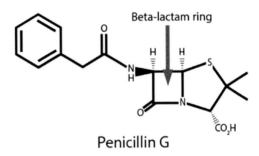

Penicillin G

Figure 6.3: Penicillin G and the location of the β-lactam ring. Bacteria that possess β-lactamases are able to cleave this ring rendering the antibiotic useless.

As discussed above, selection pressure helps to establish populations of bacteria that have the ability to survive a variety of external pressures including the actions of antimicrobials. Passing this genetic advantage to progeny ensures the continued survival of a given species of bacteria. However, this encoded advantage does not have to stay only within that species. In the big picture of antimicrobial resistance, even more important than mutations is the horizontal transfer of genetic material between bacteria, both within and across species. Horizontal transfer can occur by several means, including: conjugation, transformation, and transduction.

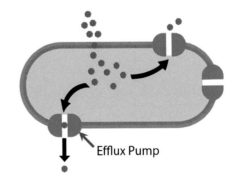

Figure 6.4: Efflux pumps aid certain bacteria by preventing the buildup of toxic amounts of antimicrobials and other substances within the cell's cytoplasm.

Conjugation

Many plasmids carry genes that confer resistance to antimicrobials. When two bacterial cells are in close proximity to each other, a hollow bridge-like structure known as a **sex pilus** forms between the two cells. As the plasmid DNA is duplicated, one copy is transferred from one bacterium to another, including the gene(s) encoding resistance. This process, called **conjugation**, enables a susceptible bacterium to acquire resistance to a particular antimicrobial agent.

Transformation

When cells die and break apart, DNA can be released in the surrounding environment. This free-floating DNA is commonly referred to as "naked" DNA. Other bacteria in close proximity can scavenge the naked DNA and incorporate it into their own DNA in a process called **transformation**. This naked DNA may contain advantageous genes such as antimicrobial resistant genes and benefit the recipient bacterial cell.

Transduction

In **transduction**, bacterial DNA is transferred from one bacterium to another inside a virus capable of infecting bacteria. These viruses are called bacteriophages or "phage," for short. When a phage infects a bacterium, it takes over the bacteria's genetic processes to produce more phage. During this process, bacterial DNA may inadvertently be incorporated into the new phage DNA. Bacteriophage infections typically end up causing bacterial death and lysis. Cell lysis releases the new phages enabling them to go on to infect other bacteria. The new phage brings along genes from the previously infected bacterium. These genes are often part of a genetic element known as a **transposon** or "jumping gene." Transposons possess the necessary machinery which allows them to not only replicate but also to "cut-out" a copy of themselves and pass that copy onto another species of bacteria. This is especially troubling, as this is one way in which different species of bacteria can acquire and share genes encoding resistance to the same sets of antibiotics. An antibiotic that was once successful at treating infections caused by many different bacteria may eventually not be effective against most or any of them!

> ## Client Education:
> ## No Resistance Here!
>
> The keys to preventing antibiotic resistance are:
> - Make sure to give the medication as directed by the veterinarian.
> - Finish the entire prescription even if the animal starts to look like it feels better.

Clinical Applications

This chapter provides an overview of the principles of antimicrobial therapy, however the application of this information must take the patient into consideration. Species, age and concurrent medical issues can render some drug choices inappropriate. Certain drugs are illegal to use in food animals. While one drug may be an excellent choice for a dog, it may kill a rabbit. Additionally, cost and the route and frequency of administration must be considered when selecting antimicrobial therapy.

Further Reading

Borzelleca, Joseph F. "Paracelsus: Herald of Modern Toxicology." *Toxicological Sciences* 53 1 (2000): 2-4.

Edlund, Thomas, and Staffan Normark. "Recombination between Short DNA Homologies Causes Tandem Duplication." *Nature* 292 5820 (1981): 269-71.

Garcia-Migura, Lourdes, et al. "Antimicrobial Resistance of Zoonotic and Commensal Bacteria in Europe: The Missing Link between Consumption and Resistance in Veterinary Medicine." *Veterinary Microbiology* 170 1-2 (2014): 1-9.

Khadem, Tina M., et al. "Antimicrobial Stewardship: A Matter of Process or Outcome?" *Pharmacotherapy: The Journal of Human Pharmacology and Drug Therapy* 32 8 (2012): 688-706.

McGowan, John E. "Antimicrobial Stewardship—the State of the Art in 2011: Focus on Outcome and Methods." *Infection Control and Hospital Epidemiology* 33 4 (2012): 331-37.

Organization, World Health. *Antimicrobial Resistance: Global Report on Surveillance.* Switzerland: World Health Organization, 2014.

Wright, Gerard D. "Bacterial Resistance to Antibiotics: Enzymatic Degradation and Modification." *Advanced Drug Delivery Reviews* 57 10 (2005): 1451–70.

Part II:

Veterinary Bacteriology

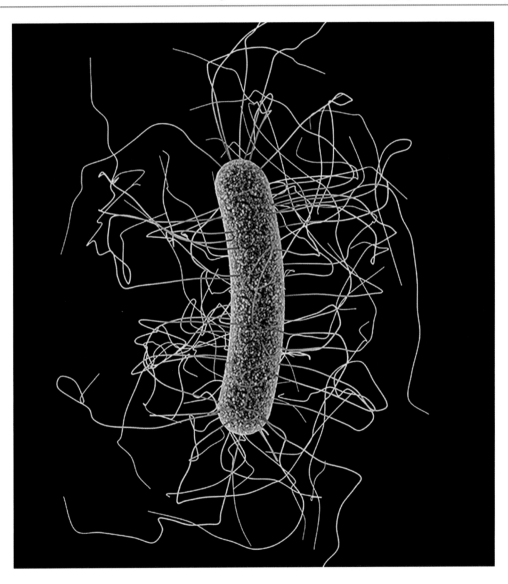

Chapter 7:

Gram-Positive Cocci – *Staphylococcus, Streptococcus,* & *Enterococcus*

Introduction

The bacteria in this chapter have many common attributes beyond their cell morphology and gram staining characteristics. For one, the members of these three genera are very widely distributed in the environment making it impossible to avoid contact with them. Many of the species are considered commensal organisms (Table 7.1). Yet, under particular circumstances, each is capable of causing significant and sometimes deadly disease.

Table 7.1: Terms to know

Term	Definition
Pathogen	Any disease-producing agent or microorganism; Also known as a "primary" or "frank" pathogen
Opportunistic pathogen	A microorganism that does not ordinarily cause disease but becomes pathogenic under certain circumstances
Commensal organism	Living on or within another organism, and deriving benefit without harming or benefiting the host

Staphylococcus

Staphylococci are spherical (coccoid), gram-positive bacteria approximately 0.5-1.5 µm in size. Inside the host and in liquid culture, staphylococci occur in irregular "grape-like" clusters, pairs, or short chains (Figure 7.1, top panel). When plated on artificial solid media, such as a blood agar plate, the colonies produced are white to off-white, smooth, and butyrous ("butter-like") (Figure 7.1, middle panel). An exception to this is *Staphylococcus aureus* which produces golden colored colonies due to the production of carotenoid pigments (Figure 7.1, bottom panel). Staphylococci are catalase-positive. This is an important test used to differentiate staphylococci from streptococci, which are catalase-negative.

Where Do Staphylococci Come From?

Staphylococci are ubiquitous, meaning that they can be found just about anywhere. They inhabit the skin of humans and animals. When we bathe, we may remove a small portion of these staphylococci, but they very quickly multiply and once again cover the surface of our skin. Staphylococci survive very well in the environment - on the ground, on the table, and on the end of that pencil you just finished chewing on nervously during the big test!

If Staphylococci Are All Around Us, Why Don't We Get Sick?

Normally, staphylococci don't cause disease. This is because of the extensive protection our bodies possess in the form of the immune system. Even biting on that pen cap and ingesting a few staphylococci is no match for our mucosal immune system. So, staphylococci need a little "help" in entering the host before they can cause much in the way of disease. This help could be in the form of a cut on the skin or a viral infection that causes a sore and inflamed throat.

Biochemical Characteristics

Staphylococci are facultative anaerobes capable of producing variable amounts of capsule. Several biochemical tests can be used to help distinguish staphylococci from other bacterial species. One of the most useful is the catalase test. **Catalase**, an enzyme that can break hydrogen peroxide down into oxygen and water, is useful for differentiating staphylococci (i.e., catalase-positive) from streptococci (i.e., catalase-negative). For more on the catalase test, see Chapter 22. Further biochemical tests, such as the coagulase test, lead to identification of the particular species of staphylococci.

Hardiness

Staphylococcal isolates are known to be fairly hardy. For example, they withstand drying inside wounds or pus for several weeks. Many staphylococci possess a plasmid-encoded penicillinase rendering them impervious to the β-lactam antimicrobials. For this reason, it is often necessary to use a combination penicillin (e.g., penicillin combined with clavulanic acid) to treat staphylococcal infections. Exchange of the penicillinase-containing plasmid from staphylococci to other bacteria results in transference of this bacterial resistance mechanism to other bacterial species, such as streptococci and bacilli.

Clinical Conditions: General

As mentioned previously, colonization of the exterior portions of the body does not result in infection. Immune defenses, such as the integrity of the skin, must be breached (e.g., a cut or wound) before disease results. The majority of staphylococcal infections result in a suppurative (i.e., pus-forming) immune response. Microscopically, neutrophils inundate the area of the wound. Small gram-positive cocci could be found both extracellularly and intracellularly (e.g., neutrophils phagocytosing bacteria).

Rarely, another clinical condition may develop called **botryomycosis**. This condition is a more

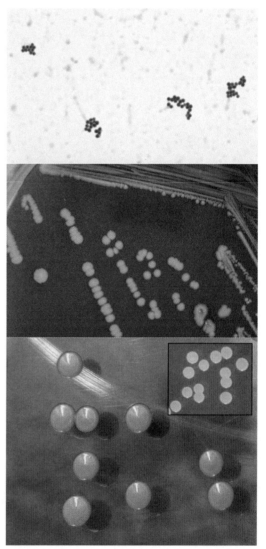

Figure 7.1: The genus *Staphylococcus*. Top panel: *Staphylococcus aureus.* The gram-positive, grape-like clusters characteristic of the genus can be seen on Gram stain. **Middle panel:** Colonies of *Staphylococcus epidermitis* showing white colonies. **Bottom panel:** Colonies of *Staphylococcus aureus.* The golden color is a result of the production of carotenoid pigments. Top and middle photo © the authors. Bottom photo courtesy of Hans Newman and used with permission.

frequent presentation in certain species (e.g., mice) but is rare in most veterinary species. Botryomycosis refers to the chronic granulomatous reaction consisting of neutrophils and activated macrophages, present as multinucleated giant cells that surround the infection. Botryomycosis in mice usually occurs with skin infections and manifests itself as a hard lump just under the skin.

Dogs and Cats

Staphylococcal infections in dogs and cats can take many forms; however, they are almost always suppurative. Examples include conjunctival, ear, skin, uterine, and bladder infections. The primary isolate recovered from these infections is *Staphylococcus pseudintermedius*.

**Remember this:
A Chink-in-the-Armor**
If your skin and mucous membranes function like body armor (*Think: King Arthur!*), then it takes a "chink-in-the-armor" to allow staphylococci into your body.

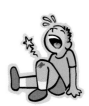

Pyoderma (literally meaning: pus in skin) resembles the acne of human adolescence. Small red inflamed pustules (i.e., "pimples") may be localized to one area like the abdomen or may be distributed over the entire body. Pyoderma is most common in dogs and there is usually an underlying or predisposing factor, such as atopy or trauma, involving the skin. **Atopy** is a condition where individuals are predisposed to develop allergic reactions to allergens that are inhaled or contact the skin. Atopy is thought to be an underlying factor in a number of skin infections.

External ear infections (i.e., otitis externa) are often secondary to atopy. Patients with atopy are extremely itchy. When they scratch the skin, their claws can cause abrasions in the skin and provide an entryway for bacteria such as *Staphylococcus* species to enter and cause infection. In cases of otitis externa, staphylococcal infection often occurs in the presence of another commensal organism, the yeast *Malassezia*. Treatment should take into account the likelihood of dual infections.

More serious, but thankfully less frequent, infections can occur such as osteomyelitis (i.e., infection of the bone). In an open fracture, such as after a hit-by-car accident, the bone is forced through the skin when it fractures. The skin staphylococci can then travel down the bone and get access to the bone and deeper tissues. Other infections in which *Staphylococcus* species may be involved include mastitis and urinary tract infections.

Changing Nomenclature:

Our knowledge about microbes is always improving. Sometimes, we discover that a bacterium is actually more closely related to another genus or species and thus the bacterium undergoes a name change.

That is the case with *Staphylococcus pseudintermedius* (formerly *S. intermedius*). These species are so similar that it takes special DNA sequencing to tell them apart. Unless proven genetically, most isolates from dogs and cats are likely to be *S. pseudintermedius* and not *S. intermedius*.

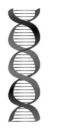

Guinea Pig & Avian Species

"Bumblefoot" is the laymen's term for the condition pododermatitis, a condition that occurs in rodents, guinea pigs, and some avian species. **Pododermatitis** literally means "inflammation of the skin of the foot," but it also implies that the inflammation results from infection. In the case of guinea pigs and birds, most often *Staphylococcus aureus* is to blame for the infection. Predisposing factors consist of anything causing nicks, scratches, and irritation to the bottom of the feet. This often includes poor footing (e.g., rough wooden perches for birds and wire bottom cages for guinea pigs). Poor husbandry and failure to keep the environment clean also contribute substantially. Once the staphylococci enter the irritated skin of the foot, an abscess can form. Infection can occasionally spread and affect the joints of the foot causing further disability.

Ruminants

Staphylococci-induced **mastitis** (i.e., inflammation of the udder) affects cattle, sheep, and goats (Figure 7.2). *S. aureus* causes severe, contagious mastitis and is always bad news when it appears on milk culture reports. Other bacteria such as *E. coli*, *Mycoplasma* sp. and *Streptococcus agalactiae* may also cause mastitis, the latter two are also classified as agents of contagious mastitis. Like other staphylococcal infections, the predominant inflammatory response is purulent with subsequent abscess formation. The condition may occur both as a low-level chronic or a peracute infection. Peracute infections can lead to **gangrene**, a serious complication that can result in the necrosis and loss of part of the udder; it may even require euthanasia of the cow. Mastitis-related decreases in milk production cause significant losses in profit. Predisposing factors to mastitis include damage to the teat sphincter and canal; improper cleaning and sanitization of the milking equipment; and an abnormally high vacuum pressure within the teat cups of the milking machine. A diagnosis of contagious mastitis results in culling of infected cows, whereas a diagnosis of environmental mastitis results in heightened awareness of milking practices, especially cleanliness.

Horses

Infections in horses usually consist of mastitis or trauma-induced abscesses caused mainly by *S. aureus*. The pectoral region, spermatic cord (e.g., after castration), and skin are all sites where staphylococci can localize after trauma to those areas. Predisposing factors to infection include trauma, surgery, and, in the case of mastitis, teat injury.

Swine

Staphylococcus hyicus causes a clinical condition in swine known as "greasy pig disease." Greasy pig

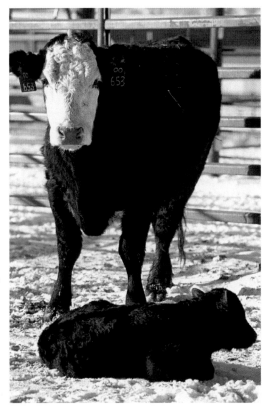

Figure 7.2: Cow with calf. *Staphylococcus aureus* is one of many species of bacteria that can cause mastitis in a variety of domestic species. The USDA is performing research on a vaccine against *S. aureus* mastitis in cattle. Photo courtesy of the Animal Research Service, United States Department of Agriculture, ARS Image Bank (#K10366), date unknown.

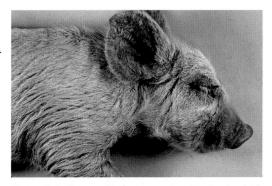

Figure 7.3: Greasy pig disease, swine. Notice the thick exudate that covers the surface of this piglet giving it an extremely unkempt appearance. Courtesy of Dr. Alan Doster, University of Nebraska-Lincoln.

disease (Figure 7.3) occurs in very young pigs and is characterized by a rapidly fatal systemic infection. The most prominent clinical sign occurs as a thick, grey brown exudate extending over most of the skin, but especially around the face and ears making the pig appear greasy. It is from this presentation that the disease gained its name. There is a wide spectrum of disease with some pigs exhibiting extremely greasy and encrusted skin to those showing very little clinical signs at all. Transmission occurs from sows to their offspring via parturition (i.e., birthing process) as *S. hyicus* colonizes the sow's vaginal tissues.

Diagnostics

Staphylococci can be cultured using standard blood agar. Alternatively, it may be cultured using selective media such as Mannitol Salt or Staph 110 agar. Gram stain, catalase, and coagulase tests can help confirm the presence of staphylococci. (For more on how to perform and interpret these tests see Chapter 22). Staphylococci are catalase-positive. The different species of staphylococci vary in their coagulase test results. For example, *S. aureus* and *S. pseudintermedius* are coagulase positive, while *S. hyicus* is coagulase negative. Because of the increasing resistance to multiple antibiotics, once an isolate is determined to be of the genus *Staphylococcus*, it is important to perform antibiotic susceptibility testing. In addition to standard microbiological testing, an ELISA is available that can be performed on milk samples to determine the presence of staphylococci in cases of bovine mastitis.

Treatment, Control, and Prevention

Treatment consists of prescribing antibiotics based on culture and antimicrobial susceptibility testing. Because penetration of antibiotics is poor in large abscesses, it may be necessary to drain the abscess surgically prior to initiating antibiotic treatment. While the prevention strategy of vaccination has been tried, antibodies are short-lived and not protective; to date, there is no commercial vaccine available. The client can do much to improve the chances of preventing new infections and controlling the spread of already existing infections. These methods include ensuring good husbandry and performing preventive maintenance on equipment (e.g., milking machine). Good husbandry practices consist of improving and maintaining sanitary conditions, reducing stressors to the animal(s), and **biosecurity** (see callout box, below).

Client Education: Biosecurity

Biosecurity consists of operations or procedures designed to decrease the likelihood of a disease entering an area of animal housing. This could be a livestock yard, a cow-calf farm, or a dog breeding facility. The principles are the same.

Owners of these facilities should limit people and animal traffic to only those individuals that need to be in the animal housing area. In addition, they may ask that persons who have recently visited other farms not enter or, alternately, that they shower and change into fresh, clean clothes prior to entering. This is to decrease the likelihood that pathogens able to cling to hair, skin, and clothing cross into the housing area with a chance of infecting the animals.

Methicillin-Resistant *Staphylococci* (MRS)

Read the newspapers and you may come across a disturbing trend; cases of methicillin-resistant *Staphylococcus aureus* (MRSA, pronounced "*MUR-sah*") appear to be on the rise. MRSA refers to *S. aureus* bacteria that have acquired resistance to not only methicillin, but multiple antibiotics such as oxacillin, penicillin, and amoxicillin. MRSA gets its ability to resist destruction by antibiotics from a penicillin-binding protein (PBP2a) that penicillin is unable to bind. The gene encoding this altered protein is located on a **transposon** (see "Genetic Transfer" in Chapter 6).

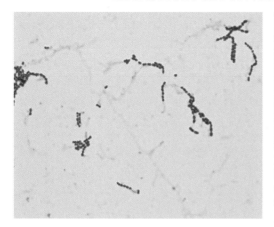

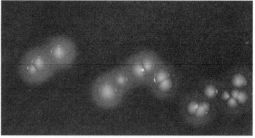

Figure 7.5 *Streptococcus pyogenes* on blood agar exhibiting a mucoid colony appearance due to the production of polysaccharide capsule. Different species of streptococci produce varying amounts of capsule.

Figure 7.4: Cellular morphology and arrangement of streptococci. Streptococci most often appear as chains (seen here). However, they may also be seen as singles or in pairs.

Other staphylococci besides *S. aureus* can carry the penicillin-binding protein. There are methicillin-resistant *S. pseudintermedius* (MRSP) and *S. epidermidis* (MRSE). MRS are considered zoonotic and the transmission appears to be bidirectional. There is circumstantial evidence that humans infected or colonized with MRSA can serve as a reservoir for infections in pets. In Denmark, MRSA infections in humans have been traced back to pigs in large production farms.

Screening for MRS isolates
The best choice of sampling sites for a clinical dermatologic case is the site of the lesion. Occasionally, the veterinarian may suspect that an individual animal is serving as an asymptomatic carrier of the infection. Samples to take from asymptomatic carriers include nasal and rectal swabs as these sites are most likely to test positive in carrier animals. Additionally, any suspicious lesions present should also be swabbed, plated on agar, and any isolates identified.

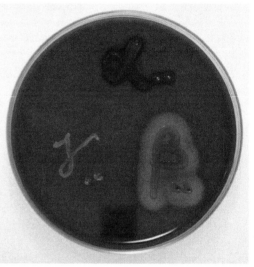

Figure 7.6: Hemolysis patterns of streptococci, blood agar plate. When a bacterial isolate exhibits alpha (α) hemolysis the agar immediately next to the colonies takes on a greenish tinge. Beta (β) hemolysis results in complete hemolysis of the RBCs in the blood agar thus appearing as a transparent zone of clearing. Gamma (γ) "hemolysis" does not actually result in any hemolysis; the designation is used to separate these isolates out from α- and β-hemolytic isolates. A lightbox was used to illuminate the back of the agar plate so that the hemolytic patterns would be more prominent and aid in classification. The same effect can be achieved simply by holding the plate up to a light bulb.

Streptococcus
Anyone who has been diagnosed with "strep throat" is well acquainted with this genus. Streptococci are gram-positive, non-motile facultative anaerobes that are circular or ovoid in shape. The genus *Streptococcus* contains over fifty species (both pathogenic and nonpathogenic). Streptococci divide in a single plane leading to the creation of single, pairs, or long chains of cocci in the host or in liquid culture (Figure 7.4). Streptococci are catalase-negative, an attribute which separates them from staphylococci. The different species of *Streptococcus* produce varying amounts of capsule. Species producing larger amounts of capsule exhibit a mucoid appearance when plated on artificial media such as blood agar (Figure 7.5).

Reservoir, Transmission, and Pathology

Streptococci are widely distributed throughout the environment. They readily colonize the skin, gastrointestinal, genital, and upper respiratory tracts. Transmission is usually by one of four methods: direct contact, **fomites** (see sidebar), ingestion, or inhalation. Like staphylococci, the primary pathologic lesion occurring in streptococcal infections is abscess formation. In chronic infections an outer fibrous capsule may develop and surround the abscess.

Client Education: Fomites

Fomites are inanimate objects that can harbor and transmit microbial infections.

Fomites of veterinary interest could include:
- Grooming supplies, e.g., curry brush
- Leashes
- Riding tack
- Food bowls
- Dog/cat beds
- And much more!

If a pathogen can be carried by fomites it is important to warn clients that they must clean and sanitize these objects at the same time as treatment is occurring. *Not doing this could lead to reinfection and treatment failure.*

Classification of Streptococci

There are two main systems used to classify streptococci: hemolysis pattern and Lancefield grouping. First, let us examine how hemolysis patterns classify this genus. Streptococci grown on blood agar plates will exhibit one of three hemolysis patterns (Figure 7.6). **Alpha (α) hemolysis** occurs when the streptococcal species contains an enzyme enabling it to reduce the hemoglobin within the erythrocytes immediately adjacent and touching the bacteria to methemoglobin. Methemoglobin imparts a greenish cast on the agar; the colony appears to be surrounded by a "halo" of green. **Beta (β) hemolysis** occurs upon lysis of the erythrocytes by the bacteria. The lysis results in a clearing of the agar around the colony and thus appears as a clear, rather than green, halo. Finally, the somewhat paradoxical term **gamma (γ) hemolysis** is given to those species that are non-hemolytic. Commensal and other nonpathogenic streptococci exhibit either alpha or gamma hemolysis when grown on blood agar. In contrast, most pathogenic streptococci exhibit beta hemolysis.

The second method for classifying streptococci is the **Lancefield grouping system** (Figure 7.7). This older method is a classification system based on antibodies produced against the bacterial cell surface carbohydrate antigens. The unknown bacterial sample to be classified is grown up in pure culture. Latex beads coated with a specific Lancefield group antibody are also obtained, one set for each Lancefield group to be tested. A specific amount of unknown bacteria are mixed with the antibody-labeled latex beads. If the antibodies on the latex beads recognize the carbohydrate antigens on the bacteria in the test tube, they will bind those same antigens. When multiple antibodies bind the same antigen, cross-linking of antigen occurs. This cross-linking causes **agglutination** (i.e., clumping) that can be seen by the naked eye. The Lancefield antibody present in the test tube exhibiting agglutination would be the correct Lancefield group to which the unknown bacteria belongs. Note: most of the streptococci which are able to be classified via the Lancefield method are beta hemolytic.

Streptococcal Diseases in Animals

Streptococcus pneumoniae

Streptococcus pneumoniae is the causative agent of human pneumonia. Humans infected with *S. pneumoniae* can transmit the disease to guinea pigs via aerosols (e.g., a cough or sneeze) and by direct contact. Thus the infection is considered an **anthroponosis**. The disease causes pneumonia in affected guinea pigs. In addition to guinea pigs, horses and many species of monkey (e.g., macaques) may contract pneumonia via the same route.

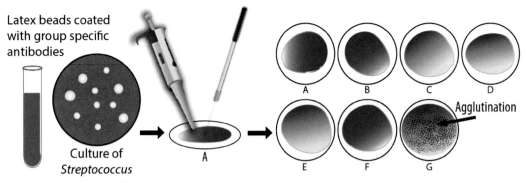

Figure 7.7: The Lancefield grouping system. Latex beads are coated with specific antibodies and mixed with a single colony of the unknown *Streptococcus*. The well showing agglutination corresponds to the Lancefield group identification.

Streptococcus agalactiae

A causative agent of contagious mastitis of dairy cattle, *Streptococcus agalactiae* is an obligate mammary pathogen. This means that the bacterium does not survive well outside of its host and particularly outside of mammary tissue. Transmission of the bacterium between cattle may occur as a result of improper or incomplete sanitation of the teat cups between milkings or via cattle behaviors such as suckling of the teats. Identification of *S. agalactiae* is aided by use of the CAMP test (see Chapter 22). *S. agalactiae* is beta hemolytic and CAMP positive.

Once a common infection within US cattle, infection rates and disease from *S. agalactiae* drastically fell as sanitation measures in the industry improved.

Streptococcus equi subspecies equi

A beta hemolytic, encapsulated bacterium, *Streptococcus equi* ssp. *equi* causes a disease known as equine "**strangles**." Clinical signs include fever with purulent inflammation of the nasal passages, pharynx, upper airways, and guttural pouches. The large abscessed mandibular lymph nodes, from which the disease gets its name, increase in size until they eventually rupture and drain. It is the rupturing and drainage of the purulent contents which poses the highest threat in transmission of the disease to other horses. Most often the infection is localized to the upper airway and associated lymph nodes. However, occasionally the disease goes systemic; this presentation is commonly referred to as "bastard strangles". With the colonization of the guttural pouch, infection may lead to a chronic carrier state in some horses. These chronic carriers most often remain asymptomatic, yet serve as sources able to transmit the infection to naïve horses.

Good specimens to obtain for culture include nasal swabs, nasal washes, or a fine needle aspirate of the abcess. Care must be taken not to rupture the abcess and contaminate the stall or other horses. Treatment consists of antibiotics based on culture and antimicrobial susceptibility testing. Long-lasting, protective immunity develops in about three-fourths of infected horses while approximately one-fourth of the animals remain susceptible to reinfection within five years. A vaccine (i.e., **bacterin**) against strangles is available commercially.

Client Education: Strangles is VERY contagious!

Shedding of *S. equi* ssp. *equi* occurs approximately 24-48 hours after the onset of fever. Owners should separate affected horses from those that appear unaffected as soon as they suspect a case of strangles. Separation of infected from uninfected individuals is a <u>critical</u> step in stopping the spread of this disease.

Streptococcus equi ssp. *zooepidemicus*

Streptococcus equi ssp. *zooepidemicus* can cause joint and naval infections, mastitis, abortion and secondary pneumonia in horses. It can also result in a strangles-like disease in guinea pigs. Like in horses infected with *S. equi* ssp. *equi*, the guinea pigs infected with *S. equi* ssp. *zooepidemicus* have greatly enlarged mandibular lymph nodes. Treatment and control measures are much like that followed for infections in horses. The affected guinea pig should be isolated while undergoing treatment so as not to become the source of infection for other guinea pigs.

In 2003, an outbreak of severe respiratory disease in kenneled dogs was found to be caused by *Streptococcus equi* ssp. *zooepidemicus*. Similar outbreaks have been recorded in 2007, 2008, and 2009. Causing a necrotizing and hemorrhagic pneumonia, this disease can be rapidly fatal to infected dogs. Without aggressive therapy, death may occur within 24-48 hours! It remains to be seen how widespread this manifestation of *Streptococcus equi* ssp. *zooepidemicus*-induced respiratory disease in dogs will become.

Flesh-Eating Streptococci in Animals

Like a really scary horror movie, news about the so-called "flesh-eating bacteria" has seeped into our consciousness. There is something rather distressing about something that is so small you can't see it, but has the power to cause such debilitating disease. Human infections of flesh-eating bacteria are caused by *Streptococcus pyogenes*. These bacteria don't actually "eat" flesh. Once it enters the skin, *S. pyogenes* releases toxins that kill the surrounding tissues and effectively shut down the blood flow to the area. The tissue dies and the bacteria enter the bloodstream allowing the bacteria to spread further. Infections can lead to massive tissue damage, necrosis, and may lead to the death of the patient.

Fortunately for the veterinary species we nurse, flesh-eating streptococcal infections are *extremely rare*, but they have been reported in both dogs and cats and are usually caused by *Streptococcus canis*. The range of disease outcomes, from skin ulceration to septic shock and death, is similar to that seen in people. Treatment must be very aggressive in order to save patients and consists of antibiotics and supportive care (e.g., IV fluid therapy).

Enterococcus

Enterococci are gram-positive cocci occurring in pairs or chains and were formerly classified as streptococci. They are facultative anaerobes and are considered commensals of the gastrointestinal tract of many species. However, when enterococci end up in the urinary bladder or in a wound they become a pathogen. The most common species are *Enterococcus faecalis* and *Enterococcus faecium*. Enterococci are intrinsically resistant to multiple antibiotics, thus antimicrobial susceptibility results can cause concern. However, most infections respond well to treatment with ampicillin or amoxicillin with clavulanic acid (e.g., Clavamox®).

Vancomycin-Resistant *Enterococci*

While not isolated from veterinary patients to date, vancomycin-resistant enterococci (VRE) exists as a huge treatment challenge in human medicine and a concern in veterinary medicine. **Nosocomial** (i.e., hospital-acquired) infections make up the majority of human cases. The antibiotic resistance to vancomycin is located on a transposon, much like MRSA. VRE are resistant to *almost all currently available antibiotics*.

> ## Client Education:
> ## Culture and Antimicrobial Susceptibility Testing
> Our diagnostic plan includes culture and antimicrobial susceptibility testing so we can avoid the indiscriminant use of antibiotics and thus avoid *even more* antibiotic resistance.

Further Reading

Hamilton, Elizabeth, et al. "Prevalence and Antimicrobial Resistance of *Enterococcus* Spp and *Staphylococcus* Spp Isolated from Surfaces in a Veterinary Teaching Hospital." *J Am Vet Med Assoc* 240 12 (2012): 1463-73.

Pesavento, Patricia A., et al. "A Clonal Outbreak of Acute Fatal Hemorrhagic Pneumonia in Intensively Housed (Shelter) Dogs Caused by *Streptococcus equi* Subsp. *zooepidemicus*." *Veterinary Pathology* 45 1 (2008): 51-53.

Sura, Radhakrishna, et al. "Fatal Necrotising Fasciitis and Myositis in a Cat Associated with *Streptococcus canis*." *Veterinary Record* 162 14 (2008): 450-53.

Taylor, Sandra D., and David W. Wilson. "*Streptococcus equi* Subsp. *equi* (Strangles) Infection." *Clinical Techniques in Equine Practice* 5 3 (2006): 211-17.

Weese, Scott J. "Staphylococcal Control in the Veterinary Hospital." *Veterinary Dermatology* 23 4 (2012).

Chapter 8:

Gram-Positive Rods – Part I:
Actinomyces, Trueperella, & Bacillus

Introduction
The species discussed in this chapter are capable of causing significant **morbidity** in many of the classic farm animals (i.e., cattle, small ruminants, and horses) as well as other animal species. Based on their cellular morphology, all of the bacteria within these genera are classified as gram-positive rods. Some infections, like those caused by *Actinomyces* infections, result in truly memorable pathology. Others, like *Bacillus anthracis*, have the potential to kill animals and humans alike in grisly fashion. Such is the power of these tiny bacteria.

Actinomyces

Bacterium or Fungus?
The members of this genus are classified as bacteria. However, the name *Actinomyces* denotes an organism related to a fungus (-*myces* is a Greek root meaning "fungus"). Indeed, this genus shares the characteristics of both bacteria and fungi. Its radiating network of branching filaments resemble some fungi (*Actino*- means "ray" in Greek). Yet it has many bacterial elements such as lacking a nuclear membrane, inability to respond to antifungal drugs, and does respond to antibacterial drugs and substances. Remember that fungi are eukaryotic organisms and so the lack of a nuclear membrane is significant as this is a key feature of prokaryotes.

Morphology
Members of the genus *Actinomyces* appear as gram-positive rods arranged like branching filaments. These filaments may break up and appear as single bacillary ("bacillus-like" or "rod-like") or occasionally as coccoid shapes. Growth conditions for members of this group range from aerobic to anaerobic, with a few species requiring a microaerophilic environment.

Habitat
Actinomyces is part of the normal flora of the oral cavity and the gastrointestinal tract of many species of animals. The source of most *Actinomyces* infections are **endogenous**. An endogenous infection originates from within the same individual. Endogenous infections are almost always opportunistic. They require disruption of mucosal barriers by trauma (bite), rough feed, foreign bodies, or other similar actions. Disease usually occurs near sites where *Actinomyces* species colonize as normal flora.

Actinomyces bovis
Actinomyces bovis causes a condition known as "lumpy jaw" in cattle. The condition's name derives from the characteristic hard, non-movable lumps that appear on the jaw of affected animals. Once access to the submucosal soft tissues has been gained, *Actinomyces* destroys tissues and accesses the bony jaw multiplying inside the bone. As the bone is destroyed and tries to repair itself, bony

swellings appear and enlarge over the course of weeks to months. Eventually the bony lump will break through the skin and purulent discharge can be seen exiting one or more of the openings. This purulent discharge contains tiny hard yellow granules of sulfur; these granules are characteristic of the disease. *A. bovis* may also play a role in equine "fistulous withers".

Actinomyces viscosus and A. hordeovulneris

In dogs, actinomycosis usually follows puncture of the skin or mucosa by a foreign body, such as a sharp object. In many cases the offending object is a foxtail seed, the seed of certain species of grass (e.g., *Alopecurus*). The seeds possess sharp burrs or edges and this is what causes the tear or puncture in the skin or mucous membrane. Foxtail seeds have been found lodged in gingival spaces and the tonsils, presumably after the dog ate the grass. Interdigital actinomycosis may occur if seeds become lodged between the dog's toes.

Actinomyces suis

Actinomyces suis causes opportunistic mastitis infections in lactating sows. The resulting granuloma formation will contain the typical sulfur granules.

Culturing Actinomyces

Sample Selection

The best results for culture rely on methods that sample deep in the lesion, such as taking a **fine needle aspirate** (FNA). This will yield a sample that has the least chance of being contaminated by surface bacteria such as *Escherichia coli*, *Staphylococcus aureus*, and various skin commensals.

Appearance

On culture media, just as its name suggests, *Actinomyces* forms rays or sunburst like patterns.

Treatment

Considerable debate exists regarding whether or not to treat actinomycosis in cattle because treatment is rarely successful in chronic cases, especially if the bone is extensively involved. Relapses occurring after the cessation of the treatment are common. It is best to discuss this with clients so that they may be well-informed prior to making decisions on treatment. Better outcomes are seen in dogs treated for actinomycosis.

Trueperella

Trueperella pyogenes inhabits the mucous membranes of the body including those associated with the respiratory, gastrointestinal, and urogenital tracts. Microscopically, *Trueperella* appears as small gram-positive rods. *Trueperella pyogenes* is the current recognized name of this species; former names of this pathogen include: *Arcanobacterium pyogenes*, *Actinomyces pyogenes*, and *Corynebacterium pyogenes*.

> **Remember this: Never Swab a Draining Tract!**
>
> Draining tracts or wound are always contaminated with surface bacteria and fungi. This will make identifying the real culprit impossible.
>
> Sampling methods such as a fine needle aspirate offer superior sample quality and dramatically increase chances of finding the cause of disease!

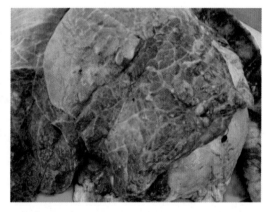

Figure 8.1: Pneumonia in a cow caused by *Trueperella pyogenes*. The dark portion of the lung (cranioventral) is affected by severe pneumonia. In addition several abscesses can be seen in the lung tissue. The trachea (clinically normal) can be seen in the lower right of the image. From: Scott, Philip R. "Clinical Presentation, Auscultation Recordings, Ultrasonographic Findings and Treatment Response of 12 Adult Cattle with Chronic Suppurative Pneumonia: Case Study." *Ir Vet J* 66 1 (2013): 5. Open access.

Trueperella pyogenes is an opportunistic pathogen most commonly affecting cattle, sheep, goats, and swine. Like *Actinomyces*, establishment of a *Trueperella* infection requires trauma or some other predisposing factor that disrupts the integrity of the mucosa allowing entry of the bacteria. Dissemination of *Trueperella* results in suppurative infections. Sequelae of *Trueperella* infections include liver and lung abscesses, polyarthritis, and abortions (Figure 8.1). *Trueperella* is a common contributor to summer mastitis of dry cows.

Diagnostics and Treatment
Clinical signs alone are not enough to distinguish *Trueperella* from other opportunistic pathogens. Diagnosis is made after growth of the organism on standard microbiological media. *T. pyogenes* appears as small, grey-white, convex colonies that exhibit β-hemolysis on blood agar. *T. pyogenes* is predictably susceptible to β-lactam antibiotics.

Bacillus
Members of the *Bacillus* genus include both pathogenic and nonpathogenic species. They are gram-positive rods, appear as long chains or in pairs, and are capable of forming endospores. Most members of the genus are motile with the exception of *Bacillus anthracis*. *Bacillus* species of veterinary importance include: *B. anthracis*, *B. cereus*, *Geobacillus* (*Bacillus*) *stearothermophilus*, and *B. subtilis*. The vast majority of *Bacillus* isolates cultured in veterinary diagnostic labs are environmental contaminants and of no clinical significance.

Bacillus Spores
Just how hardy are the endospores formed by *Bacillus* species? Perhaps the best and most notable example of survival against-all-odds is seen with *Bacillus anthracis*. These spores are widespread in nature and can survive *over one hundred years* in the soil! Like many spores, *B. anthracis* spores are resistant to desiccation, high temperatures, and many chemical disinfectants. Transmission to animals occurs when the animals are grazing and inhale or ingest these spores.

Bacillus anthracis
The causative agent of anthrax, *B. anthracis* affects all mammals including humans. Anthrax is endemic in some parts of the world such as Central and South America, sub-Saharan Africa, Central and Southwestern Asia, and southern and Eastern Europe. Cattle and other ruminants are highly susceptible to infection and disease caused by *B. anthracis*. Pigs and horses are moderately susceptible while carnivores are comparatively resistant. Resistance in avian species can be linked to their higher basal body temperatures when compared to mammals.

Transmission and Disease
Transmission of anthrax occurs in one of three ways: inhalation, ingestion, and via wounds. By far, the most deadly form is inhalation anthrax. When cattle or other animals inhale *Bacillus anthracis* spores, the spores germinate releasing vegetative cells. These cells quickly multiply. The disease results in a rapidly fatal **septicemia** with cattle dying quickly thereafter even if antibiotic treatment is instituted very soon after the animal is infected. Ingestion and wound anthrax cause less pathology and are less likely to be fatal if antibiotic therapy is instituted.

When Should You Suspect Anthrax?
Anthrax infection should be suspected in carcasses of recently deceased animals exhibiting:

- No signs of rigor mortis
- Blood coming out of most orifices (e.g., mouth, nostrils, or anus)

Hemorrhaging occurs as a result of the **disseminated intravascular coagulopathy** (DIC) that occurs subsequent to the overwhelming sepsis. (Note: DIC is almost always fatal, despite aggressive treatment).

Anthrax is a serious and potentially fatal zoonotic disease. If you see the above signs, you should

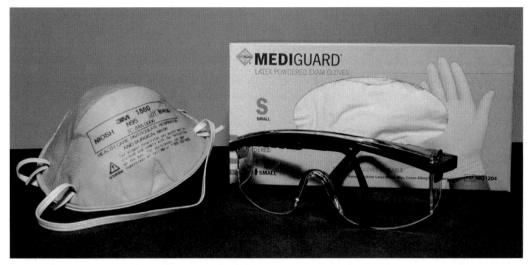

Figure 8.2: Personal protective equipment (PPE) that should be worn when working with potential zoonotic infections: N95 mask, eye protection, and gloves. An N95 *must* be fitted to the individual by a qualified respiratory specialist. Eye protection can consist of special high density plastic protective eyeglasses (shown), goggles, or a face shield. Exam gloves should always be worn when a zoonotic infection is suspected. Latex gloves are shown. Nitrile gloves are another excellent option, particularly for those individuals that have a latex allergy.

immediately contact your regulatory veterinarian (this is usually the State Veterinarian). Take care to protect yourself from inhaling any spores present. Do not handle the animal. Once the state or federal veterinarian arrives, note the PPE they don: at a minimum, gloves and respiratory protection, in the form of an N-95 mask (Figure 8.2) or full-face respirator, should be used. Carcasses suspected of being contaminated or infected with anthrax should *never* be necropsied in the field as this would result in the release of spores. Necropsy of suspected cases may only be performed in specialized facilities.

Treatment and Prevention
Antibiotic treatment is available for affected animals. Additionally, vaccines are available to prevent anthrax in cattle and other livestock.

> **Tourist Alert!**
>
> Some incidents of human anthrax have been traced back to animal products (e.g., African drums made with cow hides) brought back by tourists from endemic areas of the world. Sampling the animal products revealed the presence of *B. anthracis* spores.
>
> Animal products legally imported into the United States must undergo examination by the Department of Agriculture to ensure they are not harboring such pathogens.

Cleanup After an Anthrax Case
Given the extreme hardiness of *B. anthracis* spores, exactly how does one clean and disinfect an area, such as a farm, after diagnosing a case of anthrax? First, isolate the sick animal(s) as well as those which are in-contact with the affected animal(s). If an animal dies from anthrax, incinerate the carcass. Never open up the carcass; this will release spores into the air and the surrounding environment. An alternative to incineration is to bury the animal deep into the ground – at least 8-10 feet – ensuring that the site chosen is away from any water sources, including aquifers. Finally, disinfect everything that can be disinfected (e.g., medical instruments, walls, floors). Read the label of the disinfectants carefully and verify the activity against *B. anthracis* including activity against its spores. The owner should be informed that elimination of *B. anthracis* from the pasture is not possible.

Anthrax and Bioterrorism
In 2001, a flurry of activity could be seen outside of several federal office buildings in Washington, DC. People clothed head-to-toe in Tyvek® coveralls (DuPont™) and wearing full-face respirators

rushed in and out. The reason? Letters addressed to several members of the United States Congress were found to be laden with anthrax spores in an act of domestic terrorism. The anthrax had been altered to make them more likely to cause disease (e.g., "weaponized"). Inhalation of the anthrax spores caused a total of five deaths and dramatically changed the way in which the United States viewed domestic bioterrorism.

As a result of the "anthrax attacks" of 2001, *Bacillus anthracis* is considered a potential bioterrorism agent and its scientific use in diagnostic and research laboratories is severely restricted. Special federal permits are required before beginning any work. Due to the risk of aerosol exposure, laboratorians must conduct all work involving *B. anthracis* in a special biosafety cabinet.

Clinical Correlation: Using *Bacillus* to Our Advantage

We tend to think of most microbes in terms of what damage they cause. However, *Bacillus* species can definitely be used to our advantage. The two species used most often are *Geobacillus stearothermophilus* and *Bacillus subtilis*.

The validation of autoclaves involves the use of *Geobacillus stearothermophilus* (a microbe related to and formerly under the genus *Bacillus*). Commercially-prepared *G. stearothermophilus* spores are sealed inside a specially constructed plastic vial. The vial design allows for steam penetration without direct contact with any items against which the vial may rest. The vial is placed in the center of an autoclave load or surgical pack. This is the area least likely to get adequate penetration of steam. The autoclave is allowed to run its normal cycle. In a fully functional autoclave, the heat and humidity should penetrate the vial and kill the spores. The vial is removed and the contents are streaked onto an appropriate agar plate. If the autoclave achieved the proper temperature, humidity, and cycle length there should be no growth on the plate. Given the labor-intensive nature and the time needed to incubate the plates, this method is used less frequently. Most laboratory facilities would use this testing method at a frequency of weekly or monthly.

For daily validation of the autoclave's performance, temperature verification testing strips are most often used. These commercially available strips are sensitive to high levels of moist heat (e.g., 180°C). The testing strip is added to the inside of a clean item, such as a surgical pack. The surgical pack is packaged normally and loaded into the center of the autoclave load. The autoclave cycle is allowed to run its normal course. When adequate temperature, humidity, and pressure are achieved the steam will penetrate the surgical pack and cause a color change on the strip. When the veterinary technician opens the surgical pack during surgery, the technician checks the indicator to ensure that the color change has occurred. If the strip did not change color, the surgical pack cannot be used and must be re-autoclaved.

Whenever there is a biological or temperature indicator failure, the veterinary technician should examine the autoclave log and determine why the indicator failure occurred. **Possibilities for the failure include:** the wrong autoclave cycle was used, the autoclave is unable to achieve the set temperature and needs to be adjusted or repaired, or the testing strips are out-of-date and should be replaced with new strips.

Bacillus cereus

A much less deadly member of the genus, *Bacillus cereus* is a foodborne pathogen in people. Like *B. anthracis*, *B. cereus* is a spore-former. Foodborne illness is associated with the ingestion of products like sticky rice served on buffets. Usually, the rice is prepared ahead by cooking it in bulk at a high temperature in a rice cooker. The high temperature is sufficient to kill any vegetative *B. cereus* contaminating the rice, but is not high enough to destroy any spores present. The rice is then transferred, as needed, to the buffet where it is kept on a warmer. Here the reduced temperature allows for *B.*

cereus to sporulate and release the vegetative form which then proliferates. If the rice is not cleared off of the buffet and replaced with new rice, the *B. cereus* in the original batch has time to produce enough vegetative cells to cause illness. This is why it is important for restaurant and food service workers to follow correct procedures with regards to how long food can be kept on warmers before it must be discarded. When the contaminated rice is eaten, the individual ingests the vegetative form of *B. cereus* as well as some spores. Clinical signs are seen approximately 12 hours after ingestion and are due to the proliferation of toxins within the gastrointestinal tract. The toxins cause gastrointestinal stress in the form of vomiting and diarrhea. Infection is usually self-limiting and most individuals recover uneventfully. However, a few may require hospitalization to correct dehydration from the fluids and electrolytes lost via vomiting and diarrhea. While this disease is not common in domestic animals, it is good to keep this disease in mind as many owners still feed table scraps to their pets.

Further Reading

Day, Thomas G. "The Autumn 2001 Anthrax Attack on the United States Postal Service: The Consequences and Response." *Journal of Contingencies and Crisis Management* 11 3 (2003): 110-17.

Ribeiro, Márcio G., et al. "*Trueperella pyogenes* Multispecies Infections in Domestic Animals: A Retrospective Study of 144 Cases (2002 to 2012)." *Veterinary Quarterly* (2015): 1-6.

Scott, Philip R. "Clinical Presentation, Auscultation Recordings, Ultrasonographic Findings and Treatment Response of 12 Adult Cattle with Chronic Suppurative Pneumonia: Case Study." *Ir Vet J* 66 1 (2013): 5.

Chapter 9:

Gram-Positive Rods – Part II:
Listeria, Corynebacterium, Dermatophilus, Nocardia & *Erysipelothrix*

Introduction
The diseases produced by infection with the genera discussed in this chapter are varied. *Dermatophilus, Nocardia,* and *Erysipelothrix* infections each result in significant disease accompanied by characteristic skin lesions. In contrast, *Corynebacterium* targets the urogenital system and the lymphatics. *Listeria* tends to cause systemic illness and is a particular zoonotic concern of pregnant women. Like the genera covered in the previous chapter, these all share common cell morphology and staining characteristics; they are all classified as gram-positive rods.

Listeria monocytogenes
The most clinically important member of the genus, *Listeria monocytogenes* represents an important foodborne pathogen. *Listeria monocytogenes* is a rod-shaped, gram-positive, motile facultative anaerobe that may occur in short chains.

Reservoirs
Listeria is found in the environment as a saprophyte. *L. monocytogenes* has been isolated from the air, soil, and water. In animal agriculture settings, poor quality silage serves as a source of *L. monocytogenes* for livestock, especially domestic ruminants, which may be ingested or directly inoculated into to the eye during feeding. Silage provides a particularly amenable environment as the high pH content of poorly fermented silage coupled with pockets of aerobic microenvironments in the feed silo or bunker encourages proliferation of *Listeria*. Transmission between cattle occurs via the fecal-oral route as asymptomatic carries can contaminate the environment.

Listeria in Domestic Animals
Listeria infections cause widely varying clinical signs and outcomes. These outcomes are highly dependent upon the immune status of the host. *Listeria* infections in immune competent domestic species are usually asymptomatic (Figure 9.1, Case 1). However, ingestion of listeria contaminated silage by pregnant ruminants may cause abortion. Another clinical presentation most common in small ruminants is meningitis. In these cases, the organism crosses the oral epithelium, usually as a result of oral trauma (e.g., rough feed stuffs), and then migrates up the branches of the

> **Saphrophyte:**
> "An organism, especially a fungus or bacterium, that grows on and derives its nourishment from *dead or decaying organic matter.*"
>
> – American Heritage* Dictionary of the English Language ©2000

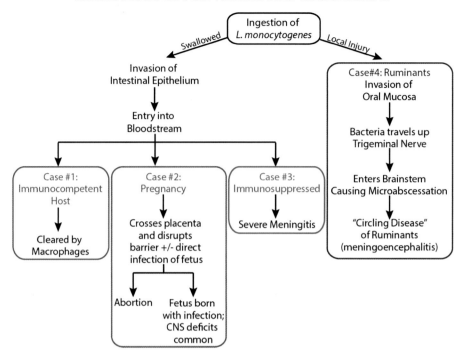

Figure 9.1: Common routes of *Listeria monocytogenes* infection and possible sequelae.

trigeminal nerve and localize in the brainstem where proliferation and formation of microscopic abscesses occurs (Figure 9.1, Case 4). *Listeria* survive intracellularly and travel from one host cell to the next by a unique mechanism whereby they hijack the host cells' cytoskeleton components and use them to propel themselves into neighboring cells. A host that is immunosuppressed cannot clear the circulating *Listeria* and the bacteria reach the brain in large numbers leading to acute (and largely fatal) meningitis (Figure 9.1, Case 3). Contaminated silage can also result in conjunctivitis due to direct inoculation of listeria into the eye during feeding.

Listeriosis in Humans: Risks in Pregnancy

Infection with *Listeria monocytogenes* poses a serious foodborne threat to immunosuppressed individuals including pregnant women (Figure 9.1, Case 2 and Figure 9.2). In food processing facilities contamination of the muscle tissue with *Listeria monocytogenes* may occur. Under normal circumstances, this does not result in infection as *Listeria* is easily killed by heat when the meat is cooked. A major risk factor for listeriosis in pregnancy is linked to consumption of deli or "ready-to-eat" meats (e.g., ham, chicken, and roast beef). The original processing of the ready-to-eat meat (e.g., salting, cooking, and smoking) is enough to kill any contaminating *Listeria*. However, if post-processing contamination with *L. monocytogenes* occurs, there is no subsequent heating or processing step to kill the *Listeria*. Ready-to-eat meats are served cold, as when making sandwiches. Making matters worse, unlike most other bacteria, *Listeria* can not only survive refrigeration temperatures, *they thrive and reproduce!* When a pregnant woman consumes a *Listeria*-contaminated ready-to-eat meat, the *Listeria* passes into the bloodstream as a septic infection and enters the placenta which results in abortion (usually late-term) of the fetus. Other risk factors of listeriosis during pregnancy are consumption of soft (unpasteurized) cheeses; raw, unpasteurized milk; improperly smoked seafood; and undercooked wild game fowl.

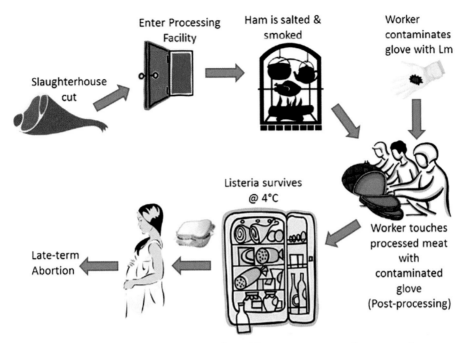

Figure 9.2: Product flow of deli meats, points of possible contamination, and outcome of consumption of *Listeria monocytogenes* (Lm) contaminated meats during pregnancy.

Diagnostics

Methods for identifying *L. monocytogenes* in culture include Gram-staining and standard biochemical tests such as the CAMP test. In addition, *Listeria* is a motile organism. Performing motility testing, by either the hanging drop method or the stab tube method, aids in identification and classification of the organism. For more details on motility testing and the CAMP test, see Chapter 22.

Treatment and Prevention

The choice of antibiotics is based on antimicrobial susceptibility testing of culture isolates. Amoxicillin, ampicillin, and aminoglycosides are all good first-choices. Prevention of listeriosis in livestock can be achieved via vaccination and attention to the condition of silage being fed to a herd.

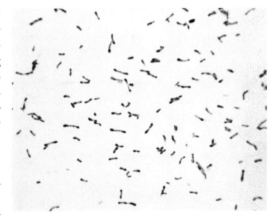

Figure 9.3: Diptheroidal or "club-shaped" appearance of *Corynebacterium diptheriae*. Courtesy of the Public Health Image Library, PHIL #12163, Centers for Disease Control and Prevention, Atlanta, 1965.

Client Education

Clients should be made aware of the risk factors associated with feeding poor quality silage to livestock, especially ruminants. Clients concerned about the role of ready-to-eat meats during pregnancy should be counselled to consult their physician.

Corynebacterium

Corynebacterium species exist as non-spore-forming gram-positive rods that appear pleomorphic.

They assume coccoid as well as "club-shaped" (i.e., **diphtheroidal**) cellular morphologies (Figure 9.3). The term diphtheroidal derives its name from the species *Corynebacterium diphtheriae*, the causative agent of human diphtheria, a pathogen causing serious childhood illness and high **mortality** in the pre-antibiotic era. The cell walls of corynebacterial organisms contains coryne-mycolic acids. Evidence suggests that this adaptation enables *Corynebacterium* to survive intracellularly as a **facultative intracellular pathogen**, similar to but by a different mechanism than *Listeria*. The genus contains many species; the ones most commonly considered pathogens of domestic animals will be discussed here. Several excellent reviews detailing the entire genus should be consulted for a more comprehensive exami-nation of the genus (See "Further Readings" at the end of this chapter).

Corynebacterium renale Group

The *Corynebacterium renale* group encompasses three species of veterinary importance. These are *C. renale*, *C. cystitidis*, and *C. pilosum*. Members of the group constitute normal flora of the lower urogenital tract in most domestic species; disease results from opportunistic infection. The most studied species in the group is *C. renale*. Discussion of the group will therefore focus primarily on this species. Transmission occurs when normal flora ascend the lower urogenital tract and gain access to the upper tract (i.e., bladder, ureters, and kidney). Therefore, infection requires direct contact. Venereal transmission is postulated to be a secondary method of inoculation. Additionally, *C. renale* survives well in soil allowing for possible indirect transmission although adequate evidence is lacking.

> **Facultative Intracellular Pathogen:**
> A pathogen that can survive and proliferate inside phagocytic cells, yet survive outside of them as well.

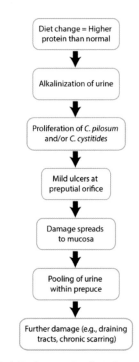

Figure 9.4: Pathogenesis of pizzle rot caused by *C. pilosum* and *C. cystitides.*

Disease in Cattle: Pyelonephritis

C. renale infection in cattle presents most often as **cystitis** and may lead to ascending **pyelonephritis**, infections of the bladder and the kidneys, respectively. Incidence of infection in cattle herds occurs at a rate of 1-5%. Risk factors associated with infection are related to problems that predispose the pooling of urine. These factors include the shortness of the female urethra; damage to the urethra and related structures during parturition; anatomical abnormalities such as diverticula and fistulas; and urinary tract obstruction. Affected animals may present with signs of acute or chronic pyelonephritis. In cases of acute pyelonephritis, fever, anorexia, increased frequency of urination with blood or pus, and an arched back indicating renal pain may occur. Chronic pyelonephritis is characterized by anorexia, weight loss, and a decrease in milk production. Other species capable of causing cystitis and pyelonephritis in cattle are *C. cystitidis* and *C. pilosum*, respectively.

Pizzle and Sheath Rot

C. renale group disease in small ruminants consists of two conditions known in laymen's terms as "pizzle rot" or "sheath rot," referring to the damage sustained to the penis and prepuce, respectively. Infections result in preputial ulcerative dermatitis in males and ulcerative vulvovaginitis in females.

The condition can be quite painful and even mimic **urolithiasis** (i.e., bladder stones). Preputial damage may be so severe that the prepuce scars down and prevents normal retraction of the prepuce thereby affecting ability to breed. In both males and females, severe damage to the penis or vagina may alter ability to void urine normally. Transmission occurs via direct contact. The major risk factor for opportunistic infections with these species relates to ingestion of a high protein diet resulting in significantly alkaline urine (Figure 9.4). While herbivores, such as cattle, normally produce slightly alkaline urine, extreme alkalinity can be very caustic to the urogenital epithelium.

Diagnostics
Aerobic culture coupled with biochemical testing is the best way to diagnose these conditions. Samples may be obtained from either urine or affected tissues, such as the kidneys.

Treatment of *C. renale* Group Infections
Cystitis and pyelonephritis require treatment with antibiotics, such as penicillin or trimethoprim-sulfa. In addition to administering antibiotics, pizzle rot may require surgery depending upon the extent and nature of the scarring

Prevention
As the agents involved are commensal organisms, they cannot be eliminated. Therefore, prevention strategies should focus on improved management, especially in avoiding sudden dietary changes, and on decreasing herd stressors.

Corynebacterium pseudotuberculosis
The disease caused by *Corynebacterium pseudotuberculosis* in small ruminants is called **caseous lymphadenitis** (CLA). Sheep and goats serve as the obligate hosts. Transmission between individuals occurs as a result of either direct contact with abscessed materials or via fomites. Common fomites include sheep dip, wool shears, and feeders with rough edges

Disease in Ruminants
Entry into the skin usually occurs as a result of trauma (e.g., shearing accident), but often the moment of introduction is obscure and goes unnoticed until disease develops. Bacteria replicate locally at the site of trauma. Macrophages move into the area and phagocytose the bacteria. *C. pseudotuberculosis* escapes killing via the phagolysosome and survives within the macrophage. As the macrophage leaves the area, it carries the bacteria with it. During this time, the bacteria replicates within the macrophage

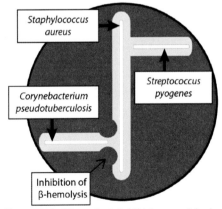

Figure 9.6: **β-hemolysis inhibition test** (also known as the Reverse CAMP test). *Corynebacterium pseudotuberculosis* produces a substance that inhibits β-hemolysis of the RBCs in the blood agar by the β-hemolytic *Streptococcus agalactia*. *Streptococcus pyogenes* is included as a negative control for this test. See Chapter 22 for more details.

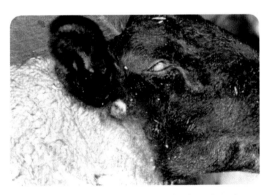

Figure 9.5: *Corynebacterium pseudotuberculosis* abscess formation in parotid lymph node. From: Malone, Frank E et al. "A Serological Investigation of Caseous Lymphadenitis in Four Flocks of Sheep." *Ir Vet J* 59.1 (2006): 19–21. Open access.

to such a large extent that it causes the eventual death of the macrophage. When the macrophage dies, *C. pseudotuberculosis* is released allowing for dissemination of the bacteria to other distant sites.

Disease is first noticed as subcutaneous abscesses (Figure 9.5), but abscesses can also be internal and therefore unnoticed by the naked eye. Internal abscesses are more common in sheep than goats. The primary pathologic lesion seen in CLA is **caseous necrosis**. Caseous necrosis appears "cheese-like" when viewed grossly. Viewed microscopically, neutrophils are surrounded by macrophages and a layer of fibrin. In chronic CLA, the necrosis may be surrounded by a tough, fibrous capsule.

Affected herds may experience high infection rates with up to 30-50% of sheep within the flock infected. This rate may increase with the advancing age of the herd. The disease takes a chronic course ending in systemic wasting known as "thin ewe syndrome." Eventually affected animals will become so thin that death ensues.

Diagnostics
Samples from animals showing clinical signs must be cultured. Culture and antimicrobial susceptibility testing form the basis of diagnosis. The β-hemolysin inhibition test (also known as the Reverse CAMP test) aids in positively identifying cultures of suspected CLA infections (Figure 9.6). Serologic tests to detect antibody in serum are available and useful for screening herds or testing an animal before introducing them to a CLA free herd. Serologic tests are not appropriate for clinically infected animals. Animals with CLA abscesses may test negative on serologic tests, whereas culture would reliably identify *C. pseudotuberculosis* as the causative agent.

Treatment
Affected animals must be isolated from healthy animals. Antibiotics show poor penetration into large, caseous abscesses. Therefore, nursing care consists of lancing and flushing the abscess while avoiding environmental contamination. Occasionally surgery must be performed to open and remove abscessed and necrotic debris. Antibiotics are prescribed based on culture and antimicrobial susceptibility testing.

Prevention
Disinfection of potential fomites (e.g., shearing blades) is critical to preventing the introduction of CLA into a herd as well as breaking the cycle of infection in an affected herd. Best management practices rely on culling chronically infected individuals. Prevention may also be realized through effective vaccination, though the safety and efficacy of vaccination is questionable and vaccinated herds can no longer be screened by serologic tests, as vaccinated animals will test positive for *C. pseudotuberculosis* -specific antibodies.

Zoonotic Potential
To date, approximately twenty cases of zoonotic infection from *C. pseudotuberculosis* have been reported. Veterinary care staff should take precautions (e.g., wearing examination gloves) while handling sheep and goats suspected of having CLA.

Client Education:
The High Cost of CLA
Abscesses and disease resulting from CLA costs the producer!
- Carcass condemnation at slaughter
- Decreased wool and milk production
- Scarring of the hide decreases value of leather
- Decreased reproductive performance
- Decreased life expectancy

Dermatophilus

These gram-positive aerobic, branching, filamentous rods were once thought to be fungi. Subsequent testing confirmed their classification as bacteria. However, some of the terminology describing their lifecycle (e.g., "spores") still retains links to fungi. The name *Dermatophilus* means "skin-lover" (from *dermato-* [skin] and *-philus* [love]). The species of most interest clinically in domestic animals is *Dermatophilus congolensis*, a pathogen occurring mostly in tropical and subtropical climates.

> **Zoospore:**
> A motile (usually *flagellated*) asexual spore especially of algae or lower fungi
>
>

Lifecycle and Transmission of Dermatophilus

Dermatophilosis is usually associated with rain and very wet conditions. *D. congolensis* is an obligate parasite and thus unable to multiply in the environment. Transmission between animals occurs by direct contact, arthropods and fomites. Superficial infections make up most of the clinical disease seen in domestic animals. *Dermatophilus* reproduces via motile cocci called **zoospores**. These spores settle into a traumatized piece of tissue or skin and proceed to elongate into rods (Figure 9.7). Division occurs in multiple planes and may appear like a flat mat consisting of multiple rows and columns of rods. To disseminate to other areas of the skin, the rods again form into zoospores and disperse enabling them to infect additional distant sites.

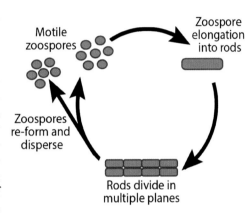

Figure 9.7: The lifecycle of *Dermatophilus congolensis*.

Risk Factors for Infection

The main risk factor is subjecting hosts to a very wet, warm environment such as that found in the tropical and subtropical regions of the world. Immunosuppression (i.e., via ticks & other causes) and mechanical trauma (e.g., scratches or fly bites) increases the risk for infection.

Clinical Disease

Many domestic species may be clinically affected by infection with *D. congolensis* including ruminants, horses, dogs, and cats. Germination of the zoospores and asexual reproduction occurs within a wound, scratch, or bite. Dividing in multiple planes the rods then grow through the epidermis of the skin. Clinically affected animals show matting of hair or wool as well as scab and crust formation. Areas covered in scabs may be substantial in chronic cases leading to the loss of hair/wool and even the underlying skin. Lesions tend to resolve without treatment in about four weeks. In wooled species, such as sheep, the disease is known as "lumpy wool disease." Other names for the condition include: "rain rot" and "strawberry foot rot."

Nursing Care

Scabs should be removed with mild soap and water followed by topical application of iodine or copper sulfate. Most infections are self-limiting, but severe infections may require systemic antibiotics.

Client Education

Clients should be informed that the clinical course of disease can be quite long, on the order of several weeks. There is no vaccine available, but thankfully reinfection does not occur.

Nocardia

A gram-positive bacteria, *Nocardia* cellular morphology is extremely pleomorphic. *Nocardia* may appear in the form of rods, cocci, and diphtheroids. A non-motile strict aerobe, *Nocardia* is a saprophyte preferring environments such as soil, decaying vegetation, animal feces, and water. As with *Dermatophilus*, *Nocardia* was originally classified as a fungal organism. The species of most concern in domestic animals is *Nocardia asteroides*.

Disease Progression and Clinical Signs

Nocardiosis may be acquired by inhalation of, ingestion of, or direct contact via a traumatic injury with environmental sources. In cases of skin infection, inoculation from the soil into the skin begins the disease process. As the immune response to *N. asteroides* develops, a hard nodule or pustule develops. Over time, the pustule ruptures releasing the bacterial-laden pus. Multiple nodules connected by small channels or "sinus tracts" may develop as the infection progresses. Most infections remain localized to the skin and subcutaneous tissues. However, occasionally the infection becomes systemic and affects multiple organs (e.g., lung, heart, and central nervous system) as a result of hematogenous spread. When the organism is acquired by inhalation, pulmonary disease is the primary clinical sign. Bovine mastitis due to *Nocardia* can be spread via fomites and by the people working in the dairy. Disseminated disease resulting in abortion, though rare, has been reported in equine, swine and ruminant species.

Diagnostics

A fine needle aspirate of an intact nodule (i.e., one that is not ruptured) constitutes the best sample choice for culture of *Nocardia*. Remember that draining tracts and wounds are commonly contaminated and will yield very poor culture results. *Nocardia* will grow on blood agar and, unlike *Dermatophilus*, will also grow on Sabouraud's Agar. Incubation on blood agar is prolonged requiring at least two weeks before colonies can be seen with the naked eye. Stains used in visualizing *Nocardia* are the Gram and acid-fast stains. *Nocardia* spp. are variably acid-fast. Additionally, the acid-fast stain is useful in distinguishing between *Nocardia* (acid-fast) and another filamentous gram-positive rod, *Actinomyces* (non-acid-fast).

Treatment

Treatment consists of prescribing antibiotics, with sulfonamides being the drug of choice. Culling infected animals, along with thorough disinfection of facilities and fomites, is recommended for cases of nocardial mastitis of cows.

> ### Client Education:
> ### *Nocardia* – in it for the long haul!
> Clients should be made aware that long-term antibiotic therapy (i.e., several weeks) may be necessary to eliminate the infection. Some patients won't respond to antibiotics and may require more intensive therapy.

Erysipelothrix

The main species of veterinary concern is *Erysipelothrix rhusiopathiae*. *E. rhusiopathiae* exists as a non-motile, gram-positive, facultative anaerobic bacterium that forms short rods. Infection with *E. rhusiopathiae* causes disease in swine, turkeys, and humans. Reservoirs for *E. rhusiopathiae* include the environment and the alimentary tract and lymphoid tissues of many healthy wild and domestic animals and the exterior slime layer on fish. In the fisheries industry, scorpion fish and lobsters are two important natural reservoirs for *E. rhusiopathiae*.

Transmission

Transmission of *Erysipelothrix rhusiopathiae* among swine occurs via two main routes: ingestion and infected wounds. Feces, food, and other materials colonized with *Erysipelothrix* are ingested and thus infect naïve animals. Wound-derived infections happen in a number of ways. Pigs within a herd attempt to assert and maintain their dominance within the group hierarchy. They do this with both play and aggressive actions, such as nipping and biting. Common areas that receive bites are the ears and tail. Also, rooting (a normal behavior of swine) often results in small scratches or cuts, particularly if the pen flooring and gating have sharp edges on them. It is through both these intentional and unintentional bites and scratches that the protective barrier of the skin is breached allowing for the entry of environmental and alimentary *Erysipelothrix* into the bloodstream and deeper tissues.

Clinical Disease in Swine

After ingestion or inoculation via trauma, the bacterium gains access to the bloodstream where it begins to reproduce. Large numbers of bacteria within the bloodstream lead to septicemia. In the case of young animals, many affected piglets die acutely. Pigs infected at an older age tend to develop a chronic infection. Clinical signs of chronic swine erysipelas depend upon where the bacteria, after traveling through the bloodstream, end up lodging and causing harm. Most often, chronic infections result in arthritis (i.e., lodge within joint cavities), endocarditis (i.e., attach and disrupt heart valve function), and abortion (i.e., cross the placenta and infect the fetus).

One of the most striking and outwardly apparent signs of swine erysipelas is the occurrence of what is called "diamond skin" (Figure 9.8). Diamond skin consists of red, slightly raised diamond- or rhomboid-shaped skin lesions occurring anywhere on the pig's skin. The lesions may occur singly or may be numerous. The reason for the striking and clear diamond shape is thought to result from blood clots (i.e., thrombi) that lodge in the skin, however the definitive pathogenesis of the skin lesions has not been established.

In addition to infection with *E. rhusiopathiae*, swine carry *E. tonsillarum* asymptomatically.

Treatment and Prevention

Antibiotic treatment is prescribed for affected swine (e.g., penicillin). Prevention is achieved through vaccination using a bacterin. Sows and gilts are typically

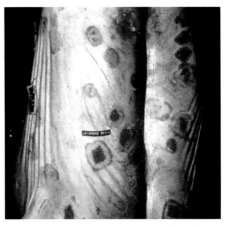

Figure 9.8: Swine carcass presented at slaughter showing characteristic diamond skin lesions caused by *Erysipelothrix rhusiopathiae.* The skin lesions may be square, diamond, or rhomboid-shaped and are usually slightly raised. Pigs may have only one or two skin lesions or they may be numerous as is the case with the carcass in this photo. Photo courtesy of the United States Department of Agriculture - Food Safety Inspection Service (USDA-FSIS).

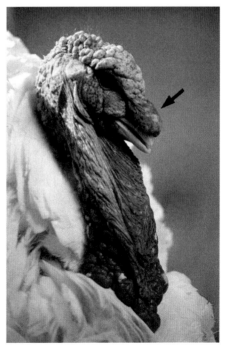

Figure 9.9: Turkey with a snood (black arrow). It is the snood which can become swollen in turkey erysipelas. Photo courtesy of the Agricultural Research Service, United States Department of Agriculture ARS Image Bank (#K8098-2), date unknown.

vaccinated prior to breeding. Vaccination of boars occurs twice annually in most swine operations. Grower pigs (i.e., those going to market) should also receive a vaccination against erysipelas.

Clinical Disease in Poultry

The only other common domestic species affected by erysipelas is the turkey. Turkeys infected with *E. rhusiopathiae* show clinical signs consistent with sepsis. Often the snood (Figure 9.9) of infected turkeys becomes swollen. This clinical sign will not be present in turkeys that have had their snood previously removed as a part of the normal husbandry procedures of some poultry farms. Infection usually results in death or necessitates euthanasia. Chronic infections result in endocarditis and arthritis, similar to swine.

Erysipelothrix in Other Domestic Species

E. rhusiopathiae infections have also been reported in sheep, dogs and dolphins. Sheep most commonly present with arthritis of multiple joints (polyarthritis). Canines experience endocarditis and arthritis due to *E. rhusiopathiae*. *E. tonsillarum* has also been reported in cases of canine endocarditis.

Zoonotic Alert: Erysipeloid

"Fish-handler's disease" occurs as a result of handling oceanic species that carry *E. rhusiopathiae*, such as scorpion fish or lobsters. Aquatic veterinarians and veterinary technicians, abattoir workers, and fish handlers are all at risk for the disease which is termed "erysipeloid" infection (i.e., "erysipelas-like"). Handling the rough surface of the scales of fish or the exoskeleton of shellfish with bare hands results in tiny cuts or scrapes whereupon *E. rhusiopathiae* enters the bloodstream. Infection most often remains local to the primary entry point of the pathogen. Consequently, most cases are confined to the hand. Redness and swelling may be seen surrounding the area of entry. Rarely, the infection can cause sepsis and, as a result, systemic disease.

The "*Other*" Erysipelas

To be frank, not all naming systems make a lot of sense. Enter the term "**human erysipelas**" – a name given to the skin infection (usually of the hands) usually caused by Group A *Streptococcus* – not *Erysipelothrix*. A form of cellulitis, typical symptoms of this streptococcal infection are blisters, painful red skin, and a skin sore. Fever and chills may accompany infection.

Client Education:
Management Decisions Affecting Swine Erysipelas

Erysipelothrix rhusiopathiae preferentially infects young, immunologically naïve animals. Because of this, two management decisions can mean the difference between prevention of disease – or suffering an outbreak of erysipelas!

- **Age-segregation:** This practice keeps same-age nursery piglets together as a group until they reach market age. No older animals (a possible source of chronic erysipelas) can enter the group and spread disease.

- **All in-all out:** Once a set of piglets are placed in a barn (e.g., as weanlings), they are kept there until it is time to go to market. No new additions to the barn are made. When they leave to go to market, every pig in the building leaves. The building is then thoroughly cleaned and disinfected. Any pathogens, including *Erysipelothrix*, will be destroyed. Only then will the producer introduce the next set of weanlings to the barn. This disinfection process is designed to "break" the cycle of infection.

Further Reading

Díaz-Delgado, Josué, et al. "Fatal *Erysipelothrix rhusiopathiae* Septicemia in Two Atlantic Dolphins (Stenella Frontalis and Tursiops Truncatus)." *Diseases of Aquatic Organisms* 116 1 (2015): 75-81.

Gouletsou, Pagona. G., and G. C. Fthenakis. "Microbial Diseases of the Genital System of Rams or Bucks." *Veterinary Microbiology* (2015).

Rosenbaum, Amir, et al. "Slaughterhouse Survey of Pyelonephritis in Dairy Cows." *Veterinary Record* 157 21 (2005): 652-55.

Chapter 10:

Acid-Fast Rods:
Rhodococcus, & Mycobacterium

Introduction

The bacteria in this chapter cannot be classified by gram staining characteristics as they cannot retain the crystal violet stain. This is due to differences in their cell wall constituents. Their cell walls contain mycolic acid and large amounts of waxes and complex lipids rendering them quite resistant to most staining dyes. In order to stain these cells for identification, carbolfuchsin is used as the stain, a compound which contains phenol; the phenol helps the stain penetrate the cell wall. The penetration of the stain is further aided by the addition of heat during the staining process. For a more complete discussion on the acid-fast staining procedure, see Chapter 22.

Rhodococcus

Rhodococcus equi is a gram-positive coccobacillus (Figure 10.1) that stains weakly with acid-fast stain due to the presence of mycolic acid in the cell wall. The term **coccobacillus** refers to very short rods that can be mistaken as cocci during microscopic examination (Figure 3.5). On agar, colonies appear mucoid producing pink to reddish pigment after several days of incubation. It is this pigmentation that gives the bacterium its name; "rhodo-" is Greek for "rose". Like many other **facultative intracellular pathogens**, *R. equi* possesses the ability to survive and reproduce inside immune cells such as macrophages.

Environmental Conditions
Favoring Transmission

Manure and nasal discharge from animals infected with *Rhodococcus equi* is a major source of environmental contamination. Certain environmental conditions enhance the spread of *R. equi* organisms throughout the environment and thereby increase the chance of infection to young naïve foals, the definitive host of *R. equi*. Foals less than 6 months of age are at highest risk of infection and disease. High summer temperatures, sandy soil, and dusty conditions all help the organism to spread to potential hosts via aerosolization. Less commonly infected animals include swine, cattle, goats and immunocompromised humans.

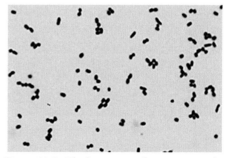

Figure 10.1: *Rhodococcus equi* demonstrating the coccobacillus cellular morphology. From: Mackowiak, Philip A. "Photo Quiz." Clinical Infectious Diseases 32 6 (2001): 929-29. Black and white photo. Used with permission.

Clinical Disease

R. equi infection in foals causes a slowly progressive lower respiratory infection characterized by difficulty breathing (dyspnea), loss of appetite, and fever. Diarrhea may develop due to organisms being coughed up and swallowed. Other signs that may be present are nasal discharge coming from both

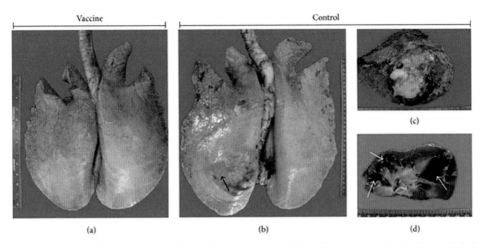

Figure 10.2: *Rhodococcus equi* in foals. The lungs of a normal foal (a) are compared with those of a foal infected with *R. equi*. A pyogranulomatous lesion can be seen on panel (b) (black arrow) and in panel (c). The kidney (d) has sustained injury due to an infarction of *R. equi* lodged in capillaries causing loss of tissue oxygenation and tissue death). From: Erganis, Osman, et al. "The Effectiveness of Anti-*R. equi* Hyperimmune Plasma against *R. equi* Challenge in Thoroughbred Arabian Foals of Mares Vaccinated with *R. equi* Vaccine." *Scientific World Journal* (2014): 480732. Open access.

nostrils and coughing. Gross lesions seen on necropsy include pneumonia with extensive abscesses throughout the lung tissue (Figure 10.2). Abscessation in swine and cattle is usually more localized to a particular lymph node, while goats most commonly present with multiple liver abscesses.

Diagnostics: Choosing the Right Sample

Sample choice must be made with the patient's potentially compromised ability to breathe in mind. Procedures that stress the foal can worsen the dyspnea and cause the foal to collapse and even die. A nasal swab is the easiest and least stressful sample to obtain. However, nasal swabs will pick up normal respiratory flora and do not accurately represent bacteria in the lungs. Alternately, the veterinarian may choose to perform a tracheal aspirate or a transtracheal wash. These samples carry less chance of contamination and are highly predictive, but they are inherently riskier to collect; the transtracheal wash carries the highest risk to the foal in terms of stress, airway compromise, and death. Every attempt to keep the foal calm during these procedures is of the utmost importance.

It is useful to interpret culture results alongside cytology. Small samples of the tracheal aspirates and washes may be stained using cytological stains (e.g., Wright's) and the smear examined for the presence of organisms, usually found within macrophages. A separate aliquot of the aspirate or wash can be grown on bacterial agar and processed further for genus and species identification.

Treatment

Treatment of foals infected remains challenging due to the fact that *R. equi* is an intracellular pathogen. Its localization within immune cells helps it hide from the same immune system that is trying to kill it! Long term treatment (i.e., anywhere from 4-10 weeks in duration) using a combination rifampin and a macrolide (e.g., clarithromycin) is recommended. Clients should be made aware of this fact prior to starting treatment. Unfortunately, many times, the disease is not recognized until it is well advanced making treatment and recovery difficult. Early diagnosis is key to a good recovery, and simply monitoring temperature of high risk and/or high dollar foals can be very useful for detecting early infections. Despite effective treatment of acute disease, the infection can have long term effects (see "Prognosis" sidebar).

Prevention

Unfortunately, to date, there is no vaccine against *R. equi*. Prevention focuses on decreasing exposure to *R. equi*. This can be accomplished through husbandry measures designed to decrease the formation of dust. Additionally, there are *Rhodococcus equi*-specific hyperimmune plasma (HIP) commercially available products which when administered to foals at approximately 25 days of age provides enhanced passive immunity. While the up-front cost of the commercial products are typically high, it may be financial advantageous when compared to the cost of treating up to 30% of the foals on the farm every year.

Client Education:
Rhodococcus equi Infections - Prognosis

Almost 70-90% of foals recover from *R. equi* especially if the infection is caught early. However, there is some debate regarding the long-term impact of the infection on the respiratory system and, hence, on the future athletic ability and performance of the foal as it becomes an adult. Racing depends on good lung function to enable the horse to draw large breaths during galloping. Owners of racing horses and foals should be made aware of the potential impact of *R. equi* beyond the initial illness.

Mycobacterium

The *Mycobacterium* genus contains well over 100 species. Most of these exist as facultative intracellular pathogens or saprophytes. Some of the species infecting animals of veterinary importance are summarized in Table 10.1. In this section, we will confine the majority of our discussion to four of the most common pathogens infecting domestic animals. These are *M. tuberculosis*, *M. bovis*, and *M. avium* ssp. *paratuberculosis*.

Table 10.1: Selected *Mycobacterium* species of veterinary importance*

Species	Main Host(s)	Sometimes Infected	Disease
M. tuberculosis	Primates	Dogs, cattle, birds	Tuberculosis
M. bovis	Cattle	Deer, badgers, dogs possums, humans, cats; sheep, goats, pigs	Tuberculosis
M. avium complex	Birds (exception: psittacines (e.g., parrots))	Pigs, cattle	Tuberculosis
M. avium ssp. *paratuberculosis*	Cattle , sheep, goats, deer	Other ruminants	Johne's Disease
M. marinum	Fish	Humans, aquatic spp.	Tuberculosis
M. leprae	Primates	Armadillos	Leprosy
M. lepraemurium	Rats, mice	Cats	Feline leprosy
Novel species (cannot culture these)	Dogs, (cats)	Range of spp.	Canine Leproid Granuloma
M. phlei	Cats, (dogs)	Range of spp.	Panniculitis Syndrome (skin disease)
M. chelonae *M. fortuitum*			Tuberculosis of aquatic and amphibians

*Species in **bold** are those that are covered in this book.

Pathogenesis of Mycobacterial Infections

How is it that mycobacterial organisms can cause disease? Like *Rhodococcus equi*, *Mycobacterium* survives inside phagocytic cells, especially macrophages. On necropsy, the inflammatory response is visible as caseous necrosis and the formation of **granulomas**. Because killing an intracellular organism is very difficult, granulomas form in an attempt to "wall-off" the disease from the rest of the body and thereby preventing further spread of the organism. Histologically, a granuloma contains a center of caseous necrosis (Figure 10.3). The caseous material contains macrophages filled with *Mycobacterium*. Occasionally, in longstanding granulomas, the caseous material may become calcified giving it a gritty feel. Surrounding the caseous center is a layer of lymphocytes attempting to clean up the caseous center. The outermost layer is the thick, fibrous capsule made of tough fibroblasts; this is the "wall" preventing spread of the organisms. Most mycobacterial infections develop over long periods of time. It may take several months, or even years, for clinical signs to develop.

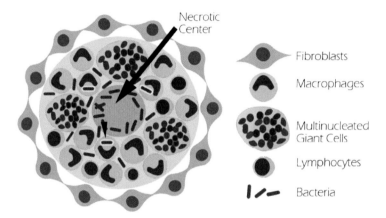

Figure 10.3: Cell types involved in caseous necrosis and granuloma formation. Infection with bacteria, like *Mycobacterium*, attract cells like macrophages, multinucleated giant cells (activated professional phagocytes in the macrophage cell line), and lymphocytes. In long-standing infections, the body creates layers of fibroblasts in an attempt to "wall-off" the infection and prevent further spread of the bacteria to other adjacent and/or distant sites.

Mycobacterium tuberculosis

The most well-known species of *Mycobacterium*, *M. tuberculosis* (Figure 10.4) causes the lung disease tuberculosis (TB). The disease is estimated to cause the deaths of over 2 million people per year with new infections acquired *at a rate of 1 per second!* The transmission of tuberculosis is most often via person-to-person aerosol transmission.

As the only reservoir host, it is humans who infect animals with tuberculosis – another example of an anthroponosis (see also Chapter 7, *Streptococcus pneumoniae*). This is especially true for nonhuman primates, like monkeys and the great apes. Epidemiology studies show that nonhuman primates with little to no exposure to humans, like those living in the deepest portions of the Amazon

> ### *Mycobacterium tuberculosis* complex
> This term refers to several tubercle-producing *Mycobacterium* that includes *Mycobacterium tuberculosis* and *M. bovis*.
>
>

rainforest, do not acquire tuberculosis. Rather *it is their exposure to people* that results in aerosol transmission of *M. tuberculosis* to them.

Because humans are the reservoir host, members of the animal care and veterinary teams working with nonhuman primates (e.g., zoos and research facilities) are asked to provide proof of a negative TB test. This testing is usually mandated periodically (e.g., annually) before a member of the team will be allowed access to the primate facilities. The test is usually performed on the person's forearm (i.e., intradermal skin test). The intradermal test in people has largely been supplanted by a blood test. Because TB can also be spread from person to person, many schools and colleges in the US require students to provide proof of a negative TB test before attending their first day of class.

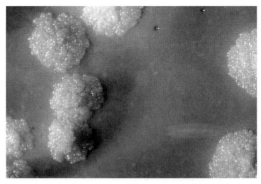

Figure 10.4: Close-up of *Mycobacterium tuberculosis* colonies. Courtesy of the Public Health Image Library, PHIL #4428, Centers for Disease Control and Prevention, Atlanta, 1976.

Dogs and Cats

Most tuberculosis infections in dogs are a result of transmission from humans to dogs. Dog-to-dog transmission is extremely rare. Therefore, the risk of dogs acquiring tuberculosis parallels that of the human population. That is to say that a dog's risk of developing tuberculosis is much higher in *M. tuberculosis*-endemic areas than those living in non-endemic areas (e.g., US). Even within countries where *M. tuberculosis* is endemic, cases of canine tuberculosis usually center on areas of dense human population (e.g., urban) rather than more sparsely populated rural areas. Tuberculosis in dogs mimics that seen in humans. Respiratory signs predominate and multiple granulomas form throughout the lung tissue.

Even though there have been no reports of transmission of TB from dogs to owners, treatment of dogs with TB remains very controversial. The veterinarian will counsel the owners on the relative risks of treating a dog with TB. Many follow-up visits and testing will likely be necessary to ensure that the dog does not constitute a substantial risk to public health.

Cats are much less susceptible to infection by *M. tuberculosis* than dogs.

Zoonotic Concerns

Luckily, the risk of the transmission of *M. tuberculosis* from dogs and cats to their owners is extremely rare. Case-in-point, a California couple adopted a rescue dog that was subsequently diagnosed with *M. tuberculosis*. The couple never became TB-test-positive despite cohabitating with the dog for over a year prior to the diagnosis! (It is likely that the dog acquired TB from another human either at or prior to entering the rescue.) However, the veterinarian will want to ensure that a given patient is not a public health risk prior to release from the clinic or hospital.

Members of the veterinary team, however, should take heed. In 2011, transmission of *M. tuberculosis* to several veterinary professionals occurred during the necropsy of a dog *that was not previously suspected of having tuberculosis*. While this is currently the only published case, it highlights the need for vigilance. Veterinary professionals should remember to always wear appropriate PPE, especially when performing an invasive procedure such as necropsy.

Nonhuman Primates

Clinical signs in nonhuman primates closely resembles those found in humans. Lung infections result in multiple granulomas throughout the lung tissues. As the disease progresses, animals have difficulty breathing. Unfortunately, nonhuman primates are very good at disguising when they are not feeling well. As a result, it is not uncommon for the first sign of tuberculosis infection in primates to be sudden death with no prior signs of illness. To identify infected primates before such a dire turn of events, institutions perform periodic TB testing in their nonhuman primate populations.

Mycobacterium bovis

Tuberculosis caused by *Mycobacterium bovis* is a reportable disease. The main hosts of *M. bovis* are cattle and buffalo. These animals also serve as the reservoir for infections in naïve animals. Transmission is via one of three routes: inhalation, ingestion, and (rarely) through wounds. Inhalation results in granuloma formation in the lungs whereas ingestion results in intestinal and local lymph node granulomas (Figures 10.5). Crowding and stress in herds increase the chances of transmission and disease

Incubation Period and Disease

Disease resulting from *M. bovis* infections is called bovine tuberculosis or bovine TB. Like most mycobacterial species, *M. bovis* infections smolder undetected for months before symptoms develop in infected individuals. Infections can remain dormant for years and reactivate during periods of stress or age-related immune system dysfunction. Thankfully, most infected cattle are identified early due to routine testing and so symptomatic infections are uncommon. In those that show clinical signs, the disease presents with chronic debilitation and progressive emaciation.

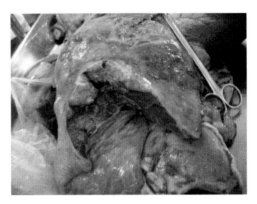

Figure 10.5: Caseous granulomatous material in the lung and draining lymph nodes of a cow during routine slaughterhouse surveillance in the Namwala District, Zambia. Lesions are consistent with *Mycobacterium bovis* infection. From: Munyeme, Musso, and Hetron Mweemba Munang'andu. "A Review of Bovine Tuberculosis in the Kafue Basin Ecosystem." *Vet Med Int* 2011 (2011): 918743. Open access.

Disease in Dogs and Cats

Cats are more susceptible to *M. bovis* than *M. tuberculosis* infections. Transmission is through ingestion of raw, contaminated milk or beef. However, the incidence of *M. bovis* infections in cats within the US is relatively low. This is due, in part, to the federal *M. bovis* eradication program in place for cattle. Cats may also acquire the infection through ingestion of *M. bovis*-infected rodents. Therefore, outdoor and barn cats are at higher risk than "indoor-only" cats. *M. bovis* infections result in tubercular lesions that can occur in the gastrointestinal tract, lung, skin, and other organs. Antibiotics, such as rifampin or quinolones have been used to treat infections. Dogs appear less susceptible to *M. bovis* infection than cats.

Zoonotic Alert: M. bovis!

While humans do not serve as the reservoir host, they are still susceptible to infection with *M. bovis*. Ingestion of contaminated materials leads to localization of the *M. bovis* bacteria in the cervical lymph nodes (i.e., located on either side of the jaw line). The cervical lymph nodes become enlarged and inflamed. Via the lymph nodes, *M. bovis* can move to other tissues including the joints and bones. For this reason, *members of the veterinary team should exercise caution during sample collection.* Any

Remember this: M. bovis and Pasteurization

The minimum temperature needed for the pasteurization of milk was originally set with the elimination of *M. bovis* in mind!

granulomas suspected to contain *M. bovis* should be sent to an approved reference laboratory for further evaluation.

Diagnostic Procedures

Herd Testing

Veterinarians use a simple intradermal skin test to diagnose bovine TB. This test is shown in Figure 10.6 and must be done by a veterinarian specially trained in the procedure. The test results are reported to the United States Department of Agriculture (USDA). This testing procedure can be done on whole herds and is thus used as a screening test. The bovine TB test is very similar to the intradermal skin test used to test people for *Mycobacterium tuberculosis*, mentioned in the previous section.

Regulatory Alert!

Both *Mycobacterium bovis* and *Mycobacterium avian* ssp. *paratuberculosis* are "**reportable diseases.**" This means that suspected and confirmed cases of *M. bovis* **must** be reported to the USDA.

Suspected Cases of Bovine TB

For individual animals suspected of bovine TB, direct smears from clinical samples may be stained with an acid-fast stain, such as the Ziehl/Neelsen stain, and visualized for the presence of mycobacterial organisms. In culture medium, *Mycobacteria* grow slowly and so cultures are incubated for at least eight weeks. In addition to standard laboratory techniques, DNA tests (e.g., PCR) are available for the identification of *M. bovis* from tissue and fluid samples.

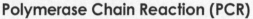

Clinical Correlation:
Polymerase Chain Reaction (PCR)

PCR is a molecular method that is increasingly being used in veterinary medicine for diagnostic testing. The method is based on the ability to replicate small, unique sequences of a pathogen's DNA from a clinical sample (e.g., blood, organ tissue, feces) to the point that they become detectable. The unique sequence of the pathogen must be known so that it can be targeted – otherwise, the results would be very non-specific. The replication reactions are carried out in a very small test tube and a special sensor detects the presence of the target DNA.

Because it tests for the presence of nucleic acids (e.g., DNA), PCR testing cannot distinguish between live and dead organisms.

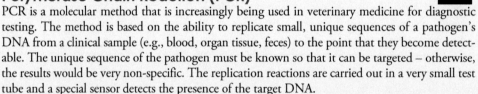

Treatment

In the US, bovine TB is not treated. Early in the last century, the Federal Government adopted a policy of eradicating bovine TB from all agriculture animals; this policy is still in effect. Only test-and-slaughter techniques are guaranteed to eradicate tuberculosis from domesticated animals. All animals that test positive on the intradermal herd screening test are tested again to confirm that they are indeed positive (i.e., some false-positives do occur with the skin test). Any confirmed positive animals are euthanized humanely.

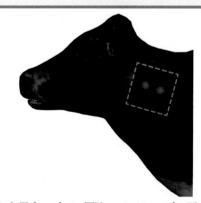

Figure 10.6: Tuberculosis (TB) testing in cattle. There are several different testing methods that are acceptable to the federal government. The test shown here is the comparative cervical test. The intradermal injections are shown (light grey circles) inside the area of the neck usually chosen for the test (dotted blue box).

Treatment of small animals diagnosed with tuberculosis is discouraged, but antibiotics may be used immediately post exposure in an attempt to prevent disease.

Mycobacterium avium subspecies avium

Currently, a member of the *M. avium* complex is the most common cause of swine mycobacteriosis. Swine may also be infected with *M. bovis* and *M. tuberculosis*. Infection is typically asymptomatic and does not appear to cause any health issues in the swine. However, economic losses are incurred at slaughter due to USDA food safety requirements that swine showing infections in multiple lymph nodes or other evidence of systemic mycobacteriosis must be **condemned**, thus completely excluding them from the human food supply. Thankfully, current biosecurity and management practices of modern indoor swine operations have greatly decreased the incidence of *M. avium* ssp. *avium*. However, swine producers raising swine out-of-doors or in facilities where birds can gain access should be aware that these same birds can serve as a source of *M. avium* ssp. *avium* to their herds. Methods to exclude birds from gaining access to swine should be devised.

M. avium ssp. avium infects birds, gaining entry through the oral route and then spreading to the liver and spleen. Many avian species, including domestic poultry, are susceptible (Figure 10.7). On the contrary, psittacine birds such as parrots are resistant to *M avium* ssp. *avium*, while remaining sensitive to *M. tuberculosis*. Granuloma formation in multiple organs is the hallmark of this disease. Progression of the disease is very slow. However, eventually, birds will become anorexic and weak. The pathogen can access bone and joints, causing lameness. Disease in flocks is best dealt with by concentrating on strategies aimed at exclusion rather than treatment.

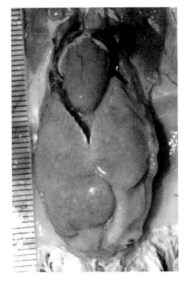

Figure 10.7: A budgerigar experimentally infected with *Mycobacterium avium* ssp. *avium* (pheasant isolate) **showing severe infiltration of the liver.** From: Ledwoń, Aleksandra et al. "Experimental Inoculation of BFDV-Positive Budgerigars (*Melopsittacus Undulatus*) with Two *Mycobacterium Avium* Subsp. *avium* Isolates." *BioMed Research International* (2014): 418563. Open access.

Mycobacterium avium subspecies paratuberculosis

The disease caused by this agent is known as Johne's disease (pronounced "*YO-nees*") (Figure 10.8). The disease affects ruminants like cattle, sheep, and goats. Non-domestic ruminants such as bison, antelope, and gazelles are also susceptible to infection and disease. Transmission of Johne's disease occurs via fecal-oral route, usually to very young animals. Incubation within the host may continue for months to years prior to recognition of clinical signs. During this time, asymptomatic individuals shed the organism intermittently. *Mycobacterium avium* ssp. *paratuberculosis* (MAP) is resistant to environmental conditions and can survive on pastures up to a year.

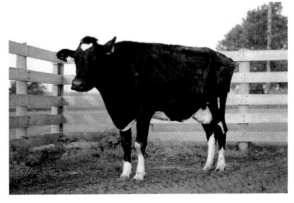

Figure 10.8: Chronic wasting leading to emaciation in a cow with chronic Johne's disease (*Mycobacterium avium* subspecies *paratuberculosis*). This cow experienced profound weight loss and had watery diarrhea – both typical for this disease. Photo courtesy of Peggy Greb © National Animal Disease Center.

Is Johne's Disease Zoonotic?

A hypothesis exists linking MAP as the causative agent in the human medical condition of Crohn's disease. However the data is conflicting. Crohn's disease is an inflammatory condition causing chronic enteritis of unknown etiology. The clinical signs, diarrhea and wasting, closely mimic those of Johne's disease. More research is needed to definitively establish causation between Johne's and Crohn's disease.

Diagnostics

Culture and PCR can be performed using feces and infected tissues. Incubation of cultures may take up to 2 months before visible colonies appear, so PCR is quickly becoming the testing method of choice. Serologic tests to detect the presence of specific antibodies in blood are also available for herd screening. The sensitivity of all testing methods mentioned here improves greatly in cases of clinically infected animals, compared to apparently healthy animals. In other words, subclinical infections of MAP can be difficult to diagnose.

Treatment

Currently, no treatment for Johne's disease exists. Infected animals should be humanely euthanized. As with bovine TB, Johne's is a reportable disease. Young animals should be kept in a clean, manure-free environment, to prevent exposure.

> ### It's all Greek to Me!
> "Chelone" is the Greek word for tortoise. Chelonia is an order of reptiles which includes turtles and tortoises.
>
>

Other Mycobacterial Species

Mycobacterium Associated with Aquatic and Amphibian Species

Mycobacterium marinum, M. fortuitum, M. cheloniae, and *M. xenopi* are found most often in the wet environments inhabited by aquatic and amphibian species. *M. marinum* and *M. fortuitum* are perhaps the best studied of the group. They are capable of causing disease in many aquatic and amphibian species and are both zoonotic pathogens of some significance. *M. xenopi*, so named because they were first isolated from African clawed aquatic frogs (genus *Xenopus*), has been isolated from zebrafish, a striped fish used in research and made popular as a pet by genetic engineering which allows them to glow fluorescent colors (GloFish®, Yorktown Technologies, L.P.). *M. cheloniae* can infect turtles, frogs, and a variety of fishes.

The clinical signs of mycobacteriosis in aquatic and amphibian animal species is generally the same as their terrestrial/non-amphibian counterparts. Namely, the main pathology observed is granuloma formation in a variety of internal organs; these include the respiratory, gastrointestinal, and integumentary tracts, to name just a few.

Each of these species has zoonotic potential. Most infections are transmitted by contact and usually requires abraded or cut skin to cause localized disease. Localized infection, often termed "fish-handler's disease" or "fish tank granuloma", results in granulomatous infections of the skin. Systemic infections are thankfully rare and are usually associated with patients who are immunosuppressed. People with aquaria should be counseled to use latex or nitrile gloves to protect their hands whenever cleaning or working with the tank and its related equipment (e.g., fish nets, filtration system). Additionally, persons with skin cuts, abrasions, or other wounds on the hands or arms should not attempt to clean the tank until these wounds are completely healed. To cut down on the transmission of mycobacterial diseases between aquarium tanks, fish nets can be disinfected. However, care must be taken as these disinfectants must be thoroughly rinsed off as they can damage the delicate mucous layer present on fishes and amphibians. While a direct link between aerosol production (e.g., created by the water turbulence in an aquarium tank) and *Mycobacterium* infections has yet to be definitively established, it is best for persons to take care to limit aerosol exposure.

Mycobacterium leprae

Mycobacterium leprae is the causative agent of leprosy. Humans are the definitive host. The reservoir host is the armadillo, so one should avoid catching armadillos by the tail bare-handed. There is no true leprosy in domestic animals.

Mycobacterium lepraemurium

A disease termed feline leprosy is caused by *Mycobacterium lepraemurium,* whose primary host is rodents. Other mycobacterial species are being investigated as other causes of the same clinical disease. The classic presentation involves ulcerated nodules of the skin, usually limited to the head, neck and forelimbs. Treatment includes surgical excision and long term antibiotic therapy.

Other Acid-fast Organisms

Nocardia

Nocardia spp. are variably acid-fast. The acid-fast stain is useful in distinguishing between *Nocardia* (acid-fast) and another filamentous gram-positive rod, *Actinomyces* (non-acid-fast). Members of the genus *Nocardia* are covered in Chapter 9.

Further Reading

Gauthier, David T. "Bacterial Zoonoses of Fishes: A Review and Appraisal of Evidence for Linkages between Fish and Human Infections." *The Veterinary Journal* 203 1 (2015): 27-35.

Gauthier, David T., and Martha W. Rhodes. "Mycobacteriosis in Fishes: A Review." *The Veterinary Journal* 180 1 (2009): 33-47.

Ghodbane, Ramzi, and Michel Drancourt. "Non-Human Sources of *Mycobacterium tuberculosis*." *Tuberculosis (Edinb)* 93 6 (2013): 589-95.

Pesciaroli, Michele, et al. "Tuberculosis in Domestic Animal Species." *Res Vet Sci* 97 Suppl (2014): S78-85.

Posthaus, Horst, et al. "Accidental Infection of Veterinary Personnel with *Mycobacterium tuberculosis* at Necropsy: A Case Study." *Vet Microbiol* 149 3-4 (2011): 374-80.

Pusterla, Nicola, et al. "Diagnostic Evaluation of Real-Time PCR in the Detection of *Rhodococcus equi* in Faeces and Nasopharyngeal Swabs from Foals with Pneumonia." *Vet Rec* 161 8 (2007): 272-5.

Shrikrishna, Dinesh, et al. "Human and Canine Pulmonary *Mycobacterium bovis* Infection in the Same Household: Re-Emergence of an Old Zoonotic Threat?" *Thorax* 64 1 (2009): 89-91.

Sykes, Jane E., et al. "*Mycobacterium tuberculosis* Complex Infection in a Dog." *J Vet Intern Med* 21 5 (2007): 1108-12.

Chapter 11:

Gram-Negative Rods – Part I: The Family Enterobacteriaceae

Introduction
This family of bacteria contains species which inhabit the intestinal tract of animals and humans. They also exist in and contaminate vegetation, soil, and water. The family can be divided into frank and opportunistic pathogens. Of the frank pathogens, this chapter will deal with *Escherichia*, *Salmonella*, and *Yersinia* species. Opportunistic species include *Klebsiella* and *Proteus*.

Escherichia coli
Escherichia coli are gram-negative motile rods. They possess peritrichous flagella which aids in their motility. In addition to flagella, *E. coli* possess numerous antigens used for classification of the species. The two main antigens used are the O- and H-antigens. The O-antigen originates in the lipopolysaccharide of the cell wall while the H-antigen forms part of the flagella. For example, *E. coli* O157:H7 is a major human foodborne pathogen contaminating items such as beef hamburgers.

Diseases Caused by *E. coli*
Most *E. coli* are considered commensal organisms. Of these, the bulk make up part of the normal flora of the gastrointestinal tract. Disease from isolates of *E. coli* results from opportunistic infections as well as virulent isolates capable of acting as frank pathogens. Diseases caused by *E. coli* infection include both enteric infections, such as gastroenteritis, as well as non-enteric infections.

Examples of non-enteric infections include:

- Urinary tract infections (UTI)
- Septicemia
- Pneumonia
- Meningitis
- Mastitis

Enteric Disease
Several forms of *E. coli* are capable of causing enteric disease. These include: enterotoxigenic *E. coli*, enteropathogenic *E. coli*, and enterohemorrhagic *E. coli*. As the name suggests, strains of enterotoxigenic *E. coli* (ETEC) cause disease through the production of toxins after first colonizing the gut. These toxins are responsible for the oversecretion of fluids into the gut lumen resulting in diarrhea. Enteropathogenic and enterohemorrhagic *E. coli* (EPEC and EHEC, respectively) destroy gut tissues and cause diarrhea through a process called "attachment and effacement" and are thus both commonly referred to in the literature as **attaching and effacing *E. coli*** (AEEC). Both EPEC and EHEC colonize the gut and proceed to damage the villi of the gut epithelial cells, resulting in diarrhea due to malabsorption. EHEC

diarrhea is often hemorrhagic due to toxin production. *E. coli* O157:H7 is one example of EHEC occurring in humans. In the case of ETEC, EPEC, and EHEC, once *E. coli* gets access to the bloodstream the infection can become systemic and multiple organs can become involved.

Diarrhea constitutes the common clinical sign of most *E. coli* infections. Enteric **colibacillosis** refers to *E. coli* infection resulting in diarrhea and dehydration and can affect young calves and piglets. ETEC is responsible for neonatal calf colibacillosis, while EPEC caused diarrhea in older calves. **Colisepticemia** occurs when *E. coli*-induced inflammation of the colon leads to infection of the blood and septicemia.

Edema disease, an ETEC, causes substantial disease and death in pigs. Piglets acquire the ETEC from either the sow or the environment. Colonization with ETEC and toxemia develop approximately 1-2 weeks after weaning. Clinical disease results in edema (especially of the face and throat) and flaccid paralysis leading to the death of the animal. Some piglets may die suddenly with only slight edema.

Nonenteric Disease
The two main nonenteric infections caused by *E. coli* are urogenital infections and mastitis. All of the common domestic species are susceptible to these *E. coli*-associated infections.

Urogenital Infections
Strains of *E. coli* originating from normal gastrointestinal flora cause urogenital infections as a result of contaminating the external genitalia. The bacteria access and ascend the urethra and localize in the bladder causing a local bacterial infection (i.e., **cystitis**). If the bacteria ascend further up into the ureters and kidneys, pyelonephritis develops.

Uterine infections (i.e., **pyometra**) are caused by bacteria such as *E. coli* ascending the vaginal canal, through the cervix, and into the uterus. Uterine infections can be open (e.g., purulent discharge is draining from the uterus and vagina) or closed (e.g., no discharge is seen). Pyometras can be life-threatening.

Mastitis
The pathogenesis of mastitis proceeds similarly to that of cystitis. Both environmental and host gastrointestinal *E. coli* are possible sources for infection. Normally, the teat canal remains closed and impervious to colonization from *E. coli*. However, teat injury and damage to the teat sphincter provide the opportunity for the bacteria to ascend the teat canal and access the deeper tissues of the udder. Infection results in local inflammation of the udder, called coliform mastitis. Coliform mastitis may affect one or more quarters. Severity of the infection can be mild or may result in the functional loss of one or more quarters.

Human Health Alert: Hemolytic Uremic Syndrome
EHEC O157:H7 is a foodborne pathogen capable of causing significant morbidity and some mortality in people. The designation "O157:H7" refers to the specific O- and H-antigens present on the pathogen's surface. These antigens are useful both in diagnosis and in determining the likely severity and prognosis of the disease. Ingestion of undercooked beef, particularly hamburger, is a big risk factor for acquiring an infection of *E. coli* O157:H7. Immunocompetent adults may be asymptomatic or may develop moderate gastrointestinal distress in the form of diarrhea. The very young, aged, or immunocompromised, however, are at risk of developing hemolytic uremic syndrome (HUS). HUS is a form of acute renal failure which can cause mortality. Those that survive may suffer from chronic kidney disease and dysfunction for the rest of their lives.

Diagnostics
Initial culture can be performed on both blood and MacConkey's agar (Figure 11.1). *E. coli* is a lactose fermenter and will produce pink colonies when grown on MacConkey's agar. Other selective and differential media may be used in specific situations. For example, **chromogenic agar** media (e.g., CHROMagar™, Rainbow® agar) are often used in suspected cases of *E. coli* O157:H7 infection. Chromogenic agar changes color depending upon the type of bacteria grown on its surface, thus aiding in the identification of the organism. In veterinary diagnostic laboratories, *E. coli* 0157:H7 is

of little interest since it does not cause disease in animals. Therefore blood and MacConkey agars are adequate for recovery of *E. coli* from veterinary clinical specimen.

Feces, tissues, milk, and urine may be collected and cultured for the presence of pathogenic *E. coli*, depending on the clinical presentation. Additionally, swabs of purulent material from suspected cases of uterine infections can be used for culture and isolation. Care should be taken to avoid contamination of the swab with commensal organisms of the skin.

Biochemical and Molecular Tests

An experience technician can identify *E. coli* based on its colonial appearance on blood and MacConkey agars and a positive spot indole test. Ruminant and porcine enteric isolates from young animals can be tested by PCR for the presence of toxin genes to allow classification of the isolates as ETEC, EPEC or EHEC.

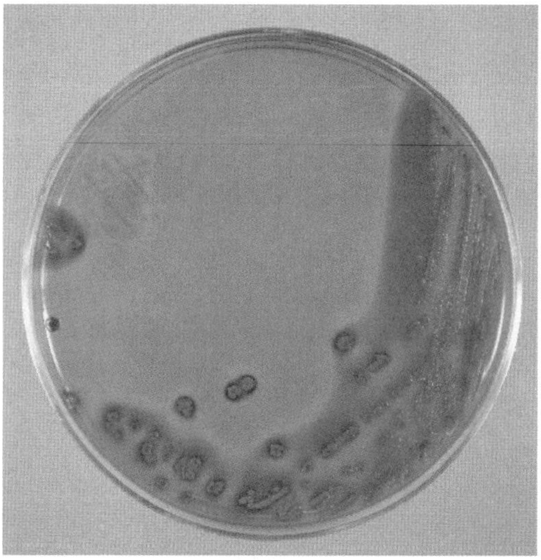

Figure 11.1 *Escherichia coli*, MacConkey's agar (MAC). *E. coli* possesses the ability to ferment lactose to lactic acid. The accumulation of lactic acid. The agar media contains a pH indicator (neutral red) that changes from yellow to red when the pH is below 6.8. The neutral red is absorbed by the bacterial colonies turning them pink.

Treatment

Treatment of animals with colibacillosis is supportive and focused on correcting fluid and electrolyte imbalances. The use of antibiotics is controversial in these cases. Non-enteric *E. coli* infections should be treated with antibiotics based on antimicrobial susceptibility results.

Prevention

Vaccination of dams prior to calving can ensure that calves receive adequate colostral antibodies against the *E. coli* strains of concern. Prevention efforts should also focus on husbandry, such as the practices for removing fecal material from the environment. A clean environment can help prevent colibacillosis and mastitis.

Salmonella

The genus *Salmonella* contains well over 2,500 serotypes. Within a single species of bacteria, groups of isolates may possess distinctive surface characteristics that can only be distinguished by serological identification methods; these distinct groups are known as **serotypes**.

All members of the genus *Salmonella* are motile via peritrichous flagella. Additionally, members cannot ferment lactose, a property that separates them from *Escherichia coli*. Most of the veterinary pathogens belong to *S. enterica* ssp. *enterica*. The host range and types of infection caused by *Salmonella enterica* infections is quite diverse (Table 11.1). Within this subspecies are a number of different important serotypes, such as *Salmonella* Typhimurium.

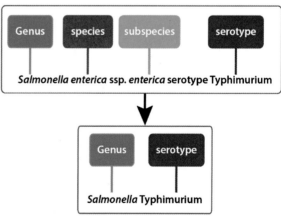

Figure 11.2: Proper nomenclature for *Salmonella* serotypes. The full nomenclature is shown in the top panel. When correctly shortening the name, the species and subspecies designations are dropped leaving only the genus and serotype designations (bottom panel). The genus, species, and subspecies should always be italicized with the genus being capitalized. Serotypes are capitalized but not italicized.

The genus *Salmonella* utilizes a special "nickname" system (Figure 11.2). Note that the serotype is capitalized but not italicized.

Table 11.1: Selected *Salmonella* serotypes, preferred (main) host, and disease manifestations

Serotype	Preferred Host	Typical Disease in Preferred Host
S. enterica subsp. *enterica*		
Abortusequi	Horses	Abortions
Abortusovis	Sheep	Abortions
Cholerasuis	Swine (young)	Septicemia with rapid death
Dublin	Cattle	Mastitis; septicemia; stillbirths
Enteritidis	Poultry	Lethal septicemia
	Human	Enteritis (e.g., eggs)
Gallinarum	Poultry	Septicemic disease (fowl cholera)
Pullorum	Poultry	Septicemic disease (pullorum disease)
Typhi	Humans	Typhoid fever
Typhimurium	Calves	Enteric disease
	Poultry	Asymptomatic carriage (zoonotic)
	Swine	Enteric disease
S. enterica subsp *arizonae*	Turkey poults	Diarrheal disease; septicemia; meningitis
	Reptiles	Asymptomatic carriage
S. bongori	Reptiles	Asymptomatic carriage

Habitat and Transmission

Salmonella is a natural inhabitant of the intestinal tract of many species including birds, reptiles, turtles, insects, and farm animals. Sources of infection for animals and humans include water, soil, animal feeds, raw meat and offal, and vegetables. By far, the most common route of infection is through ingestion of contaminated materials. Infections through inhalation, leading to upper respiratory tract infections, and conjunctiva are minor modes of transmission.

In poultry, such as layer hens, one or both ovaries may be infected by *Salmonella enterica* (e.g., *Salmonella* Enteritidis) and transmit the bacteria to the egg yolk before the shell is formed. It is because the contamination happens prior to shell formation that consumption of undercooked or raw eggs poses such a significant health risk.

Inflicting Damage onto the Host

Infections caused by *Salmonella* lead predominantly to gastrointestinal disease. In brief, once ingested, *Salmonella* invades the epithelial layer of the intestines. Damage to the epithelial cells initially occurs as a direct result of the bacteria breaching the epithelial layer. However, the subsequent immune response by the host also contributes to intestinal damage as these cells attempt to phagocytose and kill the invading *Salmonella*. Damage to the integrity of the epithelial barrier allows for fluids to move out of the gastrointestinal cells and into the lumen causing diarrhea. Because of the hemorrhage produced from damaged epithelial cells, the diarrhea may sometimes appear bloody. This hemorrhage also allows a conduit for the bacteria to enter the bloodstream. If this occurs, the *Salmonella* infection can become systemic causing sepsis and affecting organs of the body. Thus depending on the disease, the clinical spectrum in *Salmonella* infections can range from asymptomatic carriers of the disease to an acutely fatal septicemia. Factors affecting the severity of disease include the age of the animal, the infectious dose ingested, the serovar, and concurrent stress.

Clinical Infections

Enteric salmonellosis occurs most often in farm animals such as cattle, sheep, and goats. However, other domestic animals and pets can also be infected. Infected animals may present with fever, depression, and anorexia. Affected animals produce foul smelling diarrhea that often contains blood, mucus and epithelial cells. If the diarrhea is severe, dehydration and weight loss occur. If the animal is pregnant and the *Salmonella* becomes bloodborne (i.e., sepsis) the fetus may be aborted.

Diagnostics

Salmonella grows well on blood and MacConkey agars, and additional differential agars such as xylose lysine deoxycholate (XLD), Hecteon enteric (HE) and Brilliant Green (BG) are also available to aid diagnosis. Because fecal samples will undoubtedly contain many other types of bacteria, it is advisable to inoculate a selective enrichment broth to suppress growth of other intestinal bacteria while allowing *Salmonella* to grow. Enrichment media suitable for growing *Salmonella* isolates include Selenite F, Rappaport, or tetrathionate broth. The isolate is allowed to grow aerobically at body temperature (37°C) for 48 hours. An aliquot of the enrichment broth culture is taken at both 24 and 48 hours and subcultured onto a differential media such as BG or XLD. In contrast to *E. coli*, are non-lactose fermenters; therefore, they will appear white on MacConkey as well as being spot indole-negative. Further biochemical tests such as Triple Sugar Iron (TSI) agar are useful for identification (for interpretation of agar and biochemical results, see Chapter 22). Once an initial identification of *Salmonella* is achieved, serogrouping and serotyping should be performed to further characterize the isolate.

Treatment, Control, and Prevention

Multiple drug resistance in *Salmonella* species is a big concern. Therefore, clients should be advised that antibiotic susceptibility testing should always accompany culture of the organism. Fluid and electrolyte replacement is warranted as *Salmonella* infections often cause dehydration due to loss through diarrhea. Additionally, administration of fluids aids in maintaining blood pressure which is especially important when septicemia is suspected.

Patients infected with *Salmonella* should be considered highly infectious. Genetically-encoded resistance to multiple antibiotic drugs complicates treatment success of some cases of salmonellosis (e.g., *Salmonella* Typhimurium DT104). Prevention of disease consists of reducing the risk by reducing environmental contamination and host stress. Biosecurity is a key component of prevention as well as a method to control the spread of disease.

Public Health Alert: *Salmonella* as a Foodborne Pathogen

Salmonella infections result in a large number of foodborne illnesses each year. In the United States alone, there are over 1.2 million cases of gastroenteritis annually, including approximately 450 deaths, caused by various *Salmonella* serotypes. *Salmonella* infections from all serotypes cause approximately 3 million deaths worldwide. The risk is increased due to the common natural carriage of *Salmonella* within the intestinal tract of many species which are used as food (e.g., poultry, cattle, and swine). The sources of outbreaks of salmonellosis are numerous and include: eggs, poultry, beef, fresh fruits and vegetables, lettuce, tomato, cantaloupe, peanut butter, nuts, and pistachios. In 2012, two *Salmonella* outbreaks were traced back to the consumption of yellow fin tuna and mangos, respectively. Infections from eating meat most often occur due to fecal or intestinal content contamination of the meat during processing and a failure to cook the meat at a temperature high enough to kill the contaminating bacteria. Contamination of fruits, vegetables, and other non-animal products may occur subsequent to the application of fertilizers containing animal manure which harbors viable *Salmonella*. There are specific procedures that farmers can use to ensure that *Salmonella* and other fecal-associated bacteria do not survive in the farm's manure pit. Manure processed correctly carries a much lower risk of containing and transmitting *Salmonella* to foodstuffs.

"Madam, your ~~dinner~~ typhoid is served…"

The Case of Typhoid Mary

At the turn of the last century, Mary Mallon, an Irish-American immigrant cook-for-hire of New York City's wealthy families seemed to be very lucky. Some of the people she cooked for would get sick with Typhoid Fever, a potentially deadly infection caused by *Salmonella* Typhi, and yet she seemed to be immune to the disease. It wasn't until Dr. George Soper, a zealous sanitation expert of the then fledgling city health department, chased her down (literally) and tested her that he discovered that she was the cause of the families' illness from Typhoid Fever.

It was a strange case. She clearly shed *Salmonella* Typhi in her feces and yet she swore she had never been sick with Typhoid Fever in her life. Dr. Soper had discovered what appeared to be the first healthy human carrier of the disease. On further examination, Soper found that, of those 8 known families she had cooked for, at least one member in each of 6 of those families had become ill and 1 had died – a young girl.

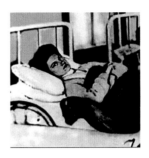

Mary Mallon on North Brother Island, 1910. (Courtesy of PBS)

Soper, a gentleman not known for having the best bedside manner, told Mary she could under no circumstances cook for people as she posed a serious health risk. A rather poor, low-skilled immigrant, Mary needed to cook to earn enough money to survive. Plus, Mary, like most other people at that time, didn't understand how a healthy person could give someone else a deadly disease. It just didn't make sense! So Mary continued to earn her meager wages by cooking for families.

In 1907, alarmed by her apparent disregard for people's health and his authority in the matter, Dr. Soper convinced city health authorities to take the unthinkable step of forcibly incarcerating her on nearby North Brother Island. She was freed on 1910 on the condition that she will never work as a cook again. But how was a low-skilled single female to survive at the turn of the century if she couldn't do the thing she was good at? She changed her name to "Mrs. Brown", worked as a cook again and in 1915 she was associated with another outbreak Twenty-five people became ill and two of them died. Mallon was again sent to North Brother Island.

In all, it is estimated that she was responsible for infecting forty-seven people, three of whom died. Eventually, other healthy carriers of *Salmonella* Typhi were identified, but they were not incarcerated. Despite the obvious double standard, Mary was never freed. She remained on the island until her death in 1937. Many experts today agree that her harsh treatment was due, in part, to the unfair and extreme prejudice of the day against Irish immigrants as "dirty" and "less intelligent."

The actions of the New York City health department shocked the community and highlighted a dilemma in health issues. When, if ever, is it okay to sacrifice someone's liberty for the "greater good" of the public's health and safety? The answers continue to be debated even today.

Klebsiella

Klebsiella is unique among the coliforms in that it is the only species that is non-motile. Infections are usually opportunistic. *Klebsiella* is found commonly in nature (e.g., soil, water, and plants) and is a commensal organism in the gastrointestinal tract of many mammals. The two species of highest importance clinically to veterinary medicine are *Klebsiella pneumoniae* and *K. oxytoca*.

Clinical Disease

Klebsiella infections can cause a variety of opportunistic infections in domestic animals. Examples include:

- Pneumonia in calves and foals (*K. pneumoniae*)
- Urinary tract infections in dogs (*K. oxytoca*)
- Endometritis in mares (both species)
- Coliform mastitis in cows (both species)

Diagnostics

Klebsiella species produce large mucoid colonies on blood agar due to the abundant capsule formation (Figure 11.3). This attribute helps distinguish *Klebsiella* from other coliforms. They are lactose-fermenters and thus form pink colonies on Mac-Conkey's agar. They do not form hydrogen sulfide gas when inoculated onto TSI slants.

Treatment

Treatment should be based on antimicrobial susceptibility results.

Proteus

Proteus mirabilis and *P. vulgaris* are both ubiquitous in the environment. Like other coliforms, they appear as gram-negative, motile rods. They are urease-positive which can help distinguish them from other urease-negative coliforms, such as *Escherichia coli*.

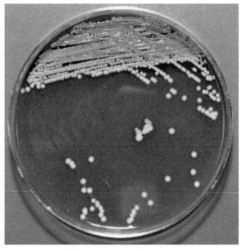

Figure 11.3. *Klebsiella* on blood agar. Colonies appear shiny due to the abundant capsule formation.

Opportunistic Infections

Both *P. mirabilis* and *P. vulgaris* can cause a variety of opportunistic infections including infections of the:

- Urinary tract
- Ear
- Wounds

Urinary tract infections due to *Proteus* are especially common in dogs and horses. *Proteus* gains access to the urinary tract through fecal or environmental contamination of the urethra. Once inside the urethra, the flagella help move *Proteus* up the urinary tract and into the bladder. Once inside the bladder, *Proteus* is able to break down the urea within the bladder into ammonia; the breakdown is accomplished with the urease enzyme. Ammonia is a basic compound. Increasing concentrations of ammonia cause the urine pH to rise to 8 or higher. This shift to a more alkaline pH creates an environment which is more conducive to the formation of stones within the bladder, called **uroliths**. If the bacterial infection ascends into the kidneys, kidney stones can result.

Culture

Due to its highly motile nature, *Proteus* colonies will exhibit "swarming" and appear to grow together as a lawn on solid agar (Figure 11.4). *Proteus* cannot ferment lactose and will thus appear as white, rather than pink, colonies on MacConkey's agar. This can help differentiate it from other gram-negative, motile, coliforms that are lactose-fermenters like *Escherichia coli*. On TSI agar, *Proteus* isolates produce hydrogen sulfide gas, turning the media black, which is useful in differentiating it from organisms such as *Klebsiella*.

Treatment & Client Education

Treatment of *Proteus* infections is based on culture and antibiotic susceptibility testing. In patients with both uroliths and a *Proteus* infection, the infection must be completely eliminated prior to or at the same time as treatment for the uroliths is pursued. This is because the urease enzyme of *Proteus* is a major contributing factor to urolith formation (i.e., the alkaline pH shift in the urine). Clients should be made aware that failing to properly treat the *Proteus* infection will most likely result in future urolith formation.

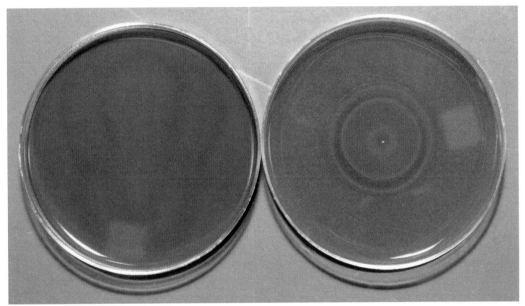

Figure 11.4. Blood agar plates with inoculated with *Proteus vulgaris* exhibiting the "swarming" motility characteristic of the genus. Swarming can be irregular (left plate) or annular (right plate).

Other Enterobacteriaceae

Yersinia

Yersinia pestis (Figure 11.5) the causative agent of the plague. A non-motile, gram-negative, facultative anaerobe, its cellular morphology resembles a safety pin when stained with a Romanowsky stain, such as Wright's Stain. The disease, first gaining infamy during the Middle Ages, is transmitted by flea-bite via rodents who harbor the fleas. When the fleas encounter a new host (e.g., humans) the infection results in two main forms of the disease: bubonic plague and pneumonic plague. Bubonic plague results in generalized lymphadenopathy – the so-called "buboes" from whence the disease gained its name. The pneumonic form causes respiratory difficulty due to pneumonia. Both forms cause fevers and are quite deadly, usually causing disseminated intravascular coagulopathy (DIC) in the end. Despite treatment, DIC is very often fatal. Reports of plague, usually in cats living in the drier climes of the Southwestern US, are occasionally reported even today. Dogs and other carnivores while certainly susceptible, appear to be less so than cats. Most large animal production species appear resistant with the exception of goats and camels, as seen from data from the Middle East. Treatment in cats consists of antibiotics (e.g., gentamicin, doxycycline) and supportive care. Antibiotics must be given for 10-21 days. Because of the zoonotic potential, cats should ideally be hospitalized during the treatment period.

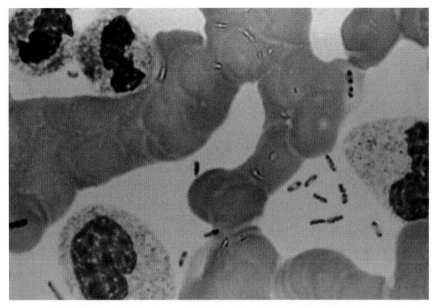

Figure 11.5: Characteristic "safety-pin" cellular morphology of *Yersinia pestis*. The sample is blood from a plague victim. Wright's stain. Courtesy of the Public Health Image Library, PHIL #2050, Centers for Disease Control and Prevention, Atlanta, 1993.

Other species of *Yersinia* of interest in veterinary medicine include *Y. pseudotuberculosis*, causing orchitis and epididymitis in rams; *Y. enterocolitica*, causing sporadic enteric or generalized infection in farm animals; and *Y. ruckeri* causing a condintion known as "red-mouth" in salmon and trout

Shigella

The members of this genus are most often associated with disease in both human and nonhuman primates. The four species within the genus are: *Shigella boydii*, *S. dysenteriae*, *S. flexneri*, and *S. somnei*. *S. dysenteriae* causes diarrheal disease, or "dysentery", among affected individuals. Humans are the only reservoir for this genus. Thus, diarrheal disease in nonhuman primates is via fecal-oral transmission from humans to primates. Members of the veterinary team should be aware of this and educate all animal handlers involved in the care of primates. Workers experiencing diarrheal disease of unknown origin should not work with primates until a diagnosis and treatment of their condition has been initiated. If proven to be shigellosis, workers should not have contact with the primates until the illness resolves.

Citrobacter

Citrobacter rodentium is the main species of concern, especially in pet and laboratory mice. Infections in adult mice are usually self-limiting, meaning that the diarrhea will occur for a time but then the immune system will eliminate the organism. However, in infant mice, the disease can lead to high mortality. Clinical signs include diarrhea, runting, rectal prolapse, and death. Disease prevention, through improved husbandry and sanitation, is best. In the midst of an outbreak, antibiotics (e.g., neomysin, tetracycline) have been used with some success.

Edwardsiella

Two species of *Edwardsiella* are most important for our aquatic veterinary species. These are: *Edwardsiella tarda* and *E. ictaluri*. Both are carried naturally in the intestinal tracts of freshwater fish and both are capable of causing skin sores on the surfaces of fish, such as farmed catfish. *E. tarda* is a zoonotic pathogen capable of causing gastroenteritis; only rarely does it cause more threatening septicemia.

Further Reading

Baker, Kate S. "Demystifying *Escherichia coli* Pathovars." *Nature Reviews Microbiology* 13 1 (2014): 5-5.

Barrow, Paul A., and U. Methner. *Salmonella in Domestic Animals.* 2013.

Brenner, Frances W., et al. "*Salmonella* Nomenclature." *J Clin Microbiol* 38 7 (2000): 2465-7.

The Most Dangerous Woman in America. 2004. DVD.

Salter, Susannah J. "The Food-Borne Identity." *Nature Reviews Microbiology* 12 8 (2014): 533-33.

Chapter 12:

Gram-Negative Rods – Part II: The Family Pasteurellaceae & Related Bacteria

Introduction
This chapter covers pathogens that can cause significant primary respiratory disease in a variety of our veterinary patients.

Bordetella bronchiseptica
Bordetella is a small, gram-negative rod. Its natural habitat is the upper respiratory tract of many species of mammals and birds. The genus *Bordetella* contains many species which cause a variety of diseases in humans and animals. In fact, humans are the host for many of the *Bordetella* species. One species of particular importance in people is *Bordetella pertussis*, the causative agent of whooping cough, which infants are commonly vaccinated against. Only the most common *Bordetella* species, *Bordetella bronchiseptica*, will be discussed in this chapter.

Dogs
Bordetella bronchiseptica is one of several organisms responsible for the condition in dogs known as infectious canine tracheobronchitis or "kennel cough." While *B. bronchiseptica* is the main pathogen involved in kennel cough, it is not uncommon to isolate *Pasteurella* (which acts together with *Bordetella* to damage the trachea and bronchi) as well.

Transmission and Clinical Signs
Dog-to-dog transmission occurs by inhaling respiratory aerosols and droplets laden with *Bordetella bronchiseptica*. Following inhalation, the organism incubates in the upper respiratory tract for 5-10 days after which there is an acute onset of clinical signs. Clinical signs include a harsh, dry, "honking" cough which is especially apparent if the neck over the trachea is pressed. Owners may complain that the cough tends to happen when the dog is excited, has been running, or enjoying other vigorous activities. In addition to coughing, dogs may occasionally gag or retch in an effort to clear accumulating mucus from within the trachea. The common name for this disease, "kennel cough", is a bit of a misnomer. *Bordetella* spreads quickly not only through dogs housed in kennels *but also any other areas where dogs are in close contact with one another* (e.g., dog shows, dog parks).

Diagnostics
Often clinical signs and history of close contact with other dogs are adequate to tentatively diagnose a *B. bronchiseptica* infection. Transtracheal washes are appropriate samples for detecting *Bordetella* in culture. Nasal swabs may collected, but these are less ideal due to the normal flora of the upper respiratory tract which is guaranteed to contaminate the sample. The organism grows readily on standard media, though their colonies are small and usually take 48 hours to appear.

Treatment and Prevention

In animals with a healthy, adequate immune system, the disease is self-limiting with the entire clinical course of the disease, from initiation to resolution, occurring in approximately 10-14 days. Recovery from the disease in most otherwise healthy dogs is largely uneventful. Because kennel cough is usually self-limiting, medical intervention often targets treating clinical signs with cough suppressants. Generally speaking, antibiotics are not indicated. If treatment of a particular patient will involve antibiotics, it's important to base drug selection on antimicrobial susceptibility test results.

Studies have shown that the organism can be shed in recovered puppies for up to 3 months after infection. These animals are a potential source of infection for naïve dogs and puppies.

Effective prevention of kennel cough is achieved via vaccination. *B. bronchiseptica* vaccines come in both parenteral and intranasal formulations. Current recommendations are for dogs to receive a yearly vaccine at a minimum. Owners of dogs with heavy dog-to-dog contact (e.g., dog parks, dog shows, kenneling often) should be vaccinated every six months.

Swine

Bordetella bronchiseptica is present to some degree in almost all swine herds. In most cases, the organism colonizes the upper respiratory tract without observable clinical signs. Rhinitis (i.e., inflammation of the nasal passages) is associated with intensive rearing conditions. Risk factors of clinical infections are poor ventilation and high stocking densities (i.e., "overstocking").

Transmission and Clinical Disease

Sows are the most common source for the infection in piglets. Transmission is through aerosol, infected droplets, and direct contact with nasal secretions. Clinical disease is seen most often in piglets of approximately 3-4 weeks of age. Signs include sneezing and nasal discharge. Co-infection of *Bordetella* with *Pasteurella multocida* causes more severe clinical signs. Toxins produced by *Pasteurella* are capable of damaging the bony nasal turbinates. Due to the damage, the snout is unable to grow straight and thus develops a characteristic bend (Figure 12.1). The condition is known as "atrophic rhinitis" and takes several months to develop in affected swine. The term "atrophic" refers to the structural degener-

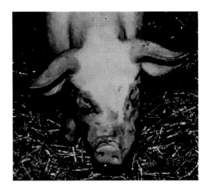

Figure 12.1: Atrophic rhinitis, swine. Co-infection with *Bordetella bronchiseptica* and *Pasteurella multocida* causes a breakdown of the cartilage and bone resulting in non-symmetrical growth of the snout, thus resulting in the conditions characteristic bent snout. Photo reproduced from Muirhead, Michael, and Thomas JL Alexander. *Managing Pig Health: A Reference for the Farm.* 2013. Used with permission.

Clinical Correlation: All-in/All-out Biosecurity

In modern swine operations, pigs are segregated into "nursery" and "grower/finisher" groups. "All-in/all-out" is a biosecurity practice where a set of grower pigs are kept in the same building from just after weaning until it is time to go to market. No new additions to the building are made at any point during this time. This prevents younger, less immune pigs from coming into contact with older pigs that may carry disease which younger pigs are more susceptible to (e.g., *Bordetella*). After the pigs within the building are sent as a group to market, the empty building is thoroughly cleaned and disinfected.

The disinfection process breaks the cycle of infection by removing or killing any pathogens that could infect the next group of weanling pigs that will be placed into the grower building. Only after this process is complete does the farmer bring in the next set of weanling pigs.

ation of the nasal turbinates. The atrophy of the turbinates results in decreased trapping of dust and infectious particles in the nasal passages thus allowing these same substances to seed deeper into the respiratory tract predisposing the pig to subsequent respiratory infections such as bronchopneumonia.

Diagnostics
Transtracheal washes or nasal swabs, though less ideal, can be submitted for *Bordetella* culture. In cases of bronchopneumonia, lung tissue should be submitted for culture.

Treatment and Prevention
In well-managed herds, emphasis is on preventing infection and the resulting atrophic rhinitis rather than on treating the disease once it occurs. Prevention can be achieved through the application of improved management practices. Stocking densities should be kept low to decrease stress among the herd. Measures to increase biosecurity, such as restricting foot traffic to only individuals who work in the swine barns and quarantining all new arrivals to the herd, will help decrease the likelihood of bringing pathogens such as *Bordetella* into the herd. All-in/all-out biosecurity measures also help maintain herd health (see sidebar). A vaccine is available and sows are vaccinated to decrease shedding to the piglets. Treatment consists of antibiotics (e.g., sulfa drugs). However, treatment may not be successful, especially after bony damage to the nose has occurred. Atrophic rhinitis predisposes pigs to many other respiratory infections. These hogs may be chronic "poor-doers" as a result.

Client Education:
Vaccine 100% Money-back Guarantee?
As a part of the veterinary medical team, veterinarians and veterinary technicians administer countless vaccines to animal patients every day. And while we'd like to believe that this means 100% of our vaccinated patients will be free from the diseases we vaccinated against, it just isn't so. This is due to a variety of reasons.

First, the individual patient may not have a healthy enough immune system that can effectively "react" to the vaccine and allow it to make a protective immune response. Second, even after vaccination, the patient may be faced with a huge overpowering pathogen load. Even the best castle can't defend itself if the invading army is just too large and too well-equipped. Finally, the components of the vaccine itself may not be the best ones to cause a fully protective response. Pathogens are very good at making proteins and other constituents that look like the host's normal cells. If we choose these parts to use in a vaccine (sometimes it's the best we have) this can fool the immune system into not mounting an immune response to the pathogen, leaving the patient vulnerable to attack later on.

What does this mean to your patients? If a vaccine is reported to have 95% efficacy, you can expect 95 out of every 100 patients to be protected when faced with the pathogen the vaccine is targeted against. What happens to the other 5%? Those patients may suffer the full range of the disease as if they had not been vaccinated at all. Or, they may get a milder form of the disease. The seasonal "flu" vaccine most of us receive each year is an excellent example of this concept. The majority that are vaccinated never get the flu, while others get milder flu symptoms which run a shorter course. It's important to let clients know that the benefits of vaccination far outweigh the risks. And while the protection the vaccines provide is often excellent – it's still not 100%.

So let clients know that while the current *Bordetella* vaccines are effective at lessening the clinical signs, such as coughing, they *may not completely eliminate them in all cases*. In that way, it is a lot like the seasonal flu vaccine we get!

Pasteurellaceae
This family of bacteria contains a number of ubiquitous, gram-negative, non-mobile, and often opportunistic pathogens affecting animals and humans. Pasteurellaceae are facultative anaerobes incapable of spore formation. Most within the family are residents of various mucous membranes of the

body (e.g., upper respiratory and gastrointestinal tract). They are susceptible to disinfectants, drying, and UV light (e.g., sunlight). However, they are capable of persisting in organic material. Two of the most important genera infecting domestic animals are *Pasteurella* and *Mannheimia*. Table 12.1 lists species of significance for veterinary species.

Host Preference and Transmission

Pasteurella infections can affect many domestic animal species including, but not limited to: dogs, cats, rabbits, pigs, sheep, goats, cattle, horses, and poultry (Table 12.1). While there are numerous species within the *Pasteurella* genus, the most clinically important of these is *Pasteurella multocida*. *Mannheimia haemolytica*, the most economically important species of its genus, mainly infects ruminants such as cattle, sheep, and goats. Transmission of *Pasteurella* and *Mannheimia* occurs via inhalation, ingestion, bites, and scratches. Many infections likely occur because of transmission between animals in the herd. These infections are **endogenous**, meaning that they originate from *within* the herd rather than from an animal outside of the herd. In addition, both pathogens are capable of contaminating and surviving in the environment and on fomites. These become additional sources of infection.

Table 12.1: Select members of the family Pasteurellaceae

Genus species	Hosts	Disease Presentations
Pasteurella multocida	Rabbits	Respiratory disease Abscesses Conjunctivitis Otitis externa Oophoritis Pyometra Septicemia
	Dogs and Cats	Bite wound abscesses Respiratory disease
	Ruminants	Respiratory disease Septicemia
	Avian species	Fowl cholera
Mannheimia haemolytica	Ruminants	Pneumonia and other respiratory diseases Mastitis (sheep)
Histophilus somni	Ruminants	Respiratory disease Abortion Septicemia (cattle) Meningoencephalitis (cattle)
Haemophilus paragallinarum	Poultry	Rhinitis, sinusitis (fowl coryza)
Haemophilus parasuis	Swine	Glasser's disease Respiratory disease
Actinobacillus pleuropneumoniae	Swine	Pleuropneumonia
Actinobacillus equuli	Equine	Septicemia (foals) Respiratory disease Abortion
Actinobacillus lignieresii	Ruminants	Wooden Tongue

Pasteurella multocida

P. multocida is often found secondary to trauma-related conditions. In these circumstances, the infection commonly presents as an abscess. Stress and another, usually viral, infection commonly precede disease manifestations of *Pasteurella* or *Mannheimia* infections. Both species commonly cause respiratory disease. Indeed, both *Pasteurella* and *Mannheimia* are part of the "**shipping disease**" complex of cattle resulting in significant respiratory disease.

Dogs and Cats

Pasteurella disease in dogs and cats is usually related to trauma in the form of bite wounds. *Pasteurella* is a common oral inhabitant of both animal species, and inflammation and abscess formation usually result when it is inoculated via a bite. *Pasteurella* may occasionally cause pneumonia and other systemic illnesses such as sepsis. *Pasteurella* is also an important complicating factor in *Bordetella bronchiseptica* infections of dogs and swine (i.e., kennel cough and atrophic rhinitis, respectively). *Bordetella* causes the initial damage to the respiratory tract allowing *Pasteurella* to come in and do even more damage.

Rabbits

Pasteurella multocida causes upper respiratory tract infections and abscesses in rabbits. Respiratory disease in rabbits is sometimes referred to as "snuffles." The infection can infect nasal passages and the sinuses. Not all rabbits show clinical signs when infected. In fact, many rabbits may be asymptomatically infected. Clinical disease is usually preceded by stress, poor management, or concurrent infections (e.g., *Bordetella*, *Pseudomonas*, or *Staphylococcus*). Occasionally, upper respiratory disease can lead to pneumonia. Pus and abscess formation are the hallmarks of *Pasteurella* infections in rabbits. Non-respiratory disease associated with infection includes: otitis, conjunctivitis, abscesses, and septicemia.

Guinea Pigs

Guinea pigs are highly susceptible to *Pasteurella*. Infection with *P. multocida* quickly leads to pneumonia which is often fatal. Because both dogs and rabbits can carry *Pasteurella* with little to no clinical signs, it is important to prevent contact of these two species with guinea pigs. Using best biosecurity practices, boarding and hospitalized guinea pigs should be located in a room entirely separate from these animal species. Veterinary staff should take care to always thoroughly wash any exposed skin after interacting with rabbits and dogs and before handling guinea pigs. If a dog or rabbit has sneezed or otherwise contaminated a staff member's lab coat or scrubs, these should be changed out for clean, uncontaminated apparel prior to handling guinea pigs.

Ruminants

Both *Pasteurella multocida* and *Mannheimia haemolytica* are capable of causing upper respiratory tract disease in ruminants. They are both part of the shipping disease complex of ruminants, particularly cattle. The upper respiratory tract infection can worsen and lead to pneumonia. Occasionally, these bacteria can escape the lung via the bloodstream and cause systemic disease usually through septicemia.

Swine

Like kennel cough in dogs, *Pasteurella* is an important complicating factor in *Bordetella bronchiseptica* infections of swine (i.e., atrophic rhinitis). *Bordetella* alone causes a transient, self-limiting infection. However, a combined infection with *B. bronchiseptica* and *P. multocida* is progressive.

Diagnostics

Pasteurella infections can be diagnosed using samples such as blood smears, exudates, and tissue impressions.

Culture

Due to special culture requirements of some species and the possibility of normal flora in samples, it is best to send samples for culture at a reference laboratory. *Pasteurella* species grow best on media enriched with serum or blood. Some *Pasteurella* require additional factors (e.g., NAD) and an enriched CO_2 atmosphere to grow. In general, *Pasteurella* species do not grow on MacConkey agar.

Pasteurella has a characteristic odor that has alternately been described as "musty" or smelling like a "wet dog".

Additional Testing
Serotyping (e.g., serological testing) can be performed at most reference laboratories.

> ## Remember this:
> ## Don't scratch and sniff in lab! ⚠
> Because we often do not immediately know what species of bacteria we have isolated from our patients, *it is not advisable to actively smell bacteria.* Aerosol transmission may occur. Remember, many of the bacteria found in animals are zoonotic.

Treatment and Prevention
Treatment relies on the judicious use of antibiotics. The choice of antibiotics should be based on the results of the culture and antimicrobial susceptibility testing. Vaccines are available to prevent disease caused by *Pasteurella* in rabbits (e.g., BunnyVac®) and swine. Additionally, poultry and swine may be fed feedstuffs mixed with antibiotics (i.e., medicated feed) as a preventive. Improved management is a key factor in the control and prevention of Pasteurellaceae infections.

Zoonotic Potential
Pasteurella can cause a variety of opportunistic infections in many animal species, including human beings. Dog and cat bites are a major source of animal-related *Pasteurella* infections in humans. *Pasteurella multocida*, a resident of cat and dog oral microflora, is inoculated into the skin and subcutaneous tissues when the dog or cat bites the person. Inflammation and abscess formation are the two most common sequelae of these animal bites.

Mannheimia haemolytica
Mannheimia haemolytica is capable of causing upper respiratory tract disease in ruminants. It is often found as a co-infection with *Pasteurella*. *Mannheimia* and *Pasteurella* are part of the "shipping disease" complex of ruminants, particularly cattle, which also includes respiratory viruses. A commercial vaccine against *M. haemolytica* is licensed in the United States for use in cattle.

For more information on the relationship of *M. haemolytica* and *P. multocida* in dual infections, see the *Pasteurella multocida* section above.

A Word about Bovine Respiratory Disease
As seen in the previous section, *Pasteurella* infections can play a significant role in respiratory disease in ruminants. Bovine respiratory disease (or "shipping fever") may occur due to multiple organisms (e.g. bacteria and viruses) and the interplay between them. Often viruses colonize the host prior to the introduction of bacteria secondarily, and thus "pave the way" for the bacteria to add to the pathology and clinical signs found in bovine respiratory disease.

Viruses involved include:
- Parainfluenza-3 Virus (PI-3)
- Bovine Respiratory Syncytial Virus (BRSV)
- Bovine Herpesvirus-1 (BHV-1)
- Bovine Viral Diarrhea Virus
- Other bovine respiratory viruses (Bovine Herpes Virus-4, Bovine Adenovirus-3, Bovine Rhinoviruses, Bovine Coronavirus)

Bacteria involved may include:
- *Mannheimia, Pasteurella, Histophilus*

Common pathogenic mechanisms involved in Bovine Respiratory Complex and that increase the severity of clinical signs include:
- Destruction/loss of ciliated epithelium
- Disruption of alveolar macrophage functions (loss of local immune response)
- Changes in the composition of mucus

Histophilus

Histophilus somni is a gram-negative coccobacilli and facultative anaerobe which lives as a resident within the urogenital organs of cattle. The bacterium can also readily colonize the respiratory tract causing significant disease. The organism is readily inactivated by disinfectants and high heat sterilization. Infections can be transmitted by aerosols and close contact. Many infections are considered endogenous. Stress often precedes infection and co-infections with other bacteria or viruses are common. Disease is usually induced when organisms reach a compromised or normally protected, sterile site, such as the alveoli. *H. somni* is part of the bovine respiratory disease complex.

Cattle

H. somni respiratory infections in cattle commonly result in pneumonia. Usually infection is complicated with the addition of other agents (see section "A Word about Bovine Respiratory Disease," above). Clinical signs become apparent especially following stress. Infection may lead to septicemia in some cases. Abortion, secondary to septicemia, may occur in pregnant cows.

Haemophilus

In addition to *Histophilus*, two closely related bacterial species of the genus *Haemophilus*, cause disease in swine and poultry.

Swine

Haemophilus parasuis is responsible for causing polyserositis and septicemia in young weanling swine. The disease is also known as Glasser's Disease. Clinical signs can include pneumonia. A characteristic finding is large amounts of **fibrinous** inflammation of many parts of the body including the pericardium, pleura, peritoneum and joint spaces.

Poultry

Infectious coryza is the name given to the acute contagious upper respiratory infection caused by *Haemophilus paragallinarum*. All ages of poultry are affected. Morbidity may be high with significantly decreased body growth and egg production. Mortality tends to be low with this disease unless complicated by additional pathogens.

Diagnostics:
General Considerations with Pasteurellaceae

Most members of Pasteurellaceae require careful specimen handling to maintain viability on the way to the microbiology laboratory. These species do not grow on MacConkey's agar. Some require additional constituents to be added to microbiological media to ensure growth. For example, *Haemophilus* species require hemin (i.e., a derivative of red blood cells) and the coenzyme nicotinamide adenine dinucleotide (i.e., NAD) to grow while *Histophilus* requires the addition of carbon dioxide in the incubator for growth.

Treatment, Control, and Prevention

Antibiotics should be instituted to treat the patient only after culture and antibi-

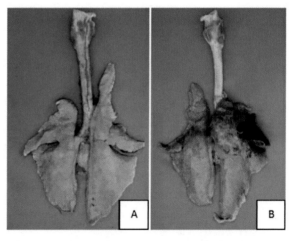

Figure 12.2.*Actinobacillus pleuropneumonia* (APP) **in swine.** Panel A shows the lungs from a health pig. The lung in Panel B is from a pig infected experimentally with APP. The lungs are swollen and there is evidence of hemorrhage. From: Zuo, Z., et al. "Transcriptional Profiling of Swine Lung Tissue after Experimental Infection with *Actinobacillus pleuropneumoniae.*" *Int J Mol Sci* 14 5 (2013): 10626-60. Open access.

otic susceptibility testing has been performed. Improved management is a key factor in the control and prevention of Pasteurellaceae infections. Commercial vaccines against *H. somni* and *H. paragallinarum* are licensed in the US for use in cattle and poultry, respectively.

Actinobacillus

Like other Pasteurellaceae, the source of most *Actinobacillus* infections is endogenous. Two species are of particular importance in food animal medicine: *Actinobacillus pleuropneumoni*a and *Actinobacillus lignierseii*. Given the similarities between them, they will be discussed together especially when considering diagnostics, treatment, and prevention.

Actinobacillus pleuropneumonia

Actinobacillus pleuropneumoniae, called "APP" for short, is considered an obligate pathogen of swine tonsils and the upper respiratory tract. There is no other known natural host. Transmission of *A. pleuropneumoniae* is via direct contact or aerosols. Infection is most common in weaning to market weight pigs (i.e., 2-6 months of age) and is characterized by acute, severe, often necrotic, pleuropneumonia. Clinical signs include fever and decreased appetite. However, this can progress to acute respiratory distress and death in heavily infected animals. Septicemia is rare, but may occur. In the chronic form of the disease, the damaged respiratory tract leads to a "failure-to-thrive" and poor growth. On necropsy, findings in chronically infected animals include scarring of the lung tissue, pleural adhesions, and, less commonly, abscess formation.

Actinobacillus lignieresii: "Wooden Tongue"

A commensal of the bovine oropharynx, infection with *A. lignieresii* leads to the formation of firm nodules in the soft tissues of the tongue, head, and neck. The nodules contain purulent material and small sulfur granules. Sulfur granules are typically yellow in color. However, they may also be white, pinkish grey or brown.

Infection with *A. lignieresii* is protracted. The nodules within the tongue and oral pharynx make the prehension and swallowing of foodstuffs difficult. Weight loss and dehydration secondary to prehension difficulties often ensues. The reduced mobility of the tongue seen in clinical cases gave rise to the lay term "wooden tongue." *A. lignieresii* can be found in the environment. Oral trauma provides access of *A. lignieresii* to the normally protected subepidermal tissues.

Diagnostics for *Actinobacillus* Species

For sample collection, a fine needle aspirate (FNA) of the nodules gives the best results. Swabs of exudates should not be used as normal oral flora will contaminate the sample making diagnosis more difficult. Exudates obtained via FNA should be Gram stained. Blood cultures (if **bacteremia** is suspected) or affected tissues may also be submitted for culture. Many *Actinobacillus* species require supplements in media (i.e., NAD) for growth. Molecular tests, such as PCR have been developed for some species of *Actinobacillus*.

Treatment and Control

Treatment with antibiotics is based on the results of culture and antibiotic susceptibility testing. Prevention and control for endogenous *Actinobacillus* infections centers on good management practices. These include decreasing the stress of the herd and improving sanitation. Prevention of exogenous sources of *Actinobacillus* requires the enforcement of good biosecurity practices.

Zoonotic Potential

While an infection with *Actinobacillus* in people is possible, the likelihood remains low. That said, transmission

> ## Remember this: Wooden Tongue vs. Lumpy Jaw
>
>
> *A. lignieresii*, the causative agent of "wooden tongue" usually affects SOFT tissue such as the tongue and spares the bony tissue. This contrasts with *Actinomyces bovis* ("lumpy jaw") which affects the HARD tissue like the bony jaw.

of *A. lignieresii* to people via bite wounds has been documented in several case reports.

Pseudomonas

Pseudomonas aeruginosa, appears as gram-negative straight to slightly curved motile rods. *Pseudomonas* forms colonies that appear blue-green in color. The color is due to production of the pigment pyocyanin ("cyan" is another word for "blue"). This color may even be seen in the exudate of clinical cases.

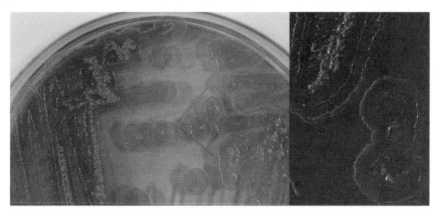

Figure 12.3: Pyocyanin pigment produced by *Pseudomonas aeruginosa.* Colonies appear blue-green due to the production of this pigment. **Left panel:** TSA agar plate streaked with *P. aeruginosa.* **Right panel:** enlargement of one portion of the same plate.

Habitat and Transmission

For the potential hosts to *Pseudomonas* infections, environmental exposure is nearly constant as the bacteria are ubiquitous in nature. *Pseudomonas* is an opportunistic infection capable of causing infection secondary to a compromised immune system. As an opportunist, the bacterium requires an underlying injury or damage to the skin or mucous membrane before accessing the body and doing damage. Most often *Pseudomonas* favors colonization in areas that are wet or moist. In an animal with a compromised immune system or a disruption of normal gastrointestinal flora, ingestion of *Pseudomonas* may lead to infection. For example, prolonged antibiotic therapy for an unrelated infection can disrupt the flora and predispose animals to secondary, opportunistic pseudomonad infections.

Clinical Disease in Animals

Domestic Animals: General Considerations

As mentioned above, *Pseudomonas* prefers to colonize surfaces, both animate and inanimate, that are warm and moist. In humans and domestic animal species, *Pseudomonas* can cause primary and secondary infections of the urinary tract, skin (i.e., pyoderma), and is a common contaminant of wounds including catheter entry sites (see Clinical Correlation, below). Because it is capable of growing in various solutions (i.e., saline, chlorhexidine) and on inanimate surfaces, it is often responsible for nosocomial (i.e., hospital acquired) infections.

Dogs

Pseudomonas has been isolated from ear infections in dogs. The combination of the relatively long vertical and horizontal canals of the dog ear provide a moist, warm, dark environment in which *Pseudomonas* can colonize and readily thrive. Dog breeds with long "floppy" ears (e.g., Cocker Spaniels) that form a sort of cover over the vertical canal are predisposed to chronic ear infections as a result. Coverage of the ear canal with the ear flap creates the moist environment that *Pseudomonas* thrives in. *Pseudomonas* has also been recovered from cases of canine pneumonia. These dogs are usually immunosuppressed. For example, in 2013, a case of multi-drug resistant *P. aeruginosa* pneumonia in a dog recovering from kidney transplantation was reported.

Rabbits

"Slobbers" is the common term used to describe malocclusion in rabbits. When the open-rooted front incisors of the rabbit are misaligned, these teeth overgrow and often begin to curl around. Eventually these overgrown teeth cause damage to the lips and the oral cavity. Such damage is accompanied by secondary bacterial infections and excessive salivation. *Pseudomonas* is one of several bacteria responsible for secondary infections and can be visualized as a bluish-green tinging to the fur where the *Pseudomonas*-laden saliva and its pyocyanin pigment have been deposited.

Diagnostics and Treatment

Samples for isolation and culture can be obtained by swabbing the area suspected of harboring *Pseudomonas*. Antibiotic susceptibility testing should be considered mandatory as a precursor for successful therapy as antibiotic resistance is common.

Clinical Correlation: Catheter Site Preparation

Good nursing care requires attention to the details of ensuring patients' health and well-being. Many patients staying in the hospital or clinic will require a catheter through which intravenous fluids and drugs will be administered. The needle stick through which the catheter is threaded provides ready access of opportunistic bacteria into the deeper tissues of the body. It is important to prevent patients from picking up these pathogens during their stay in the hospital or clinic. Common catheter contaminants include:

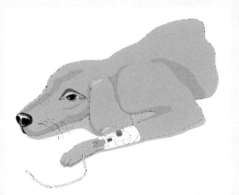

- *Pseudomonas*
- *Staphylococcus*
- Other skin commensals

For this reason it is important that veterinary care staff properly prepare the catheterization site. Hair should be closely clipped from the area over the vein to be catheterized. Next, the site is scrubbed with at least 3 cycles of alternating applications of antiseptic scrub (e.g., chlorhexidine) and isopropyl alcohol. Once the catheter is inserted and stabilized, antibiotic ointment may be applied to the catheter entry site; this last step is controversial and is not universally adopted by all clinics/hospitals. The catheter is then secured to the skin with bandage tape.

Pasterellaceae-Related Bacteria Encountered Less Frequently

Burkholderia

The species of highest interest within this genus are *Burkholderia mallei* and *Burkholderia pseudomallei*, the causative agents of glanders and melioidosis, respectively. Interestingly, *Burkholderia mallei* and *B. pseudomallei* are two of only a few bacterial species carrying two circular DNA chromosomes, rather than a single chromosome. Both are classified as potential bioterrorism agents; laboratories wishing to work with them must get special permission from the federal government and must adhere to strict safety procedures. Finding either of these bacterial species in a natural infection requires the veterinarian in charge of the clinical case to report it to state and federal veterinarians.

Burkholderia mallei (Glanders)

The only natural animal reservoirs of *Burkholderia mallei* are horses, donkeys, and mules. This gram-negative rod is capable of causing significant morbidity and mortality in these same three animal species. *B. mallei* is non-motile and requires an aerobic environment. The disease goes by a number of unusual layman's terms such as "glanders", "farcy", and "droes". Entry into the host is achieved by invasion of *B. mallei* through the mucous membranes, gastrointestinal tract, or the skin. Incubation can take weeks to months. Clinical signs seen may include fever; tiredness or decreased stamina, especially when exercised; depression; cough; anorexia; and weight loss. Ulcerative nodular ("lumpy") lesions present on the skin and mucous membranes are striking signs that may aid in raising the index of suspicion for members of the veterinary team. Diagnostically, the use of serology alone results in a significant number of false-positive test results. Best practices are to use a combination of serology and molecular detections methods (e.g., PCR) as this increases the likelihood of detecting a true *B. mallei* infection while minimizing false-positive test results. It is important to relay this need for confirmation to the client lest they consider it extravagant and unnecessary.

B. mallei has been eradicated from the US, thus it is considered a foreign animal disease. The USDA keeps a tight watch to ensure that the disease does not re-enter the country, particularly as a result of importing diseased equids. All horses wishing to enter the US <u>must</u> test negative for *B. mallei*. The disease is still found in some areas within Eastern Europe, Africa, the Middle East, and Asia. Closer to home, it is present in Mexico and South America. For this reason, if *B. mallei* infection is suspected, the veterinary technician should aid the veterinarian in taking a thorough travel history. As a foreign animal disease, any suspected cases of *B. mallei* infection must be reported to the state and federal veterinarians. Under federal regulations, *B. mallei*-positive animals must be euthanized.

B. mallei is zoonotic. Infections in people can be either acute or chronic. Inhalation results in acute fever and ulcerative necrosis of the upper respiratory tract. Lymph nodes of the neck can become enlarged. Acute disease may lead to septicemia.

Burkholderia pseudomallei (Melioidosis)

Burkholderia pseudomallei is a gram-negative rod. Unlike *B. mallei*, this species is a motile, facultative anaerobe and capable of infecting many mammalian species. This soil saprophyte is endemic to India, Southeast Asia, and the northern portion of Australia. Sporadic cases are reported in Mexico and the northwestern portion of South America. It can survive and replicate in a variety of both phagocytic and nonphagocytic cells, such as macrophages and lymphocytes, respectively. It has an environmental reservoir, preferring soil or stagnant water. For example, it is often found in rice paddies.

In people, melioidosis is characterized by a wide variety of non-specific symptoms which hampers diagnosis. The infection in some is asymptomatic. Clinical signs seen in symptomatic patients include fever, headache, cough, chest pain, muscle pain, and abdominal discomfort. The respiratory signs may even mimic tuberculosis. People who are immunosuppressed or have preexisting health issues (e.g., diabetes or liver failure) are at increased risk of disease. A history of exposure or travel to endemic areas should raise suspicions of possible transmission. Septicemic infections are rapidly fatal with a mortality rate of 40-70%. Death can occur as soon as 24-48 hours after the onset of symptoms.

Disease in animals mimics that of people. *B. pseudomallei* has been isolated from

> ### Remember this:
> ### Take a Travel History
>
> When taking an animal or herd history, it is important to remember to ask about travel outside of the state or country within at least the last 12 months. Diseases that won't seem at all likely (e.g. foreign animal diseases) will suddenly be high on the veterinarian's list of possible pathogens if we know that the animal has traveled and to which areas of the world.
>
>

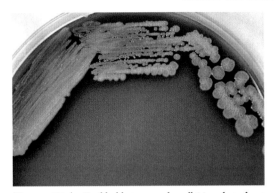

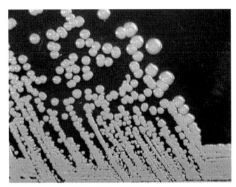

Figure 12.4: *Burkholderia pseudomallei* incubated at 37°C for 72 hours on chocolate agar. Colonies appear to have a flat "cornflower" appearance. Courtesy of the Public Health Image Library, PHIL #12279, Centers for Disease Control and Prevention, Atlanta, 2010.

Figure 12.5: *Burkholderia pseudomallei* incubated at 37°C for 96 hours on sheep blood agar. Colonies have a smooth "button" appearance. Courtesy of the Public Health Image Library, PHIL #1929, Centers for Disease Control and Prevention, Atlanta, 2002.

a variety of animal species living within endemic areas including sheep, goats, pigs, cattle, rabbits, ostriches, and various African and Asian nonhuman primates. *B. pseudomallei* is commonly called the "masquerader" or "mimicker" due to its changing colony morphology over time under incubation conditions (Figures 12.4 & 12.5.). For safety reasons, *B. pseudomallei* is only cultured in properly equipped (i.e., BSL3) laboratories. United States military dogs suffered from melioidosis during the Vietnam War.

Taylorella

Until 2008, the US was free of *Taylorella equigenitalis*, the causative agent of a condition known as contagious equine metritis. This gram-negative coccobacillus is venereally transmitted and causes short-term infertility in the mare, an asymptomatic carrier state in the stallion, and rarely results in abortion. The activity at highest risk for transmission is natural breeding – also termed "natural cover". Artificial insemination using fresh semen carries less risk than natural cover. The risk of using frozen semen has not been established.

An extensive investigation by federal regulators uncovered the most likely source of introduction of the disease as a Fjord stallion that had been imported into the US in 2000 – 8 years before the first clinical case was discovered. A nationwide search to identify any other animals infected by the original stallion ensued. A total of 28 *T. equigenitalis*-positive animals were identified. Regulators then moved aggressively to eliminate the disease from the US. In 2010, the US was once again declared free of *T. equigenitalis*. The incident highlights the need of a vigilant veterinary team and their role in ensuring the health of imported animals. This incident also demonstrates that it takes just one animal to initiate a significant outbreak.

Further Reading

Choy, Jodie L., et al. "Animal Melioidosis in Australia." *Acta Trop* 74 2-3 (2000): 153-8.

Erdman, Matthew M., et al. "Diagnostic and Epidemiologic Analysis of the 2008-2010 Investigation of a Multi-Year Outbreak of Contagious Equine Metritis in the United States." *Prev Vet Med* 101 3-4 (2011): 219-28.

Khan, Iftikhar A., et al. "Glanders in Animals: A Review on Epidemiology, Clinical Presentation, Diagnosis and Countermeasures." *Transbound Emerg Dis* 60 3 (2013): 204-21.

Limmathurotsakul, Direk, et al. "Melioidosis in Animals, Thailand, 2006-2010." *Emerg Infect Dis* 18 2 (2012): 325-7.

Park, Kyung-Mee., H. S. Nam, and H. M. Woo. "Successful Management of Multidrug-Resistant *Pseudomonas aeruginosa* Pneumonia after Kidney Transplantation in a Dog." *J Vet Med Sci* 75 11 (2013): 1529-33.

Peel, Margaret M., et al. "*Actinobacillus* Spp. And Related Bacteria in Infected Wounds of Humans Bitten by Horses and Sheep." *Journal of clinical microbiology.* 11 29 (1991).

Poester, Fernando P., Luis E. Samartino, and Renato de L. Santos. "Pathogenesis and Pathobiology of Brucellosis in Livestock." *Scientific and Technical Review of the Office International des Epizooties (Paris)* 32 1 (2013): 105-15.

Schulman, Martin L., et al. "Contagious Equine Metritis: Artificial Reproduction Changes the Epidemiologic Paradigm." *Vet Microbiol* 167 1-2 (2013): 2-8.

Chapter 13:

Gram-Negative Rods – Part III: *Moraxella, Brucella, & Francisella*

Moraxella bovis

Infectious keratoconjunctivitis, or "Pinkeye," is a costly disease in ruminant herds. Caused by *Moraxella bovis*, this disease can result in veterinary bills exceeding $100 per incident in beef cattle. It is estimated that pinkeye costs the United States $150 million *annually*. The disease affects many ruminants including cattle, sheep, and goats. Microscopically, *Moraxella bovis* appear as gram-negative short rods which normally occur in pairs. The organism is aerobic.

Transmission

Face flies (*Musca autumnalis*) act as a mechanical vector, transferring *M. bovis* from one animal to another by directly contacting the area surrounding the eye, including the conjunctiva.

Disease

Once inoculated with *M. bovis* by the fly, the animal's eye and conjunctiva becomes irritated and inflamed. Redness and some swelling of the eyelids and surrounding tissues may be seen. Upon opening the eye, redness and swelling of the conjunctiva can be seen. As *M. bovis* proliferates, the infected eye's corneal surface becomes cloudy. If not treated, damage to the cornea can become so severe that it weakens and breaks. This leads to rupture of the globe of the eye. Once the globe ruptures, they eye is beyond treatment and removal of the eye is the only option. Therefore it is imperative to recognize the clinical signs early in the disease process.

Diagnostics

A conjunctival swab should be obtained for culture of *M. bovis*. To avoid contamination of the swab by normal skin commensals, care should be taken to sample only the conjunctiva and not the surrounding skin. The pathogen grows best on agar plates supplemented with blood or serum and provided an aerobic environment. PCR testing for *M. bovis* may also be performed on the conjunctival swabs.

Treatment

Treatment must both eliminate *M. bovis* as well as protect the integrity of the eye. Antibiotics such as, oxytetracycline, are used to eliminate *M. bovis*. To prevent further mechanical damage to the eye by rubbing during the healing process, an eye patch is applied to the eye using a non-toxic adhesive. Eye patches specially fitted for cattle and other ruminants are available commercially.

Control

Because face flies are the main means of transmitting *M. bovis*, a high quality fly control program is imperative to the successful control and prevention of further infection.

Biosecurity

As members of the veterinary team, it is important that we don't act as the mechanical vector and spread *M. bovis* to other cattle. Handwashing after examining each animal suspected of harboring *M. bovis* decreases the chances of transmission. Handwashing is also important for preventing zoonotic diseases from infecting us.

Remember this: Zoonotic Conjunctivitis

While *Moraxella bovis* is not zoonotic, other causes of conjunctivitis, especially in sheep and goats (e.g., *Chlamydophila psittaci*), are zoonotic. Whenever restraining an animal with conjunctivitis take care not to infect yourself. Always wear exam gloves and don't rub your eyes.

Neisseria

While many of the microbes discussed in this textbook have a direct and serious effect on our patients, members of the genus *Neisseria* are largely commensals within their respective animal hosts, such as dogs, cats, guinea pigs, and cattle. Rather, the danger they possess is in their role as zoonotic infections. In particular, *Neisseria canis* and *Neisseria weaver*, both commensals of the dog oropharynx, may result in purulent infections in people as a result of dog bites. While the possibility exists that one dog biting another could cause infection in the dog sustaining the bite wound, opportunistic infections due to *N. canis* are currently only reported in one case report. *Neisseria iquanae* inhabits the oral cavity of iguanid lizards and is rarely the cause of opportunistic cutaneous abscesses and septicemia in these species.

Brucella

Members of the genus *Brucella* are small coccobacilli which stain gram-negative. They are capable of intracellular survival in immune cells such as macrophages, making them a facultative intracellular pathogen. They are oxidase and urease positive. *Brucella* species carry two circularized chromosomes. Species within the genus *Brucella* causes significant reproductive disease in a variety of species (Table 13.1). Infection with *Brucella* species is a major cause of abortion in domestic animals worldwide.

Table 13.1: *Brucella* species and their host-specificity.

	Target Species	Reservoir
B. abortus	Cattle	Bison, water buffalo, elk
B. melitensis	Sheep, goats	Same as target
B. suis	Swine	Feral swine
B. ovis	Sheep	Same as target
B. canis	Dogs	Same as target

Transmission

Transmission of *Brucella* occurs via three main routes: aerosol, ingestion, or venereal. Aerosol transmission is possible via bacterial-laden droplets from aborted tissues. This aerosol exposure represents the highest risk for zoonosis and occupational exposure among farmers and veterinary care staff. Ingestion of the placenta is a common practice of many mammalian mothers. The placenta of an aborted fetus is teeming with *Brucella* bacteria (over 1×10^3 organisms!). Males may become chronically infected with *Brucella* with the bacteria localizing in the testicles. In this way, the male is a reservoir for venereally transmitted *Brucella* infections of females.

Clinical Disease

Livestock

Brucella abortus infection in pregnant cows results in abortion. Infection localizes in the placenta causing significant inflammation (Figure 13.1). Ewes (*B. ovis, B. melitensis*), nanny goats (*B.*

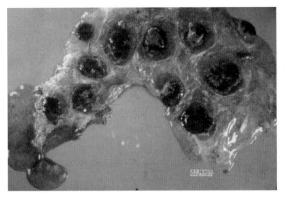

Figure 13.1: Inflammation of the placenta in cow caused by *Brucella abortus*. Notice how the circular placental attachments (i.e., cotyledons) are swollen reddened with hemorrhage. Courtesy of the Armed Forces Institute of Pathology and the Center for Food Security and Public Health. Used with permission.

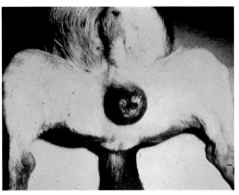

Figure 13.2: Swollen scrotum and testicles (orchitis) caused by *Brucella canis*. Dogs infected with *B. canis* shed the disease lifelong and are a significant zoonotic hazard for owners and other people coming in contact with the dog. Courtesy of the Armed Forces Institute of Pathology and the Center for Food Security and Public Health. Used with permission.

Remember this:
A Surgical Mask is NOT Protective against Zoonoses

When trying to prevent exposure to zoonotic diseases, particularly those transmitted by aerosols, often it is a good idea to wear a mask that provides respiratory protection. The choice of mask is critical. While it may be easier (and cheaper) to don a surgical mask, a surgical mask is designed to provide *patient* protection – *not protection to the user*. In contrast, a so-called "N95" mask is specifically designed and tested to filter out 95-percent of the infectious particles that may be floating in aerosols. Individuals wishing to wear the N95 mask must be fitted to ensure a proper fit so that there are no "leaks" which might lead to exposure.

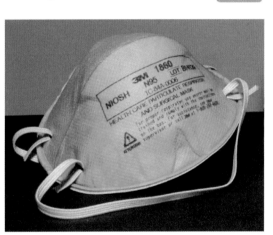

melitensis), and sows (*B. suis*) are all similarly affected with abortions occurring usually within the second half of gestation and commonly accompanied by retention of the placenta after giving birth. In those that survive until birthing, offspring are often born very weak and may not survive into adulthood; their dams typically produce a low milk yield. Infection in males causes inflammation of the genital tract resulting in epididymitis, orchitis, and prostatitis. Male infertility is a long-term sequella in many affected individuals.

Dogs
Brucella canis causes abortions at an estimated prevalence rate between 1-19% in the US. Breeding kennels are at particular risk for *B. canis* infections. Like livestock, affected bitches become bacteremic and spontaneously abort during the last trimester of pregnancy. Thick, white vaginal

discharge may also appear in infected females. Other signs that may present in females are a failure to conceive and stillbirths. Males may present for inflamation of gonadal structures including orchitis, prostatitis, and epididymitis (Figure 13.2). Brucellosis should also be on the differential list for cases of discospondylitis.

Isolation of *Brucella*

Culture

Blood, semen, urine, and other tissues (e.g., aborted fetus or placenta) can be used for culturing *Brucella* species. However, since *Brucella* is zoonotic, special precautions must be taken to prevent accidental aerosol exposure to the person(s) working with the sample. This usually requires specialized equipment, such as a **HEPA-filtered biosafety cabinet** (Figure 13.3), which are not commonly available in most veterinary clinic settings. Care should be taken when attempting to sample animals suspected of brucellosis infections. At a minimum, veterinary care staff should wear latex or nitrile examination gloves, eyewear (to prevent eye splash), and respiratory protection, such as an **N95 mask** (see sidebar).

Other Diagnostics (Non-Culture Methods)

Serum samples may be submitted for serological detection of antibodies formed against *Brucella*. Brucellosis agglutination tests (e.g., card test or slide test) as well as the *Brucella* milk ring test are diagnostic tests commonly performed on-site.

Other tests are available through commercial and reference microbiological laboratories such as: ELISA, fluorescent antibody tests, and PCR.

Treatment

Unfortunately once a dog (of either sex) is infected, it is infected for life. Due to public health concerns, euthanasia is the safest, most resposible option *and should be strongly recommended*. In owners that opt not to euthanize, therapy will require spaying/neutering, prolonged treatment using a combination of antibiotics, and lifetime monitoring. Pursuit of treatment and monitoring is therefore quite expensive. Importantly, the animal should not have contact with other canines, nor should other canines be brought onto property where the dog resides. Any other in-contact dogs should be quarantined until all are negative for three monthly tests in a row.

Prevention

Two vaccines, RB51 and Strain 19, are licensed in the US for prevention of brucellosis in cattle and goats. There is no vaccine licensed for swine or canines.

Zoonosis

Human brucellosis results from contact with infected animals or animal products. Unpasteurized milk, soft (unpasteurized) cheeses, and other unpasteurized milk products constitute the food products of high risk for the transmission of brucellosis. Occupational exposure occurs in veterinary care (e.g., helping with

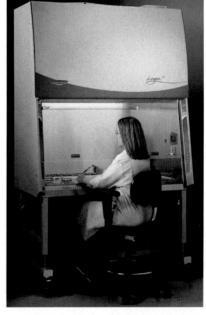

Figure 13.3: Laboratory working with bacterial cultures in a Class II, Type A2 biosafety cabinet (BSC). A biosafety has two functions. First, it provides protection to the laboratory worker. Second, it protects the cultures from contamination (e.g., airborne fungi). This is also called "product protection". A BSC should not be confused with a chemical fume hood. A chemical fume hood provides personal protection but no product protection. Therefore, a "fume" hood should not be used for culturing microorganisms. Courtesy of Labconco Corporation. Used with permission.

abortions), the meat-packing industry, and the laboratory as a result of lab-acquired infections. Patients are treated using a combination of antibiotics, such as doxycycline and gentamicin. Due to the ability of *Brucella* organisms to survive within cells like macrophages, treatment may need to be continued for some time to ensure all organisms are killed. Treatment regimens lasting several months are not uncommon.

Brucella can cause significantly debilitating disease in humans and is transmitted via aerosol. For this reason, the federal government classifies *B. melitensis*, *B. suis* and *B. abortus* as potential (terrorist) bioweapons.

Soft Cheeses and Your Health

Soft cheeses are those which are neither "aged" nor pasteurized. Cheddar, swiss, and parmesan cheeses are aged in a process that eliminates most pathogens including *Brucella*). Feta, queso fresco, and brie are examples of soft cheeses.

The Centers for Disease Control and Prevention (CDC) lists these soft cheeses as high risk for transmission of foodborne pathogens such as *Listeria* and *Brucella*. Both these pathogens are capable of causing abortion; pregnant women are strongly advised to steer clear of high risk food items like soft cheeses and raw milk during pregnancy due to the risk to the fetus.

US Brucellosis Eradication Program in Cattle and the Role of Wildlife

Once upon a time, brucellosis raged among the cattle herds of the United States causing significant losses in calves and milk production. In the mid-1930s, over one-in-ten adult cattle tested positive for brucellosis. By 1954, the problem was so great both to animals and human health that Congress appropriated funds to develop a program to rid the US of this costly disease. The eradication program consists of vaccinating all cattle between 4-12 months of age and testing all adult cattle. Cattle which test positive are euthanized (i.e., "test-and-slaughter"). The eradication program still runs today. In the year 2000, for the first time since the beginning of the eradication program, all 50 states classified as *Brucella*-free.

Despite this remarkable milestone, occasionally an individual cattle herd will test positive for brucellosis. This is due to the fact that *Brucella* is present in wild elk (Figure 13.4) and bison. Feral swine pose a similar threat for transmission of *B. suis* to domestic swine herds. Vaccination in these wildlife populations is problematic, to say the least. These wild hoof stocks constitute a continual reservoir of disease capable of infecting our domesticated livestock.

Brucellosis is a reportable disease. All animals which test positive for brucellosis must be reported to the federal government.

Francisella

Francisella tularensis is the single most important pathogen in this genus. *F. tularensis* is a small, pleomorphic facultative intracellular gram-negative rod which is endemic across much of North America. This bacteria is capable of causing significant disease, called tularemia, in rabbits, cats, dogs, and humans. Transmission of tularemia occurs through ticks that infest rabbits. These

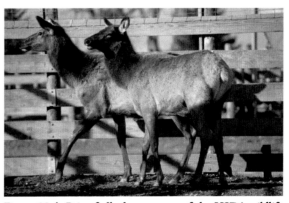

Figure 13.4: Pair of elk that are part of the USDA wildlife *Brucella* vaccination program. Courtesy of the Agriculture Research Service, United States Department of Agriculture, ARS Image Bank, K#8753-1, date unknown.

same ticks can transmit the disease to inadvertent hosts (e.g., cats). There are two subtypes of *F. tularensis*, named Type A and Type B. Type B does not cause clinical disease in rabbits, but is capable of causing disease in cats and humans; type A causes disease in all four animal species. Four species of North American ticks can transmit the disease: *Dermacentor andersoni* (wood tick), *Dermacentor variabilis* (American dog tick), *Dermacentor occidentalis* (Pacific Coast tick), and *Ambylostoma americanum* (Lone star tick). Infection within the ticks is lifelong and can be transmitted transovarially to progeny. Adult ticks are the most likely stage to transmit the disease, although all stages are capable of transmission. A secondary mode of infection for dogs and cats is the hunting and subsequent consumption of wild rabbits or hares. Disease in dogs and cats consists of bacteremia and the subsequent effect of infection to multiple organs. Cats appear to be more susceptible than dogs to more severe disease. The lungs, spleen, liver, lymph nodes, and skin are commonly effected as a result of the bacteremia. Thus, cats often present with fever, depression, generalized lymphadenopathy, splenomegaly and hepatomegaly. Treatment involves the use of antibiotics such as gentamicin.

Isolation of *F. tularensis* requires the use of enriched media for growth. It is a highly infectious zoonotic disease and only 25 aerosolized microorganisms are necessary for infection. An even smaller number (ten!) can cause disease when injected subcutaneously (e.g., bite wound or accidental laboratory needle stick). Because of this, only specialized laboratories with enhanced safety features (i.e., biosafety level 3 [BSL3] or higher) may work with *F. tularensis*. With this in mind, in a clinical setting, everyone in contact with animals diagnosed with tularemia should exercise extreme caution and should wear gloves, at a minimum. If aerosols are likely to be created, such as when cleaning skin wounds, the addition of eye and face protection should always be used. When handling an animal, especially a rabbit, that has been hunted or trapped, it is crucial to wear gloves as a minimum protection. Humans may also acquire the infection from arthropod bites, or via inhalation during landscaping.

Further Reading

Cantas, H., et al. "First Reported Isolation of *Neisseria canis* from a Deep Facial Wound Infection in a Dog." *J Clin Microbiol* 49 5 (2011): 2043-6.

Chapter 14:

Bacteria without Cell Walls

Introduction
The two bacterial genera discussed in this chapter, *Mycoplasma* and *Ureaplasma*, aren't like most other bacteria. Namely, their structure is drastically different from other bacteria in that they completely lack a cell wall. In fact, the class to which these bacteria belong, Mollicutes, means "soft skin". This lack of a cell wall means that the DNA, ribosomes, and other organelles are bound only by a cytoplasmic membrane. As a result, the cells are unusually flexible. Most other bacterial organisms can be filtered out of liquid media by passing the liquid through a filter with extremely small 0.2 μm pores. The filter works because most bacteria have a rigid cell wall and are greater than 0.2 μm in size. Conversely, because of their small size and increased flexibility, mycoplasmas can slip right through the pores. This is a problem when we are trying to eliminate mycoplasmas from liquids like intravenous fluids and, in research, cell culture systems.

Mycoplasma

General Characteristics
Mycoplasmas are very slow growing, facultative aerobes. The generation time of the average mycoplasma is anywhere from one to sixteen hours. Compare this to the average strain of *Escherichia coli* with a super speedy generation time of twenty minutes!

Transmission
Mycoplasmas are transmitted by contact directly or with infectious droplets such as those found in oral, nasal, ocular, and genital secretions. Mycoplasmas are capable of infecting many species (Table 14.1). In this section, we will focus on three of the most common *Mycoplasma* species seen in clinical veterinary practice: *M. gallisepticum, M. hyopneumoniae,* and *M. bovis.*

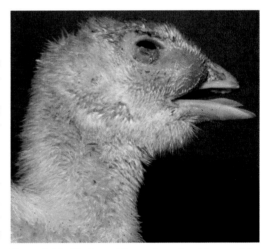

Figure 14.1: Turkey with purulent sinusitis caused by a *Mycoplasma* infection. Photo © Dr. N. Cheville, ISU, CVM, courtesy of the Center for Food Security and Public Health. Used with permission.

Mycoplasma gallisepticum
Mycoplasma gallisepticum causes respiratory disease in poultry that is usually confined to the upper respiratory tract. Clinical signs are those commonly found in upper respiratory tract infections such as nasal discharge, conjunctivitis, coughing, sneezing, and wet rasping of air in the windpipe during respirations (i.e., "tracheal rales"). Turkeys are more susceptible to infection and subsequent disease than chickens. Turkeys often develop severe sinusitis (Figure 14.1) in addition to the other clinical signs listed above. The impact of mycoplasma upper respiratory disease can be seen in the production losses in both meat and egg industries.

Table 14. 1 Mycoplasmas infecting domestic animals and the diseases they cause.

Species	Hosts	Diseases
M. agalactiae	Goats, sheep	Contagious agalactia (mastitis)
M. bovis	Cattle	Arthritis, mastitis, pneumonia, abortions, abscesses, otitis media, genital infections
M. capricolum ssp. *capricolum*	Goats, sheep	Mastitis, sepsis, polyarthritis, pneumonia
M. capricolum ssp. *capripneumoniae*	Goats	Contagious caprine pleuropneumonia
M. conjunctivae	Goats, sheep	Infectious keratoconjunctivitis
M. gallisepticum	Chickens, turkeys	Airsacculitis, sinusitis
M. hyopneumoniae	Pigs	Enzootic pneumonia
M. hyosynoviae	Pigs	Polyarthritis
M. meleagridis	Turkeys	Airway sacculitis
M. mycoides ssp. *capri*	Goats	Arthritis, mastitis, pleuropneumonia, sepsis
M. mycoides ssp. *mycoides* (small-colony variant)	Cattle	Contagious bovine pleuropneumonia REPORTABLE DISEASE
M. pulmonis	Laboratory rodents	Murine respiratory mycoplasmosis
M. synoviae	Chickens, turkeys	Infectious synovitis

Mycoplasma hyopneumoniae

The etiologic agent of porcine enzootic pneumonia, *Mycoplasma hyopneumoniae* causes high levels of morbidity, but low mortality rates. Disease due to *M. hyopneumoniae* is commonly complicated by other opportunistic bacteria and viruses. Porcine enzootic pneumonia constitutes an important economic disease affecting swine production worldwide.

Transmission

Transmission of *M. hyopneumoniae* is through direct contact and occurs when older pigs in the herd infect young, naïve pigs. Mechanical transmission is also possible. Mechanical transmission may occur via boots or other clothing not appropriately cleaned or laundered after leaving one hog building or farm and before entering another. Thus, biosecurity is important in both preventing the introduction of the pathogen and controlling its spread through the herd.

Clinical Disease

Clinically apparent pneumonia is often seen in younger (i.e., weanling to market) rather than older breeder pigs. On necropsy, the pneumonia is most apparent in the cranioventral lung lobes (Figure 14.2). Lung lesions cause respiratory difficulty which in turn affects overall productivity. Significant decreases in feed conversion and total body weight gains as well as money spent on treatment cause economic losses to the hog producer.

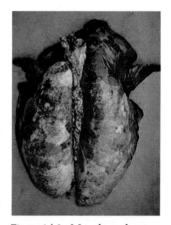

Figure 14.2: *Mycoplasma hyopneumoniae*, pig, lungs. The cranioventral lung lobes are markedly affected (darkened red and sunken) compared to the rest of the lung tissue. This is typical for the disease. Photo reproduced from Muirhead, Michael, and Thomas JL Alexander. *Managing Pig Health: A Reference for the Farm.* 2013.

Mycoplasma bovis

Mycoplasma bovis is among the most virulent mycoplasmas affecting cattle worldwide. The agent is most often associated with respiratory disease, especially bronchopneumonia. Colonization of the respiratory tract with *M. bovis* is most likely a predisposing factor for overt respiratory clinical signs due to the bovine respiratory disease complex (i.e., shipping fever). While primarily a respiratory tract infection in cattle, it is not uncommon for *M. bovis* to spread systemically. Systemic spread of *M. bovis* may lead to a variety of conditions including: arthritis, middle ear infections, mastitis, infection of the cornea and conjunctiva, and (rarely) meningitis. Infection of the reproductive tract secondary to systemic spread is not uncommon and may include: uterine (endometritis) and ovarian (oophoritis) infections, abortion, and infection of the seminal vesicles of bulls.

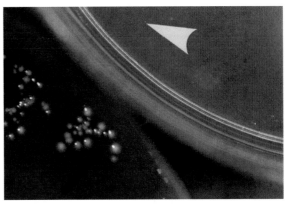

Figure 14.3: Relative size of *Mycoplasma* colonies. Both agar plates were incubated for 48 hours at 37°C. However, the colonies of Streptococcus pyogenes (black arrow; blood agar) are enormous when compared to the pin-point mycoplasma colonies (yellow arrow; mycoplasma media) that are barely visible by the naked eye.

Diagnostics: Culturing Mycoplasmas

Successfully culturing *Mycoplasma* species in the laboratory takes time and skill. Mycoplasmas require complex media and antibiotics are commonly added to the media to inhibit other bacterial contaminants. Most mycoplasmas require at least 4-5 days incubation before it is possible to see colonies (Figure 14.3). Some species take much longer – on the order of weeks!

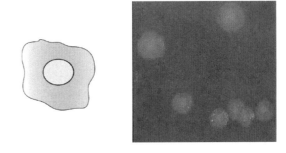

Figure 14.4: Colony morphology of mycoplasmas. Mycoplasma species, such as *Mycoplasma bovis* (right panel) typically exhibit a "fried egg" appearance. The left panel shows a simplified drawing of the colony shape.

Once colonies appear, they often have a "fried-egg" appearance (Figure 14.4). Because mycoplasmas lack a cell wall, Gram staining cannot be used for identification purposes. The stain simply won't be taken up and retained. Therefore, alternate stains, such as **Diene's Stain** are used. Instead of picking a colony, making a suspension on a glass slide, and staining it as we would with Gram staining, Diene's stain can be applied directly to the agar plate. *Mycoplasma* colonies are positive for Diene's stain and turn blue. Colonies of L-form bacteria which have temporarily failed to produce a cell wall may have mycoplasma-like colonies, but they are Dienes' stain negative (i.e., clear in color) because they take up and then metabolize the stain.

Treatment

Mycoplasmal infections are very hard to eliminate. Many species, such as the avian mycoplasmas, exhibit resistance to an increasing number of classes of antimicrobial drugs. *M. bovis* is particularly difficult to control with its increasing resistance to antimicrobial therapy and a lack of efficacious vaccines.

Prevention and Control

Prevention and control of mycoplasmal infections in a production setting benefit from management practices designed to minimize stress factors. Segregation of new animals before addition to a herd/flock, all-in-all out, and segregated early weaning management strategies also contribute to preventing the introduction of mycoplasmal infections to a herd. Medicated feeds may be used to control enzootic herd infections. There is currently no vaccine protecting against mycoplasma infections.

Some producers, such as those that produce laboratory mice for research, have such high biosecurity practices that they have been able to eliminate mycoplasmal infections from entire colonies of mice. In this setting, all materials that come into contact with the mice (e.g., food, water, and bedding) must be completely sterilized, typically by autoclaving. This level of biosecurity is high and is neither practical nor economically feasible for production herds.

Mycoplasmas Targeting Red Blood Cells (Hemoplasms)

Historically, members of this group have been placed in one of several different genera with all the members regarded as being closely related to ricketsial organisms (see Chapter 15). However, gene sequencing of the various species has led to their reclassification and placement within the genus *Mycoplasma*. To reflect their **hemotrophic** nature (i.e., all target and parasitize red blood cells) their species names often start with the prefix "*haemo-*". Like other mycoplasmas, **hemoplasmas** do not contain a cell wall. Three species of *Mycoplasma* cause disease in domestic animals: *Mycoplasma haemocanis* (formerly: *Haemobartonella canis*), *Mycoplasma haemofelis* (formerly: *Haemobartonella felis*), and *Mycoplasma suis* (formerly: *Eperythrozoon suis*). The host specificity of each is listed in Table 14.2. Transmission of the hemotrophic mycoplasmas is via an arthropod vector. In the case of *H. felis*, fleas, lice, and ticks can transmit the disease. The dog tick (*Rhicephalus sanguineus*) transmits *M. haemocanis*. With *M. suis*, vectors include lice, mosquitoes, and stable flies.

Each of the hemoplasmas targets and parasitizes the outer membrane of red blood cells. The presence of the mycoplasmal organisms marks the red blood cell as foreign and the infected red blood cell are removed from circulation by phagocytosis via splenic macrophages, thus predisposing the infected animals to anemia. The clinical signs resulting from this parasitism, however, vary widely. Dogs infected with *M. haemocanis* are often asymptomatic, only showing signs of acute hemolytic anemia after splenectomy. Cats infected with *M. haemofelis*, on the other hand, often show signs of acute hemolytic anemia even without splenectomy. While serious, life-threatening acute anemia in swine can occur, *M. suis* infection most often results in mild chronic anemia and poor growth rates in young pigs.

These species cannot be cultured like the mycoplasmas discussed in the previous section. PCR tests are available for each of the three species. All three species are susceptible to most tetracyclines.

Table 14. 2: The hemotrophic mycoplasmas and their vectors

Species	Host	Vectors
Mycoplasma haemocanis	Dogs	Ticks (*Rhicephalus sanguineus*)
Mycoplasma haemofelis	Cats	Fleas, lice, ticks
Mycoplasma haemosuis	Pigs	Lice, mosquitos, stable flies

Ureaplasma

A common inhabitant of the bovine reproductive tract, *Ureaplasma diversum* may occasionally cause a condition known as "granular vulvitis". Nodular inflammation is the most common presentation in this opportunistic infection of cattle. *U. diversum* has also been occasionally implicated in abortions and stillbirths. While *Ureaplasma* and *Mycoplasma* colonies cannot be distinguished morphologically, a simple urease test will show that *Ureaplasma* colonies are urease-positive and *Mycoplasma* colonies are not. Episodes of granular vulvitis have resolved spontaneously. Antibiotic treatments, such as intrauterine tetracycline, have been attempted with some success. As venereal transmission is postulated to facilitate transmission in the herd, artificial insemination is recommended as a control and prevention measure.

Further Reading

Hoelzle, Ludwig E., et al. "Pathobiology of *Mycoplasma suis.*" *The Veterinary Journal* 202. 1 (2014): 20-25.

Messick, Joanne B. "Hemotrophic Mycoplasmas (Hemoplasmas): A Review and New Insights into Pathogenic Potential." *Veterinary Clinical Pathology* 33 1 (2004): 2-13.

Sykes, Jane E. "Feline Hemotropic Mycoplasmas." *Journal of Veterinary Emergency and Critical Care* 20 1 (2010): 62-69.

Chapter 15:

Obligate Intracellular Bacteria

Introduction
Some bacteria have very restricted environments in which they live. They must reside not only within a host but within certain cells of the host. These species find themselves constantly under attack by the host's immune system when located, for example, in the bloodstream or other bodily fluids. They seek protective refuge from this barrage by entering into and "hiding out" within cells of the host. These bacteria are termed **obligate intracellular bacteria**. These organisms cannot be diagnosed by standard culture as they will not survive outside of cells on solid media or in enrichment broth media. Many can be propagated in cell culture lines, but this process is time consuming and not offered by most diagnostic laboratories. Special stains allow visualization of the organisms within host cells. Molecular (PCR) and serologic methods are the primary methods for diagnosing infection with obligate intracellular bacteria. This chapter deals with these obligate intracellular pathogens and the diseases they cause.

Chlamydophila
The family Chlamydiaceae is split into two genera: *Chlamydia* and *Chlamydophila*; though there are proponents for a single genus, *Chlamydia*. The species within the two genera are capable of causing disease in a number of animal species (Table 15.1). Members of the genus are gram-negative. While the cell wall contains both cytoplasmic and outer membranes, Chlamydiaceae are unique in that there is no peptidoglycan layer present. Unlike the gram-negative Enterobacteriaceae, the cell wall of Chla-

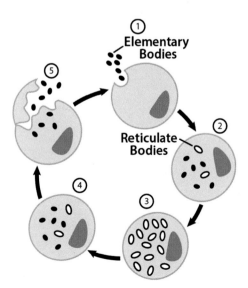

Figure 15.1: Lifecycle of chlamydiae. Elementary bodies (1) initiate infection and are taken up by macrophages. Once phagocytosed, the chlamydiae survive in the intracellular environment (2) whereupon they reorganize into reticulate bodies (3) which are capable of avoiding phagolysosome fusion. These replicate (4) until such time as there is no more space or nutrients to support replication. Once replication is complete, the reticulate bodies revert to elementary bodies and the cell ruptures (5), releasing the elementary bodies to the extracellular environment whereupon the lifecycle begins anew.

mydiaceae does not produce lipopolysaccharide (LPS), the cell constituent capable of producing endotoxic shock.

Chlamydiaceae are pathogens of mammals, birds, and reptiles. Transmission of the bacteria is mainly through two routes: direct contact or aerosol. The lifecycle of chlamydial organisms is unique from other bacteria discussed thus far in this book. The lifecycle is illustrated in Figure 15.1. Small infectious units of chlamydiae, known as **elementary bodies**, initiate the infection in the host. Elementary bodies possess spore-like qualities allowing them to survive outside of the body. The elementary bodies can be taken up by macrophages and by some non-ciliated cuboidal or columnar epithelial cells. Once inside the macrophage's cytoplasm, these elementary bodies undergo structural changes and reorganize to form **reticulate bodies** capable of avoiding phagosome-lysosome fusion. Reticulate bodies possess the ability to replicate and do so to increase their numbers within the cell's cytoplasm. Once replication is complete, the chlamydiae revert back to elementary bodies. Eventually, the burden of carrying so many elementary bodies causes the macrophage to rupture thereby releasing the elementary bodies and allowing the spread of the infection to new cells.

Table 15.1: Selected Chlamydiaceae, their hosts, and diseases produced

Genus species	Host	Disease
Chlamydophila psittaci	Birds, humans	Pneumonia, conjunctivitis, diarrhea, pericarditis, encephalitis
Chlamydophila abortus	Sheep, goats, cattle, pigs	Abortion
Chlamydophila felis	Cats	Conjunctivitis, pneumonitis
Chlamydophila caviae	Guinea pigs	Conjunctivitis
Chlamydia suis	Pigs	Diarrhea
Chlamydia muridarum	Mice	Respiratory infection

Chlamydophila psittaci

Strains of *C. psittaci* can be divided into those that are highly virulent and those with low virulence. Highly virulent strains are capable of mortality between 10-30% and morbidity in excess of 80%. Birds infected with *C. psittaci* may show signs of inappetence (anorexia), fever, and conjunctivitis. Some birds may excrete abnormal feces in the form of yellowish-green gelatinous droppings. In addition, a significant decrease in egg production may be observed in birds such as layer hens.

Both respiratory and systemic signs may be observed in *C. psittaci* infections. Respiratory lesions observed may include: air sacculitis, congestion in the lungs (pneumonia), and inflammation of the pleura which may extend to include the pericardial sac. In highly virulent strains, systemic infection is more likely and may result in a bacteremia and thus infecting multiple organs such the liver, spleen, and intestines.

Diagnostics

Identification of chylamydiae species as the cause of disease is most often done using serology to detect chlamydial antibodies. Occasionally, it may be feasible to identify chlamydial organisms on Giemsa-stained impression smears of infected animal tissue. Other methods include molecular tests such as PCR and DNA sequencing.

Treatment and Control

All infected birds should be isolated from those that are uninfected. Infected birds are treated with antibiotics (e.g., tetracycline). Once a bird with a suspected *C. psittaci* infection has completed their visit to a clinic, it is important

Table 15.2 Examples of psittacines and non-psittacines birds kept as livestock or pets

Psittacine	Non-psittacine
Budgerigars	Canaries
Cockatiels	Chickens
Cockatoos	Doves
Lorikeets	Finches
Lovebirds	Pigeons
Parakeets	Turkeys
Parrots	

to adequately disinfect the examination room and any surfaces the bird has been in contact with. *Chlamydia* is susceptible to most disinfectants, detergents, and heat. Possible disinfectants to use are products where the active ingredient is a quaternary ammonia, 70% isopropyl alcohol, a phenolic, or bleach (1:100). Personnel assigned to clean the area should use adequate respiratory protection (e.g., N95 mask) while cleaning.

Zoonotic Alert!

Recovered birds can shed chlamydiae in the droppings and nasal discharge for extended periods of time. This constitutes a significant zoonotic threat to pet and livestock owners as well as veterinary care staff. Transmission to humans usually occurs via inhalation of aerosols produced by droppings, feathers, or animal tissues of slaughtered poultry. However, there are reports of direct contact transmission via mouth-to-beak. Contact with pet birds, particularly psittacines, is a risk factor. The disease in humans can causes respiratory illness usually in the form of a flu-like illness accompanied by muscle aches. Occasionally, the disease may result in a severe, even life-threatening pneumonia. Anyone suspected of contracting a *C. psittaci* infection from a bird should be advised to go to their physician for confirmation and treatment. Thankfully, person-to-person transmission has not been documented.

Remember this: Occupational Health and Safety

Always tell your physician what animals you are exposed to during work so that they can more accurately diagnose any zoonotic infection.

For example, if you are working with birds, you should tell your doctor this so that they will consider psittacosis when symptoms fit that disease. Otherwise they may dismiss psittacosis as very unlikely, as most of the general population has very little hands-on contact with avian species.

Coxiella burnetii

This genus contains a single species of importance in veterinary medicine: *Coxiella burnetii*, the causative agent of **Q-fever**. The term "Q-fever" originates from the late 1930s when the condition was first described by Australian pathologist Edward Holbrook Derrick. The "Q" stands for "query".

Morphology and Staining

Coxiella burnetii appear as small pleomorphic rods (Fig. 15.2). Their cell membrane is similar to that found in gram-negative bacteria. However, due to the variability in cell membrane constituents among individual isolates, they appear gram-variable under normal staining conditions. Therefore, it is not advisable to use Gram staining for identification purposes. Giemsa staining can be used successfully to visualize *Coxiella* organisms. In point of fact, serology is the most common method for diagnosing exposure and illness due to *C. burnetii*.

Lifecycle

C. burnetii is an obligate intracellular bacterium capable of surviving phagosome-lysosome fusion within the host macrophage (Figure 15.3). This is rather remarkable given the powerful enzymes, such as lysozyme, found within the phagolysosome. The organism is marked as foreign once inside the host. Host macrophages are recruited to the area of infection and proceed to phagocytose the organism. As a part of normal phagocytosis, the *Coxiella*-laden phagosome is fused to the macrophage's lysosome. However, unlike other bacteria, once inside the phagolysosome *C. burnetii* replicates until a sufficient number of daughter cells are created. Then the phagolysosome and the cell

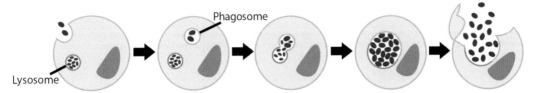

Figure 15.2: Intracellular lifecycle of *Coxiella burnetii*. *C. burnetii* (purple rods) is capable of surviving the hostile environment of the macrophage's phagolysosome (center), thus giving it an advantage in survival within the host.

lyses, releasing the daughter cells into the extracellular environment whereupon they can attach to additional cells and spread the infection.

Reservoir and Disease

The primary reservoir for *Coxiella burnetii* is ruminant species. Of these, the most common in clinical practice are sheep and cattle. The disease in ruminants is mainly restricted to reproductive problems such as abortion. Ruminants may become silent carriers of *C. burnetii*. That is, they may have circulating *C. burnetii* without showing any clinical signs. Carriers may intermittently shed the organism from a variety of biological fluids including: vaginal discharges, feces, urine, milk, and birth products (e.g., placenta, amniotic fluid).

Zoonotic Potential and Q-fever

Q-fever, the zoonotic disease caused by infection with *C. burnetii*, is a very serious threat to human health. The transmission of just *one* bacterium can result in a serious, potentially life-threatening infection! The primary route of zoonotic infections is via inhalation of contaminated aerosols. In the veterinary field, this may occur due to urine or fecal splash of infected animals. Even more likely is the transmission of *C. burnetii* organisms due to aerosols created during parturition or abortion. There is an inherent occupational risk for farmers, the veterinary medical team, and slaughterhouse/abattoir workers due to the likelihood of encountering aerosols of infected ruminants. A relatively minor, though no less serious, risk factor is the consumption of raw milk.

In most individuals, Q-fever takes one of two forms: an acute course or a chronic one. In the acute disease, upon infection with contaminated materials, an incubation period of 2-4 weeks is followed by the appearance of clinical signs. Affected individuals may experience flulike syndrome with severe headache, malaise (tiredness), fever, myalgia (muscle aches), and chills. Luckily, the disease is self-limiting and systemic complications are uncommon. Mortality is usually low in the absence of such complications. In a very few patients, usually less than 5%, chronic disease may occur. Most of the individuals that eventually develop chronic disease have preexisting conditions (e.g., heart valve damage) which increases their risk of developing the chronic form.

In pregnant women, Q-fever may cause in abortion. During pregnancy, a woman exists in a state of relative, physiologic immunodeficiency. This means her body is less able to fight off infections that it could in its non-pregnant

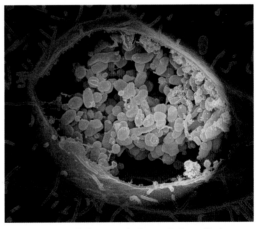

Figure 15.3 Cellular morphology of *Coxiella burnetii*, colorized SEM. Note the pleomorphic appearance of the rods (colorized green); some appear very small and blunted and others appear somewhat club-shaped. These bacteria were grown inside a special Vero cells. Here a Vero cell (colorized orange) has been fractured showing the *Coxiella* within. Photo courtesy of Robert Heinzen, Elizabeth Fischer and Anita Mora, National Institute of Allergy and Infectious Diseases, National Institutes of Health.

state. Q-fever in pregnant women is more likely to become systemic and enter into the maternal (and thus also the fetal) blood circulation causing the death of the fetus. Because there is a delay between conception and positively diagnosing pregnancy, all women of childbearing age should take precautions against Q-fever when working with ruminants. These precautions could include limiting exposure to ruminants (where possible) and wearing appropriate personal protective equipment (e.g., obstetrical gloves, N95 mask) when working with these species.

Control of Q-fever

Control efforts are directed primarily toward high risk individuals and should encompass the following elements:

- Public education on sources of infection
- Appropriate disposal of placentae, birth products, fetal membranes, and aborted fetuses
- Appropriate disposal of PPE
- Restriction of access to barns and laboratories used in housing potentially infected animals
- Pasteurization of milk and milk products before consumption

While at least one country does have an approved vaccine licensed for use in livestock (e.g., Australia), there is no vaccine approved for use within the United States.

Treatment

Antibiotics are used to treat most ruminant infections, and doxycycline is the current treatment of choice. Zoonotic infections should be reported to a physician early so proper treatment can be instituted.

Zoonotic Alert: Q-fever and pregnancy don't mix!
It's important to remember that all ruminants may potentially carry *C. burnetii*, causative agent of Q-fever. Q-fever can cause spontaneous abortion in pregnant women.

Even if an individual doesn't think she is pregnant, all woman of childbearing age should seriously consider taking precautions against transmission of Q-fever such as using appropriate PPE to protect against potential aerosol transmission.

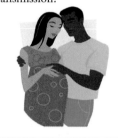

Anaplasmataceae

Members of the family Anaplasmataceae share some common characteristics. All are obligate intracellular pathogens enabled with the ability to replicate within cytoplasmic vacuoles. Cell types that Anaplasmataceae can inhabit, depending on the particular bacterial species, include: red blood cells, endothelial cells, phagocytes (e.g., macrophages), and even platelets. Most members of Anaplasmataceae require an invertebrate vector as part of their life cycle. Anaplasmataceae contains numerous species; too many to cover in this text. Therefore, we will limit our discussion to select species of high importance to the veterinary medical team. These will include select members of the genera *Ehrlichia*, *Neorickettsia*, and *Anaplasma*. Members of these three genera are often referred to as **rickettsial** organisms.

Ehrlichia canis

Ehrlichia canis is a gram-negative, pleomorphic bacterium appearing in coccoid to ellipsoid shapes. It is an obligate intracellular pathogen which can survive and multiply within the cytoplasmic vacuoles of monocytes. The bacterium is able to survive as it possesses the ability to prevent phagolysosome fusion; how it does this has not yet been elucidated. *E. canis* is the causative agent of a disease affecting dogs known as canine monocytic ehrlichiosis.

Transmission

Dogs are the main host for *E. canis* infections. *Rhipicephalus sanguineus*, the brown dog tick, serves as a

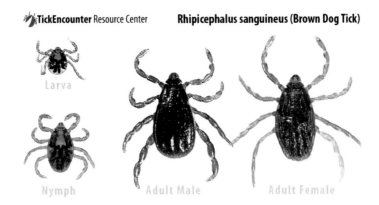

Figure 15.4: *Rhicephalus sanguineus,* the brown dog tick. All stages of the lifecycle may serve as a vector for the transmission of *E. canis* infection. Photo courtesy of the Tick Encounter Resource Center (www. tickencounter.org)

vector (Figure 15.4). All stages of *R. sanguineus* are capable of transmitting the infection via tick bite.

Disease
E. canis infections in dogs are characterized by an initial incubation period of between 8-20 days. Canine monocytic ehrlichiosis presents as a three-stage infection. In the acute stage, dogs present with fever, anorexia, depression, and enlarged lymph nodes. In the next phase, the subclinical phase, dogs do not show clinical signs (i.e., asymptomatic). It is at this stage that most dogs with a competent, fully functioning, immune system eliminate the infection. Dogs unable to clear the infection progress to the third, chronic phase. During the chronic phase, hemorrhage, particularly nose bleeds, and emaciation occur as a result of the increase in rickettsial numbers and the destruction wrought by the rickettsia on the leukocytes and endothelial cells.

Diagnostics
The easiest, and most readily available sample to use in diagnosing canine monocytic ehrlichiosis is blood. Peripheral blood can be examined microscopically, looking for the presence of the morulae (See Figures 15.6 and 15.7 for examples of morulae from a related genus, *Anaplasma*). Serology testing for antibodies to *E. canis* may also be performed. So-called "cage-side" or "snap" tests are commercially available. While time consuming, cell culture may be used to positively identify *E. canis* infection in patients. PCR, sequencing, and other molecular tests are available from some reference laboratories.

Treatment
Treatment of canine monocytic ehrlichiosis requires administration of appropriate antibiotics to combat the intracellular infection. The treatment of choice is tetracycline. However, treatment failures have occurred and clients should be warned of this possibility. Treatment may have to be extended. Sometimes additional antibiotic susceptibility testing must be performed leading to the change in the choice of antibiotic for further treatment.

Control
A keystone of prevention of canine monocytic ehrlichiosis infections is tick control (see panel below). Currently, there is no commercially available vaccine against *E. canis* infection. A related species, *E. ewingii,* is transmitted by *Amblyomma* ticks and is found in neutrophils, causing canine granulocytic ehrlichiosis.

Neorickettsia risticii
First recognized in 1979, veterinarians and horse owners in the states of Virginia and Maryland reported that a strange fever was affecting horses, particularly those that were housed near the Potomac River

basin (Figure 15.5), a large body of water that forms a natural border between the two states. The mysterious disease, which had a seasonal peak in the summer months, was named Potomac Horse Fever after the area in which it was first discovered. Potomac Horse Fever has been reported across the continental United States. The agent was originally identified as *Ehrlichia risticii*, but has recently been reclassified and named *Neorickettsia risticii*.

Morphology

Neorickettsia risticii is a gram-negative, obligate intracellular pathogen which infects monocytes. It can be found in the cytoplasm of a variety of cells including: monocytes, tissue macrophages, mast cells and glandular intestinal epithelial cells.

Lifecycle and Transmission

Like most Anaplasmataceae, the lifecycle of *Neorickettsia risticii* requires the use of a vector, in this case a trematode (fluke). The trematodes life cycle requires passage through a snail, considered the reservoir, before being released into water. Once in the water, the trematode (which is carrying the bacteria) is ingested by larvae of aquatic insects. Horses acquire the infection when they consume aquatic insects who have taken up the trematode which contains the organism. This agrees with the findings that the disease is restricted to low-lying areas of land near bodies of water. The organism preferentially targets mononuclear leukocytes (e.g., monocytes) and enterocytes (i.e., cells that line the stomach and intestines).

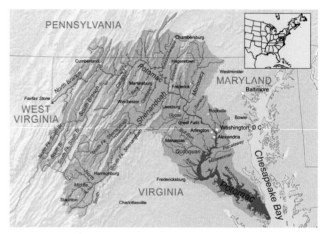

Figure 15.5: The Potomac River basin, origin of the first cases of Potomac Horse Fever (*Neorickettsia risticii*). Today, the disease may be found in all of the continental United States. Courtesy of Karl Musser.

Disease & Clinical Signs

Potomac Horse Fever results in profuse, acute watery diarrhea which results from direct damage to the host's enterocytes. This can cause a mild colic in some horses. Most also show signs of fever, depression, and dehydration. Laminitis can occur in some horses. Abortion, while rare, has occurred in infected pregnant mares. Up to thirty percent of cases are fatal if not treated early. The most common reason for fatalities is severe, irreversible laminitis.

Diagnostics

Veterinarians rely on serology or molecular methods (e.g., PCR) to diagnose this disease. Samples for PCR include blood or feces.

Treatment

Treatment of Potomac Horse Fever consists largely of a combination of supportive therapy and the judicious use of antibiotics. Supportive therapy in the form of intravenous or oral fluids, electrolyte supplements, and antidiarrheal medications are used to restore hydration and electrolytes lost from the profuse diarrhea. **Antipyretics**, such as flunixin meglumine, may be used to reduce fever. Antibiotics used to treat Potomac Horse Fever include members of the tetracycline class, with oxytetracycline being the current treatment of choice.

Prevention

There is a *N. rickettsia* vaccine licensed for use in horses in the US. However, the antibody response to the vaccine is relatively poor necessitating the need for periodic revaccination (e.g., every 6 months) especially in high risk areas such as around ponds and waterways where the snail may cohabitate. There have been reports of disease in spite of proper vaccination; these are termed **vaccine failures**.

Client Education:
Successfully Using Tick Sprays and Spot-on Treatments
It is important that clients are educated on the proper application of products designed to repel and kill ticks. Many of the newer sprays and spot-on treatments which have good tick kill-rates require the presence of the pet's natural oil layer on their skin. The oil layer ensures maximal coverage of the product over the skin of the pet. This means that the pet should not be bathed or get wet for a period extending from at least 24 hours before and 24 hours after application of the product.

Certain products may have additional requirements in order to be the most efficacious. Always check the product insert to ensure proper application of any product.

Other Anaplasmataceae

Anaplasma marginale
This tick-borne rickettsial organism targets erythrocytes (Figure 15.6). The organism gets its name because of its appearance on cytology. In Giemsa-stained blood smears, *A. marginale* appears as an intracellular purple spherical inclusion located on the periphery, or "margin", of the bovine erythrocyte. A related, also cleverly named species not discussed in this book, is *A. centrale* which can be detected in Giemsa-stained blood smears as an inclusion in the center of red blood cells. Ruminants, especially cattle, are the primary hosts.

Once the tick (e.g., *Dermacentor variabilis*) bites the host, *A. marginale* enters the bloodstream where it is taken up by erythrocytes. The organisms readily replicates in the erythrocyte cytoplasm until they are released. Following release into the blood, they proceed to infect other cells. The destruction of the erythrocyte contributes to the clinical sign of anemia. Erythrocytes may be recognized as foreign and removed from the circulation by splenic macrophages, therefore exacerbating the anemia. Other clinical signs of bovine anaplasmosis include diarrhea, fever, increased heart rate (i.e., as a result of the anemia), anorexia, depression, and cardiac arrest (i.e., late in the disease). This disease has a great economic impact by decreasing weight gain and depressing milk production. Animals 6 months to 3 years are the most seriously affected.

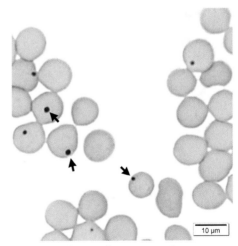

Figure 15.6: Blood smear from an *Anaplasma marginale*-infected calf. The blood smear is stained with Hema 3 stain. The arrows point to some of the intraerythrocytic *A. marginale* inclusion bodies called morulae. Courtesy of Dr. Delphine Guldner Washington State University, Pulman, WA.

Tetracycline is the most effective antibiotic against bovine anaplasmosis. Many countries rely on vaccines to decrease the severity of clinical disease, but no commercial vaccine exists in the US. However, the USDA has approved a killed vaccine as an experimental vaccine against *A. marginale* for use in many (but not all) of the states.

129

Anaplasma platys

The target of *Anaplasma platys* is the canine platelet. The disease is known as canine cyclic thrombocytopenia, and is widely distributed across the US. However, concentrations can be found along the eastern seaboard, Texas, and Washington. *A. platys* has been recovered from *Rhicephalus sanguineus* ticks, indicating that they are likely the vector. The reservoir host is also unknown. The destruction of platelets is cyclical and results in increased risk of uncontrolled hemorrhage due to an insufficiency of platelets in the clotting cascade. Treatment is similar to *A. marginale*. There is no commercial vaccine against *A. platys* for use in dogs.

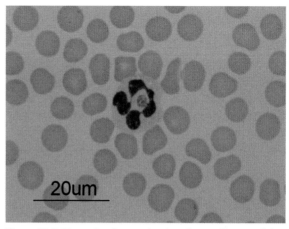

Figure 15.7: Example of a morula: *Anaplasma phagocytophilum* **morula within a neutrophil, dog.** Courtesy of Dr. Pierre Deshuillers, Purdue University, West Lafayette, IN.

Neorickettsia helminthoeca

Salmon poisoning is an acute and often fatal rickettsial disease of dogs. The causative agent, *Neorickettsia helminthoeca*, is a gram-negative coccoid bacteria endemic to the Pacific Northwest coast of the US. Transmission is through ingestion of salmonid fish which have been parasitized with the encysted form of the *Nanophyetus salmincola* fluke, which in turn harbors the bacteria, *Neorickettsia helminthoeca*. Once a dog eats a raw salmon, the cysts hatch and the fluke matures and attaches to the small intestinal epithelium. In a pathway that has yet to be firmly established, *N. helminthoeca* gains access to the cytoplasm of canine intestinal epithelium and macrophages; the bacteria are capable of surviving within the vacuoles of canine macrophages. Dogs first experience fever approximately 5-7 days after ingestion. However, hypothermia (i.e., below 100°F) may be evident in some patients, particularly those patients that are decompensating and near death. Diarrhea becomes progressively bloodier as the infection proceeds and may even resemble canine parvovirus infection. Up to ninety percent of dogs infected die from the infection. Those that survive are protected from reinfection.

Diagnosis relies on obtaining a good patient history (e.g., history of travel to the Pacific Northwest) and identification of *N. salmincola* eggs in feces using either fecal smear or sedimentation techniques. Early intervention and treatment are crucial for a positive outcome and consist of aggressive antibiotic therapy using tetracyclines (e.g., oxytetracycline) and supportive therapy.

The Family Rickettsiaeceae

Members of this family are all obligate intracellular pathogens which can cause significant zoonotic disease. Their cell walls are very similar to gram-negative bacteria; however, they stain very poorly with Gram stain. All are transmitted via an arthropod vector, although the vector(s) will differ depending upon the particular rickettsial disease in question. For most of these pathogens, domestic animals act as asymptomatic reservoir hosts. However, as in the case of *Rickettsia rickettsii*, some are capable of causing significant disease in domestic animal species.

Rickettsia rickettsii

Originally called "black measles" because of its characteristic rash, Rocky Mountain spotted fever (RMFS) is estimated to affect approximately 2,000 persons each year in the US. The causative agent of RMFS, *Rickettsia rickettsii*, has a relatively large geographic distribution that covers large portions of the Western Hemisphere including most of the United States, and also portions of southern Canada, Central America, Mexico, and South America.

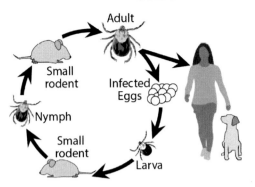

Figure 15.8: Life cycle of *Rickettsia rickettsia*. Trans-mission to humans and dogs is accidental and requires a bite from a tick vector. The organism is passed to the incidental host through the tick's mouth parts.

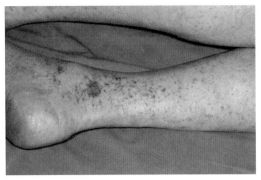

Figure 15.9: Clinical presentation of skin rash on a human patient diagnosed with RMSF. Courtesy of the Center for Food Safety and Public Health and the Armed Institute of Pathology. Used with permission.

Morphology

Rickettsia rickettsii is a gram-negative obligate intracellular organism that inhabits the cytoplasm of endothelial cells – cells for which this organism has a particular affinity. *R. rickettsii* organisms are difficult to visualize using routine staining methods, such as Gram and Giemsa staining.

Lifecycle and Transmission

Rodents serve as the reservoir host for *Rickettsia rickettsii* infections (Figure 15.8). Humans and dogs are incidental hosts and therefore only become infected if they are in contact with the vector. In this case, a number of different ticks serve as arthropod vectors of the organism including *Dermacentor* species, *Amblyoma cajennense*, and *Rhipicephalus sanguineus*. Transmission of *R. rickettsii* to dogs and humans occurs during the tick bite because the organism is present in the tick's mouth parts. Dogs serve as an important "transport host" by carrying ticks on their fur which then leave the dog and move to a human host.

Zoonotic Disease

RMSF is the most severe and frequently reported rickettsial illness of humans within the US. Initial symptoms reported in infected individuals include the sudden onset of fever, headache, and muscle pain, followed by the development of the characteristic skin rash (Figure 15.9). RMSF can be difficult to diagnose in its early stages. However, without prompt and appropriate treatment it can be fatal. It is estimated that the **case fatality rate** is approximately 3-5%. (For a discussion on the case fatality rate and how to calculate it, see side panel).

Disease in Dogs

Dogs are the only known susceptible domestic animal host to *R. rickettsii*. Disease is more common in dogs that are less than 2 years of age, purebred dogs (especially German shepherds and English springer spaniels), and during the tick season (occurring from March-October in the Northern Hemisphere). The higher occurrence of the disease in young dogs and particular breeds may indicate a lifestyle risk. Younger dogs and dogs of sporting/hunting breeds are more likely to spend extended periods of time out-of-doors when compared to older dogs or particular breeds (e.g., toy breeds). It may also indicate the genetic susceptibility of certain breeds of dogs when compared with others.

Clinical signs in dogs consist of a fever occurring approximately 4-5 days after the tick bite and a skin rash. Other non-specific signs include general joint and muscle pain accompanied sometimes by anorexia (i.e., a lack of appetite).

Diagnostics

Because of the significant human health risks associated with it, culturing *R. rickettsii* requires strict

Words to Know:
Case Fatality Rate

Case fatality rate is a term that describes how fatal a disease is within the group of individuals that actually contracted the disease. The CFR can be used to determine how deadly a particular disease is once a person becomes ill with that disease. It can be calculated using the following formula.

$$CFR = \frac{\# \ of \ individuals \ who \ died \ of \ the \ disease}{total \ \# \ who \ contracted \ the \ disease} \ x \ 100\%$$

As an example, bubonic plague, or the "Black Death" as it was commonly referred to in the Middle Ages when it ravaged Medieval Europe, **even today** has an estimated case fatality rate of 50-60% if no treatment (i.e., antibiotics) is given. In other words, one person dies of the plague for every two people

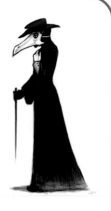

A Plague doctor

safety measures and a "high containment" laboratory (e.g., Biosafety level 3). These highly specialized laboratories are most often found only in larger reference laboratories. Serology is the most common diagnostic test used in the clinical setting.

Therapy and Prevention
Antibiotic therapy consists of the administration of a tetracycline class drug (e.g., tetracycline or doxycycline). Prevention of RMSF centers on preventing a dog's access to the vector, the tick. Therefore, topical preventives such as fipronil (Frontline Plus®, Merial, Inc.) should be used monthly during athe tick season. However, depending upon their geographic location and local weather patterns, clients may be counseled to apply the preventive to their dogs year-round, particularly in the warmer southern states of the US.

Rickettsia felis
R. felis is the causative agent of a rare zoonotic disease named "Flea-borne Spotted Fever" (also known as cat flea rickettsiosis) and is carried by arthropod vectors, most notably the cat flea (*Ctenocephalides felis*). *R. felis* has a worldwide distribution with special prominence in Western Europe, Africa, South America, and Southeast Asia. There have been isolated reports of the disease in the US in people. Cats act as an asymptomatic carrier for the disease; to date, no clinical signs have been reported.

Rickettsia typhi
The life cycle of murine typhus (*Rickettsia typhi*) consists of rodent or opossum reservoir hosts and flea vectors (e.g., *Xenopsylla cheopis*, the Oriental rat flea; and *Ctenocephalides felis*, the cat flea). Cats act as asymptomatic carriers of the fleas, and thus, the disease. People are infected with *R. typhi* after a flea bite. The disease causes fever, headache, myalgia, confusion, and a diffuse rash. Disease severity is greater in the elderly and in patients with immunosuppressive conditions.

Further Reading

Headley, Selwyn A., et al. "*Neorickettsia helminthoeca* and Salmon Poisoning Disease: A Review." *Vet J* 187 2 (2011): 165-73.

Qurollo, Barbara A., et al. "A Serological Survey of Tick-Borne Pathogens in Dogs in North America and the Caribbean as Assessed by *Anaplasma phagocytophilum*, *A. platys*, *Ehrlichia canis*, *E. chaffeensis*, *E. ewingii*, and *Borrelia burgdorferi* Species-Specific Peptides." *Infect Ecol Epidemiol* 4 (2014).

Chapter 16:

Spiral & Curved Bacteria

Introduction

Spiral and curved bacteria are so named due to their cellular shape (Figure 16.1). All the spiral and curved bacteria in this chapter stain gram-negative. Additionally, they share the characteristic of motility meaning that they can move purposefully toward nutrients or a favored niche. Likewise, they can move away from hostile environments and the host immune system. This gives them somewhat of a selective advantage over non-motile organisms that are not in control of where they end up in the body. The motility of the spiral and curved bacteria is achieved by the use of flagella. Some, like *Helicobacter pylori*, have external flagella (Figure 16.1). Others, like *Treponema pallidum* are equipped with endoflagella found within a structure called the axial filament (Figure 16.2). Contraction of the axial filament and the endoflagella within create the spiral movement characteristic of spiral organisms. The number and location of the flagella differ between genera and among different species within a single genus. Motility can aid us in detecting them as when a sample such as feces is mixed with saline and a drop is placed on a slide and examined under the microscope. The nature and direction of the motility (e.g., corkscrew, darting) can sometimes further aid in determining which genus of bacteria is present in a sample.

For a more detailed discussion of diagnostics designed to help identify motile organisms, see Chapter 22.

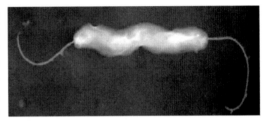

Figure 16.1: The spiral-shaped bacterium *Helicobacter hepaticus*, TEM. Note the bipolar flagellae present. *H. hepaticus* colonizes mice and can often interfere in research utilizing mice. Photo from: Falsafi, Tahereh, and Mohaddese Mahboubi. "*Helicobacter hepaticus*, a New Pathogenic Species of the *Helicobacter* Genus: Similarities and Differences with *H. pylori*." *Iran J Microbiol* 5 3 (2013): 185-94. Open access.

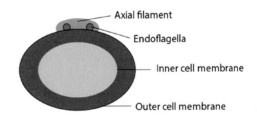

Figure 16.2: Cross-section of a spiral bacterium showing the location of the endoflagella. The endoflagella are pre-sent within the axial filament. The axial filament runs the length of the bacterium. Contraction of the axial filament and the endoflagella are what create the movement spiral movement that is characteristic of these organisms.

Campylobacter

A gram-negative, spiral, curved rod, those within the genus *Campylobacter* move in a darting, corkscrew motion. Microscopically, when two of the curved rods are in close proximity they give the characteristic appearance of Gull's wings (Figure 16.3). *Campylobacter* organisms are microaerophilic, meaning that they require lower than normal levels of oxygen, as they are poisoned by atmospheric concentrations of oxygen. Transmission of *Campylobacter* infections is most often via the fecal-oral route.

Campylobacter jejuni subspecies jejuni

C. jejuni ssp. *jejuni* lives as a commensal organism within the gastrointestinal tract of many companion and food animals. On occasion, it may cause disease in domestic animals. However it is more likely to cause zoonotic disease.

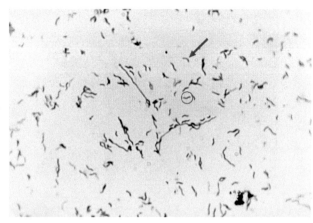

Figure 16.3: Examples of cellular morphology of *Campylobacter* species. While predominately spiral, *Campylobacter* can appear gull- (red circle) or comma-shaped (red arrow) when viewed under high magnification. Courtesy of the Public Health Image Library, PHIL #6654, Centers for Disease Control and Prevention, Atlanta, 2002.

Zoonosis

C. jejuni ssp. *jejuni* is a zoonotic foodborne pathogen. Risk factors increasing the chance of illness include consuming undercooked meats, such as chicken and other poultry, and unpasteurized "raw" milk. Clinical signs follow an incubation period of 24-72 hours and may include diarrhea which is sometimes bloody, vomiting, fever, and abdominal pain. With healthy individuals, the infection is usually **self-limiting**.

Disease in Small Animals

Most dogs and cats which ingest and harbor *C. jejuni* ssp. *jejuni* appear clinically normal. Occasionally, however, colonization may result in clinical signs relating to diarrhea and enteritis. These animals are usually young, stressed, and living under less than ideal husbandry conditions (see sidebar). Treatment is aimed at correcting any dehydration resulting from the diarrhea and may include intravenous fluids and an antiemetic to stop vomiting, if present. A veterinarian may prescribe antibiotics if the number of *Campylobacter* is sufficiently high.

Remember: this:
Shelters and Stockyards can be a little stressful

Even the best run, most well-equipped animal shelters and stockyards can be a stressful place for animals.

Within the confined space of the shelter (or stockyard) are many animals that have unknown genetics, immunity statuses, pathogen loads, and behavior profiles. An animal with a poorly functioning immune system that is stressed out by its new loud and unruly neighbors is at increased risk for contracting an infectious disease. Shelters try to minimize this by sanitizing runs and performing health checks on the animals, but this does not guarantee all animals won't get sick.

As a veterinary technician, if you are asked to help take a history on a sick animal, be sure to ask how long they've had the animal and where they obtained the animal.

Disease in Large Animals

Like dogs and cats, most food animal species which ingest and harbor *C. jejuni* ssp. *jejuni* appear clinically normal. In individuals showing signs of disease, the most common findings are diarrhea with or without mucus and blood. These signs are seen because the *Campylobacter* are infecting and causing damage to the mucosal surface of the intestines. Infection may result in abortion of pregnant females. These abortions usually occur within the first trimester and, thus, may falsely appear to the farmer as a failure to "take" (i.e., become pregnant) rather than as a recognizable abortion. Abortions are more often seen in sheep and goats as compared to pigs.

Campylobacter fetus subspecies *fetus*
C. fetus ssp. *fetus* causes late-term (usually third trimester abortions) in sheep. The ewe usually becomes infected by ingesting contaminated food or water. The bacteria circulate in the maternal bloodstream and, via the placenta, gain access to the fetus. Inflammation and infection of the fetus and related tissues leads to spontaneous abortion.

Other *Campylobacter* species
Campylobacter fetus ssp. *venerealis* is transmitted venereally and most commonly causes infertility or early embryonic death. *C. upsaliensis* and *C. helveticus* may cause diarrhea in dogs and cats in the same manner as *C. jejuni* ssp. *jejuni* (see above). *C. hyointestinalis* ssp. *hyointestinalis* was once thought to cause porcine proliferative enteropathy, a disease condition now attributed to infection with *Lawsonia intracellularis* (discussed later in this chapter). *C. hyointestinalis* ssp. *hyointestinalis* is now considered normal porcine flora. Other *Campylobacter* species and subspecies have uncertain or negligible virulence or are considered to be normal flora of the species from which it was isolated.

Remember this:
Timing is everything!

Some of the organisms discussed in this chapter have a tendency to cause abortion during a particular portion (i.e., trimester) of pregnancy. While this is not absolute, the timing of the abortion can help in identifying the most likely possible organisms responsible. The veterinarian then uses this list to decide on what further tests are needed as well as what therapy to begin while waiting for test results.

Therefore, it is important to note down in the medical records how many days pregnant the patient was when the abortion occurred.

You may be asked to help the veterinarian look through a herd's breeding records to see if other animals have had similarly timed abortions. This can help identify if others were likely infected with the same organism.

Diagnostics
Culture is most often used to identify *Campylobacter*. Culture conditions must be microaerophilic for the organism to grow. Individual *Campylobacter* species require different temperatures for optimal growth. This temperature "preference" can aid in identifying the species of *Campylobacter* causing a particular illness. For example, *C. fetus* will grow at 25°C, but not 42°C while *C. jejuni* will grow at 42°C, but not 25°C. And while it is possible to examine *Campylobacter* organisms using light microscopy, darkfield and phase contrast microscopy are preferred as they yield better visualization of the organisms.

Biochemical tests also aid in diagnosis. For example, most campylobacters are urease-negative which is useful in distinguishing them from other spiral and curved bacteria. For example, many *Helicobacter* species (covered later in this chapter) are urease-positive. Molecular tests, such as *Campylobacter*-specific PCR, are also available.

Treatment and Prevention of *Campylobacter* Infections
Treatment involves antimicrobial therapy based on the results of culture and antibiotic susceptibility

testing. Improved sanitation helps reduce the environmental load of *Campylobacter* available for animals to ingest. A commercially-available bacterin may be used to prevent disease; however, clients should be made aware that immunity is usually short-lived. Zoonotic foodborne infections can be prevented through proper food handling techniques.

Helicobacter

Numerous species of *Helicobacter* exist which infect animals and humans. This gram-negative rod can be helical, curved, or straight depending upon the exact species being observed. All species are motile and microaerophilic. Some are zoonotic. They can all be compared to the originally discovered species, *H. pylori*, in their severity of disease. Thus, we will discuss *H. pylori* first in this section.

Helicobacter pylori

Discovered in 1982 by scientists Marshall and Warren (see sidebar), *H. pylori* is one of the most researched pathogens of the current scientific era. A 2015 search in the National Institutes of Health database PubMed using the search term "*Helicobacter pylori*" retrieved over 37,000 articles!

The disease state in humans caused by *H. pylori* can range from mild chronic gastritis to gastric/duodenal ulcers to cancer. Many factors contribute to which disease state predominates in a given individual. Host factors such as genetics, the ability to mount an immune response, and the exact type of immune response generated in the face of infection. The single most important host factor which contributes to determining disease progression appears to be the host's output of stomach acid. Those producing low amounts of stomach acid are more likely to develop *H. pylori*-related stomach cancer. This trait is often found in people of the so-called "developing nations". Whether this is linked to host genetics or due to acquired "lifestyle" activities is unclear. People inhabiting "developed" countries, such as the US, are more likely to produce higher amounts of stomach acid. High acid production is a risk factor for the development of peptic ulcer disease. Clinical signs associated with peptic ulcer disease include:

- Dyspepsia
- Feelings of "heartburn"
- Melena
- Vomitus with "coffee ground" appearance due to digestion of blood leaking from ulcer
- Symptoms associated with anemia
- No symptoms ("silent" form)

Other host-related factors include whether or not a person smokes, drinks alcoholic beverages, or takes non-steroidal anti-inflammatory drugs such as acetaminophen or ibuprofen. All three of these host-related factors favor the development of chronic gastritis.

You tell 'em, Guys!

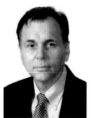 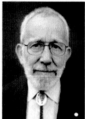

Photo: C. Northcott   Photo: U. Montan

®©The Nobel Foundation

Helicobacter pylori was first discovered in 1982 by Drs. Barry J. Marshall and J. Robin Warren. Their pioneering work led to the Nobel Prize in Physiology and Medicine in 2005.

What was so momentous about this work? Marshall and Warren established the role of *H. pylori* as the causative agent of stomach and duodenal ulcers, a condition which plagues the lives of millions of people each year worldwide. Up until the discovery, medical texts taught that stress and stomach acidity were solely responsible for the development of these ulcers.

Reaction from the medical community to Marshall and Warren's results was largely negative. *Ulcers as a result of an infection? Impossible.* Yet by using Koch's postulates, Marshall and Warren were able to disprove their opponents. Today, their work has been fully accepted and embraced by the same communities that doubted them. Their work led to the discovery of many more species of *Helicobacter* which infect animals and humans.

Helicobacter mustelae

Nearly one hundred percent of post-weanling ferrets are colonized by *H. mustelae!* Thankfully, most ferrets remain asymptomatic over their lifetime. However, serious clinical disease may occur with acute death being the first sign. This is usually due to an undetected ulcer which becomes so severe that it actually perforates (i.e., makes a hole in) the stomach wall. When this happens, the blood loss is usually sudden and severe, leading to the death of the ferret within minutes to hours. Even in the event that the blood loss does not kill them, the leakage of gastric contents and acid causes severe, life-threatening peritonitis. A few cases of MALT lymphoma and gastric cancer occurring in ferrets have also been reported. Ferrets that are free of *H. mustelae* have been successfully raised and are available for use in research.

Helicobacter heilmannii and H. felis

Estimates put the prevalence of *Helicobacter* infections in dogs and cats somewhere between 50-100%, depending on the population surveyed. The two most prevalent species are *H. heilmannii* and *H. felis*. Both have been linked to the development of gastritis using **epidemiology**. However, definitively establishing exactly just how these species cause gastritis has been more difficult. In addition, *H. heilmannii* has been linked to MALT lymphoma, a cancer of the lymphoid or immune tissue of mucosal surfaces, such as the mucosal lining of the stomach and intestines. *H. heilmannii* can infect people and is thus zoonotic.

> **Melena**
> Hemorrhagic diarrhea where the blood has been digested. Often described as "tarry" stool. Blood in the stool can be confirmed by an occult blood test.

Diagnostics

Culture

Helicobacter can be cultured on artificial media such as agar with optimal growth achieved when incubated at 37°C. Most *Helicobacter* species found in veterinary patients can also grow at 42°C. This can be useful diagnostically. *H. pylori* will not grow at 42°C, and cultures must therefore be incubated at 37°C. As this is not a common test in most veterinary diagnostic laboratories, the veterinary technician should call the laboratory prior to obtaining and sending off samples.

Urease Test

Helicobacter produces the enzyme urease which helps it to survive in the very acidic environment of the stomach. Testing for the presence of the urease enzyme helps to rule out other non-urease producing organisms that may be on the veterinarian's differential diagnosis list. The test can be performed using commercially available test strips. To perform the urease test using this method, a biopsy of the stomach lining must be obtained by the veterinarian. Today, this is usually done by using an endoscope; however, open abdominal surgery may also be performed to obtain adequate samples. Once the biopsy sample has been obtained the test is performed as described briefly below:

1. The reagent strip contains urea which must be rehydrated using a buffer provided in the test kit.
2. Place the gastric biopsy on the reaction pad. If *Helicobacter* is present in the biopsy sample, the urease produced will react with the urea on the pad and produce ammonia gas which then diffuses to the adjacent reaction pad (i.e., pH indicator paper). The ammonia gas turns the yellow reaction pad to an intense blue/purple color.

Other Diagnostics

Gastric biopsies should also be submitted for histopathology. When filling out the paperwork to send with the biopsy, be sure to record that *Helicobacter* is suspected. This is because visualization of *Helicobacter* organisms is often enhanced by the use of special stains (e.g., Warthin-Starry silver stain) not routinely used on histology samples. PCR may also be used to diagnose *Helicobacter* infections.

Treatment

Treatment of most *Helicobacter* infections relies on using the affectionately known "Triple Therapy" consisting of two antibiotics and bismuth subsalicylate (yep, that's right – Pepto Bismol!). There are many different "Triple Therapies" that have been used to treat infections in animals and people with varying success. One of the most common triple therapy regimens uses a combination of amoxicillin, metronidazole, and bismuth.

Prevention

Given the high transmission of *Helicobacter* species from dam to offspring it is virtually impossible to prevent colonization of offspring with *Helicobacter*. This has been achieved in the research setting (e.g., in ferret colonies), but is not practical for clients in a practice setting. There is no vaccine against any of the *Helicobacter* species.

Lawsonia intracellularis

Within the genus *Lawsonia*, the species of most importance to veterinary medicine is *Lawsonia intracellularis*.

Morphology and Staining

Lawsonia intracellularis is a gram-negative, curved, non-spore-forming rod. Optimal growth occurs in a microaerophilic environment. A single polar flagella allows the organism to be motile.

With histopathology tissue preparations, the organism stains a deep dark brown when a silver stain (e.g., Warthin-Starry) is used; this contrasts with the yellow stain imparted to the tissues. For this reason, *L. intracellularis* is sometimes referred to as **"argyrophilic"** (i.e., silver-loving).

> ### Common Synonyms for Lawsonia intracellularis:
> - Proliferative enteritis (preferred)
> - Proliferative ileitis
> - "Wet tail"
> - Regional enteritis
> - Terminal ileitis
> - Atypical transmissible ileal hyperplasia
>
>

Hosts and Transmission

Various animals can act as host to the organism. *Lawsonia intracellularis* is considered an endemic infection within US swine herds. Hamsters, horses, and numerous other species may also be infected. *L. intracellularis* does not appear to be zoonotic. Transmission is primarily via the fecal-oral route.

Disease Conditions

Over the years, the disease conditions caused by *Lawsonia intracellularis* have been given many descriptive names. By far the most common name the disease is referred to in hamsters is "wet tail". The term refers to the fecal soiling of the perianal and tail regions due to the extensive diarrhea present. While descriptive, this is a bit of a misnomer as many diseases other than *Lawsonia* may cause diarrhea and a "wet tail". Therefore, it is best to avoid using this term when talking to clients.

Swine

In swine herds, two different disease presentations (acute or chronic) may be seen depending upon the age at infection. The acute form of the disease, proliferative hemorrhagic enteropathy, is most often seen in older pigs (e.g. aged 4-12 months). Clinically, these pigs most often present with hemorrhagic diarrhea. The blood seen in the diarrhea is frank (non-digested) blood as the bleeding occurs

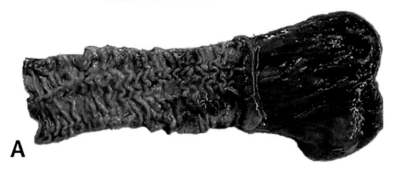

Figure 16.4: Proliferative enteropathy of the terminal ileum, foal. Experimentally-infected foal that was euthanized 24 days after the start of the infection. The mucosa is reddened with the pooling of blood in the tissues and there is diffuse and severe thickening of the intestinal mucosa. Adapted from: Vannucci, Fabio A., et al. "Evidence of Host Adaptation in *Lawsonia intracellularis* Infections." *Veterinary Research* 43 1 (2012): 53-53. Open access.

in the intestines and not the stomach. In naïve animals, the disease can result in such severe hemorrhage and diarrhea, that the pigs are left vulnerable to death from severe dehydration, anemia, and systemic bacteremia causing septic shock.

A milder, more chronic form of infection, porcine intestinal adenomatosis, typically affects young post-weaned piglets (e.g., aged 6-20 weeks). Pigs exhibit chronic, mild diarrhea with concurrent reduced rate of gain. This can result in permanent stunting of affected hogs. The disease typically lasts 4-6 weeks.

Hamsters
Disease in hamsters closely follows that seen in the chronic form of pigs and results in diarrhea, rapid weight loss, and dehydration. Severe intestinal hyperplasia occurs. However, in the later stages of disease pyogranulomatous inflammation may develop.

Horses
Equine proliferative enteropathy, caused by *L. intracellularis*, constitutes an emerging disease in the equine industry. Once confined to individual case reports and sporadic outbreaks, cases of equine proliferative enteropathy (Figure 16.4) are increasing in number. The disease mainly affects weanling foals (i.e., aged 4-7 months) causing fever, lethargy, diarrhea, colic, and weight loss. Ventral edema may be seen along the ventral abdomen, scrotum, and distal limbs.

In the laboratory, equine isolates of *L. intracellularis* have successfully infected other animal species, such as rabbits. Therefore, owners of a *Lawsonia*-infected animal should take precautions not to inadvertently spread the infection to other animals in the household. While the source of infections in horses has not been positively identified, wild (cottontail) rabbits have tested fecal-positive for *L. intracellularis* and may constitute a wild reservoir of this infection.

Diagnostics
Diagnostics rely on serology, histopathology, and molecular methods (e.g., PCR). On necropsy, swine affected with proliferative hemorrhagic enteropathy show marked hemorrhage originating from severely thickened, proliferated intestinal mucosa. In the case of pigs and horses, it is recommended that herd mates that have been in contact with affected individuals also be tested. Special stains, such as the Warthin-Starry silver stain, are often required to aid visualization of the *Lawsonia* rods on histopathologic sections of tissue.

Treatment
Treatment in the various species consists of a combination of antimicrobial therapy and supportive care. Antimicrobials of the macrolide class are most often employed. However, various combinations

therapies are also used. Supportive care in the form of IV fluids, plasma transfusions, parenteral nutrition (i.e., diseased gut has decreased absorptive capacity), and anti-ulcer drugs (e.g., sucralfate, H2-blockers) is instituted concurrently with antimicrobial therapy.

Prevention

A vaccine licensed for use in pigs is available in the US. Field trials of an avirulent live EPE vaccine given intrarectally to foals has shown some promise in preventing disease, however, more studies are needed to characterize its overall effectiveness. Purchasing hamsters from a reliable vendor which regularly tests for a variety of pathogens, including *Lawsonia*, is recommended.

Brachyspira hyodysenteriae

As the genus designation suggests, the organism is a slender, gram-negative **spirochete**. *B. hyodysenteriae* is motile; its mobility takes on a helical path, highly characteristic of the spirochetes. This organism is responsible for the disease known as "swine dysentery".

> ### Spirochetes
> **Spirochetes** are thin, highly flexible, helically coiled ("hair-like") bacteria. Some are so slender that it is difficult to resolve them using light microscopy. In that case, dark field or electron microscopy must be used to visualize an individual bacterium.
>
>

Synonyms

The genus of this organism has undergone several name changes due to increased knowledge of its genetics. Historical names include: *Serpulina hyodysenteriae* and *Treponema hyodysenteriae*.

Host and Transmission

Swine, usually limited to grower/finisher pigs, are at risk for swine dysentery. Infection is transmitted between swine via the fecal-oral route.

Disease Conditions

While relatively uncommon in the United States, swine dysentery can cause significant morbidity (up to 90%) and moderate mortality (0-30%). Two forms of the disease exist. The more severe form consists of mucohemorrhagic diarrhea characterized by extensive inflammation and necrosis of the small intestine. Severe dehydration, emaciation, red blood cell loss, and secondary sepsis (i.e., due to movement of gut bacteria from the damaged intestine and into the bloodstream) contribute to the mortality seen with this form of the disease. A less severe, more chronic form occurs when there is less intense intestinal inflammation and necrosis. This form is characterized by gradual weight loss and mild unthriftiness. Mild diarrhea is seen on presentation.

Diagnostics

Culture

Brachyspira hyodysenteriae is challenging to grow in culture, but some diagnostic laboratories do offer specialized culture procedures for *Brachyspira*. A slow grower, it can take up to 10 days to see evidence of growth. Identification can be pursued using dark-field microscopy and biochemical tests. PCR can be performed on clinical specimen including biopsies of the cecal and colonic mucosa or feces.

Other Diagnostic Methods

Mucosal scrapings using a rectal swab can be used for cytology. Direct fecal exams may also be performed. The fecal sample is diluted in saline, rolled onto a glass slide and Gram stained. However, this method is not reliable when a patient is shedding low numbers of organism in the feces.

Treatment and Control

Antimicrobials, such as tiamulin or lincomycin, are used therapeutically as well as prophylactically (e.g., herds where *Brachyspira* is prevalent). Improved management and biosecurity on swine farms are effective means to prevent the introduction of *Brachyspira* to naïve herds. A commercial bacterin is available in the US; however, it is not highly or reliably effective.

Leptospira

Members of the genus *Leptospira* are gram-negative spiral rods. Historically, the genus *Leptospira* has been divided into 2 species. The species *Leptospira interrogans* contains the pathogenic strains, while *Leptospira biflexa* contains mainly saprophytes and environmental strains. *Leptospira interrogans* can be divided into numerous serovars; only a few of these are of importance to the veterinary team (Table 16.1).

Table 16. 1: Major serovars of veterinary importance.

Serovar	Host(s)	Disease manifestation
L. autumnalis	Canine	Kidney and liver disease (Suspected, but not proven)
L. bratislava	Equine	Abortion
L. canicola	Canine	Kidney and liver disease
	Swine	Abortion; systemic disease
L. grippotyphosa	Canine	Kidney and liver disease
	Racoons, Skunks	Reservoir host
L. hardjo	Cattle	Abortion; infertility
L. icterohaemorrhagiae	Rat	Reservoir host
	Cattle, Swine	Abortion
	Canine	Sepsis
L. kennewicki	Horses	Abortion
L. pomona	Swine, Bovine, Equine	Abortion

Proposed New Taxonomy

With whole organisms' genomes being sequenced (e.g., human, dog, mouse), DNA sequencing has become a fast, reliable method for species identification. Thus, there is a movement in the diagnostic laboratory world to use genetic typing to identify bacterial species. A new system providing more accurate identification and naming of *Leptospira* species, called "genomospecies", has been developed using DNA sequencing technology. Currently, methods for genomospeciation are not widely available. Therefore, diagnostic laboratories will most likely use the older, serologic typing system for some time. However, members of the veterinary team should be familiar with the newer taxonomy (Table 16.2).

Hosts and Transmission

Leptospira interrogans colonizes both the liver and kidney of affected individuals. Colonization of the kidneys leads to excretion of the bacteria in the urine. This excretion can happen over extended periods of time. Some (reservoir) hosts do not show clinical signs. This carrier state can be lifelong. Reservoir hosts can include raccoons, skunks, feral swine. Diseased and carrier individuals transmit leptospirosis through contact with their infected urine. A major environmental source of infection are

Table 16. 2: Proposed "genomospecies" classification of *Leptospira*

L. alexanderi
L. biflexa
L. borgpetersenii
L. fainei
L. inadai
L. interrogans
L. kirschneri
L. meyeri
L. noguchii
L. parva
L. santarosai
L. weilii
L. wolbachii

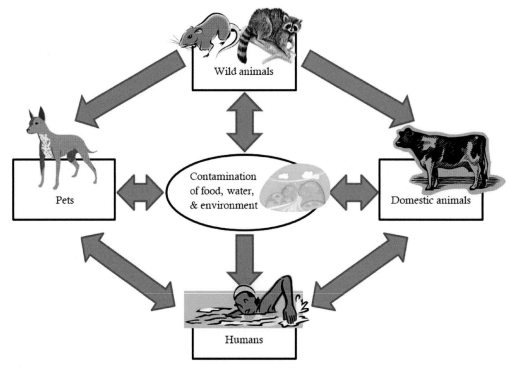

Figure 16.5 *Leptospira interogans* reservoirs and potential modes of transmission.

water sources, such as ponds and streams. Diseased and carrier animals urinate into these water sources and thus contaminate them with leptospiral organisms (Figure 16.5). Venereal transmission, while possible, plays a minor role in the spread of leptospirosis.

Pathogenesis

Entry into a new host begins with exposure of the mucosa, conjunctiva, or broken skin to water, food, or environment contaminated with *Leptospira*. The bacteria invade these tissues and quickly access the blood stream where upon they replicate (i.e., leptospiremia) and disseminate to multiple organs in the body, such as the liver, kidneys, spleen, and meninges. Venereal transmission can result in reproductive disease such as abortion in pregnant animals.

Disease Conditions

Leptospirosis results in various non-specific signs making it, arguably, one of the most difficult diseases to diagnose. Generally, due to its **tissue tropism** for the liver and kidney, signs are related to damage to these two organ systems. Signs related to kidney damage and/or failure that may be seen include: increased thirst; increased urination; pale, dilute urine; blood-tinged urine; and painful kidneys on palpation. The hallmark of marked liver damage and possible liver failure is **icterus**. Leptospirosis should be a differential in cases of bovine abortion.

Diagnostics

Culture

Culture is not offered as a routine diagnostic test due to numerous challenges, including the short-term survivability of the organism in clinical samples. It is possible to culture the organism if samples are inoculated into special media immediately upon collection, so culture is often used in research settings.

Serology

Serology is commonly used to detect anti-leptospira antibodies in serum. The standard testing method is the microscopic agglutination test (MAT). The MAT combines live cultures of several serovars with the patient's serum at multiple dilutions. The lowest dilution of serum that causes agglutination of the leptospira serovar represents the endpoint of the test. Agglutination is due to the presence of specific antibody in the serum sample binding to the test organism. The inverse of that dilution is the titer. Like with any serologic test, it is best to collect two samples approximately 4-6 weeks apart, to determine if titers are changing due to an active infection.

Fluorescent Antibody Testing

A leptospira-specific antibody conjugated to a fluorescent molecule can be used to detect *Leptospira* on direct preparation of clinical material. Samples may include urine or tissues (ex: fetal tissues, kidney, liver) that are applied to a glass slide. A microscope capable of detecting fluorescence is used to examine the slides for the presence of the organism.

Cytology

Urine specimens may be examined for the presence of the spirochetes (Figure 16.6). However, due to their small size, this often requires the use of darkfield microscopy which is usually only available at a reference laboratory. When sending off urine samples of animals suspected of harboring *Leptospira*, the urine can be mixed with 10% formalin (i.e., ratio of 20 mL of urine to 1.5 mL 10% formalin). The addition of formalin preseves the morphology of the leptospiral organisms.

Remember this: Identifying Icterus

Icterus is a yellowing of connective tissue as a result of a backup of bilirubin. This occurs when the liver cannot properly process bilirubin in a timely manner.

The best places to examine an animal and confirm icterus in the live animal are the:

- sclera of the eyes
- gums
- mucous membranes

In darkly pigmented animals, it may be difficult to determine if icterus in the gums and mucous membranes as these tissues are often also heavily pigmented.

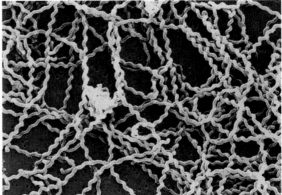

Figure 16.6: *Leptospira interogans,* colorized SEM. Courtesy of the Public Health Image Library, PHIL #138, Centers for Disease Control and Prevention, Atlanta, 1998.

Zoonosis

Leptospirosis is strongly environmentally-associated. That is, most human infections are strongly linked to exposure to *Leptospira*-contaminated ponds, streams, or other places traversed by the mammalian reservoir hosts. Rodents and other wildlife, such as skunks and racoons, can carry the pathogen and shed it in their urine, resulting in contamination of water bodies. Transmission to humans can be via direct or indirect contact between the person and the reservoir host. Precautions must be taken when caring for a pet with leptospirosis or working with farm animals experiencing abortions due to leptospirosis. The disease varies among affected individuals. Leptospirosis may present as a mild, flu-like illness. A more severe manifestation of the disease may lead to acute pulmonary hemorrhage with liver and renal failure.

Treatment

Antibiotics are used to treat leptospirosis. The choice of antibiotics is based on culture and antibiotic susceptibility testing. Additionally, the choice of antibiotics may be altered based on whether they are kidney or liver "sparing" (i.e., gentler on these organs). While antibiotics will kill *Leptospira*, clients should be warned that these drugs will not reverse any existing liver and kidney damage caused by the bacteria. This damage can be quite severe. In addition to antibiotics, supportive care is instituted to mitigate the liver and kidney dysfunction and to help to prevent/treat disseminated intravascular coagulopathy (a potential complicating factor).

Control and Prevention

Rodents, cattle, and swine may all serve as carriers of *Leptospira*. Animals diagnosed as chronic carriers should be humanely euthanized as they pose a potential source of the infection for other animals in the herd. Care should be taken to cleanup any environmental contamination. Where practical, ponds located within pastureland should be fenced off or drained. Rodent control in and around barns should also be instituted. Whether dogs and cats can serve as longterm reservoir carriers is currently open to debate. More research in this area is needed before recommendations can be made.

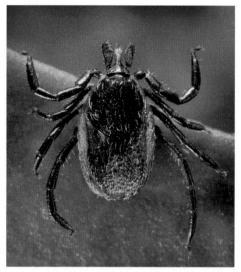

Figure 16.7: *Ixodes pacificus*, the Western black-legged tick, an insect vector of Lyme disease (*Borrelia burgdorferi*). Courtesy of the Public Health Image Library, PHIL #8686, Centers for Disease Control and Prevention, Atlanta, 2006.

Commercial vaccines are currently available in the US against leptospirosis and are labelled for use in cattle and for dogs. The vaccine label designates how many serovars of *Leptospira* the vaccine protects against. A "2-way" vaccine protects against two serovars while a "4-way" protects against four serovars. Care should be taken to explain to clients which exact serovars of *Leptospira* an individual vaccine preparation protects against. Should an animal be infected with a serovar <u>other</u> than the ones used in the vaccine, little to no cross-protection will be provided to the animal and the animal may become infected and show clinical signs of leptospirosis. The vaccine should be administered yearly. Vaccination cannot eliminate the carrier state. There is no vaccine licensed for horses.

Borrelia burgdorferi

A member of the family Spirochaetaceae, *Borrelia burgdorferi* is the causative agent of **Lyme disease**, a systemic tick-borne disease that results in chronic degenerative joint disease and lameness in both dogs and humans.

Morphology

B. burgdorferi is a small, thin gram-negative spirochete. Measuring 25 um long and only 0.2 um in diameter, they are too small to be reliably identified using light microscopy. This necessitates the use of dark field microscopy for visualization. The spirochete's endoflagella creates the wavelike motion that characterizes their motility.

Lifecycle and Transmission

Transmission of *B. burgdorferi* is via *Ixodes* ticks, such as the black-legged deer tick (*Ixodes scapularis*) and the Western black-legged tick (*Ixodes pacificus*) (Figure 16.7). Geographic distribution of ticks differs by species with *I. scapularis* inhabiting the eastern half of the US. As its name suggests, the location of *Ixodes pacificus* is mainly restricted to the western states of Washington, Oregon and California with additional pockets in Utah and Nevada. The larval and nymph stages of these ticks feed on small mammals and birds. Adult ticks feed on larger mammals, such as deer. Incidental hosts for *Ixodes* ticks include humans, dogs, and cats.

It is estimated that approximately 50% of North American *Ixodes* ticks are infected with *B. burgdorferi*. Given the geographic distribution of *Ixodes* and other species of ticks, a thorough travel history should be taken in pets suspected of having been bitten by a tick (especially if the owner cannot show you the tick) or tests positive for *B. burgdorferi* (see Diagnostics). If the pet has not traveled, it is likely a "local" tick. This can help the veterinarian narrow down what tick-borne diseases may have been transmitted to the animal.

Transmission of *B. burgdorferi* is not immediate. The spirochete is transmitted from 1-4 days after a tick bites and feeds on the host. Interestingly, a protein in the tick's saliva is thought to protect *B. burgdorferi* against attack from the host's immune system. How the spirochete localizes to joints is still not clear, but dissemination via the bloodstream is likely.

Disease in Dogs

Asymptomatic infections

The majority, up to 95%, of naturally exposed dogs remain asymptomatic. However, there is some evidence from experimentally infected dogs that microscopic synovial (joint) lesions occur even in the absence of observable clinical signs.

Symptomatic Disease

In the infections that become symptomatic, two main disease manifestations may present: lameness and kidney disease. Only a minority of naturally-infected dogs eventually show clinical signs. The immediate signs are mild, non-specific, and most often missed or dismissed by owners. Fever, tiredness, mild lameness, and swelling of lymph nodes (i.e., those located near the site of the tick bite) may occur, but generally resolve after several days. Due to the apparent transient nature of the initial signs, owners may not seek medical attention for their pets.

Lameness and Arthritis

As the infection becomes chronic and *B. burgdorferi* organisms spread throughout the body, the hallmark signs of Lyme disease begin to appear. The most common and striking clinical finding is lameness which may occur in one joint (e.g., right stifle), only to reappear several weeks later in another joint (e.g., left hock). This is termed **shifting-leg lameness** (see sidebar). Dogs will show signs of pain in the affected joints. Periods of lameness typically last up to 5 days. These bouts of lameness may occur weeks to months after the initial infection.

Remember this: Shifting-leg Lameness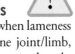

Shifting-leg lameness occurs when lameness appears to be localized in one joint/limb, then resolves, only to reappear several weeks later in *a totally different joint/limb*.

While there are other diseases that can result in shifting-leg lameness, this clinical sign is helpful to the veterinarian in forming a list of potential causes of disease in a lame pet. If a client complains that their dog is limping, it is not only important to ask which leg it is, but also if other limbs have been affected in the past weeks-months.

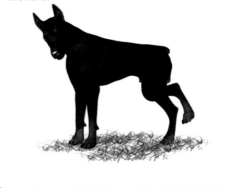

Kidney Disease

Fatal and progressive kidney failure has been reported in certain dog breeds; the majority were Labrador or golden retrievers. Importantly, it should be noted that while these dogs were antibody-positive for *B. burgdorferi*, no live organisms could be cultured. Experimentally infecting laboratory beagles did not result in kidney disease. Therefore, it has not be definitively established that *B. burgdorferi* directly caused the kidney disease. More research in this area is needed. In 2013, the number of cases was estimated to occur at a rate of less than 1-2% of all Lyme-positive dogs. Therefore, members of the veterinary team should be careful not to overstate the risks of kidney disease to avoid unduly alarming clients.

Diagnostics

In-clinic testing relies on antibody-testing. Commercially available "SNAP" tests (SNAP®, IDEXX Laboratories, Inc.) are available to test a patient's blood for antibodies to *B. burgdorferi*. These SNAP tests are often designed to test for multiple pathogens using only a single blood sample. Dogs that test positive for *B. burgdorferi* antibodies should have their infections confirmed as false positives do occur. A more specific antibody test is the C6 antibody test, currently only available at commercial or reference laboratories. This confirmatory test is designed to look for antibodies to a protein region of *B. burgdorferi* called C6. PCR testing is available. However, currently, the rate of false negative results is high.

Treatment

In dogs with clinical signs, long-term (i.e., 31-day course) of doxycycline is the current gold standard to eliminate *B. burgdorferi* infections. Amoxicillin is cheaper and has a good cure rate (though not as high as doxycycline. Recently, a long-acting injectable cephalosporin, cefovecin (Convenia®, Zoetis), has been successful in treating experimentally infected beagles. Its success in natural infections has not been adequately established.

Treatment of asymptomatic serologically-positive dogs is somewhat controversial. The veterinarian will evaluate each dog and decide if treatment should be pursued. The treatment regimen is the same as that of symptomatic dogs.

Prognosis

The majority of *Borrelia*-infected dogs remain asymptomatic throughout and after treatment. In the 5% showing clinical signs, the prognosis for recovery from lameness due to Lyme disease is generally good. Joint disease existing at diagnosis cannot be reversed. However, treatment eliminates the organism thereby decreasing inflammation, stopping disease progression, and preventing a worsening of the lameness. When caught early, most dogs return to (nearly) normal function. Lyme nephritis carries a poor prognosis, especially in dogs that are dehydrated and have elevated kidney blood chemistry values (i.e., high blood urea nitrogen (BUN) and creatinine).

Control and Prevention

Prevention of Lyme disease centers on a strict tick control program. Topical, "spot-on", and chewable oral preventives are available commercially. Veterinary technicians should familiarize themselves with the various products available so as to be in a position to best help clients choose a tick preventive that best fits the pet's and client's needs (see sidebar).

Cats and *B. burgdorferi*

While cats can be experimentally infected, to date there have been no natural infections of *B. burgdorferi* reported in cats.

Zoonotic Potential

Because transmission of Lyme disease requires a tick bite, direct transmission of the disease from dogs to humans cannot occur. However, a *Borrelia*-infected tick can bite and take a blood meal from a person. This is the method of transmission of human Lyme dis-

Remember this: "Treating" a Pet's Lifestyle

For every patient that laps up that chewable heartworm preventive begging for more, there's always one that turns up its nose - "yuck!"

While most medications may come in only one formulation, some medications come in multiple forms. Medications, such as tick preventives, need to fit the pet's (and owner's) lifestyle.

Dog hates to swallow pills? Try a chewable formulation. *Owner can't get the dog to take any oral medication?* Offer a topical or "spot-on" treatment.

Because medication can't work
if it can't get there!

ease. Prevention of human Lyme disease consists of preventing the tick bite in the first place. Ticks tend to inhabit grassy or wooded areas. While in or near these areas, wearing protective clothing (e.g., long pants, long socks) that maximizes coverage of skin plus the use of topical insecticides, such as those containing N,N-diethyl-meta-toluamide (DEET), are useful in prevention of tick bites and attachment.

Other Spiral Organisms Encountered Less Frequently

Treponema species

Treponemes are members of the family Spirochaetaceae. *Treponema paraluiscuniculi* (Formerly: *T. cuniculi*) is the causative agent of rabbit syphilis. It is also referred to as "vent disease". *T. vincentii* contributes to lameness in sheep. A related species, *T. pallidum*, causes human syphilis.

Disease in Rabbits

T. paraluiscuniculi is transmitted between rabbits both directly and through venereal contact. The disease is largely self-limiting. Asymptomatic carriers occur and aid in the spread of disease. Lesions occur on the epithelium and are usually found in the perianal or genital region. However, lesions may occur anywhere on the body (e.g., face). Lesions begin as red, raised swollen area that are covered with sparse or no hair. These lesions eventually break open and ulcerate. Finally, lesions will scab over. Rabbit syphilis causes decreased reproductive rates and the death of kits.

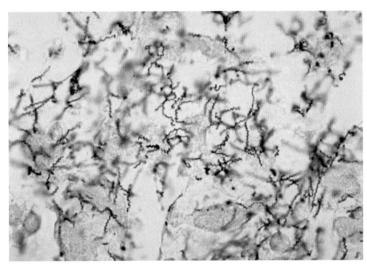

Figure 16.8: Example of a silver stain used to highlight spiral organisms such as *Treponema* spp. Modified Steiner silver stain. Organisms, such as *T. palladium* pictured here, that take up the elemental silver of the dye stain brownish-black while all other cells stain a yellowish color. Courtesy of the Public Health Image Library, PHIL #836, Centers for Disease Control and Prevention, Atlanta, 1986.

The best diagnostic sample is a skin biopsy containing the lesion(s). Veterinary technicians should be sure to explain to the histopathology lab that *T. paraluiscuniculi* is suspected as identification is aided by the addition of a special (silver) stain (Figure 16.8). Serological tests are also available. Treatment consists of antibiotics given subcutaneously or intramuscularly. Oral antibiotics are best avoided as the rabbit's gastrointestinal microflora are exquisitely sensitive to killing by broad-spectrum antibiotics. Life-threatening diarrhea from *Clostridium difficile* (see Chapter 17) and other opportunist bacteria that colonize the gut after antibiotic administration can kill a rabbit.

Disease in Sheep

Treponema vincentii has been identified as the causative agent of an emerging disease known as contagious ovine digital dermatitis (CODD). Unlike classical foot rot in sheep (covered in Chapter 17) which causes inflammation and "rot" on the underside of the hoof, CODD infections start at the coronary bands and eventually causes sloughing of the entire hoof from the soft underlying tissues of the digits. Currently, CODD appears to be geographically limited to the United Kingdom. However, members of the veterinary team should remain vigilant in case the disease appears in US herds.

Vibrio

Although this pathogen does not cause clinical disease in domestic animals, *Vibrio parahaemolyticus* is nonetheless an important spirochete in that it is a significant cause of animal-related foodborne illness. Many sea animals consumed as seafood can carry the pathogen asymptomatically. These animals include: mackerel, tuna, sardines, crabs, shrimp, and bivalve mollusks (e.g., mussels, oysters, clams). According to the Centers for Disease Control and Prevention (CDC), approximately 4500 people are infected with *V. parahaemolyticus* annually. People become ill, usually within 24 hours, after eating one or more of the aforementioned tainted seafood items. Common clinical signs are gastrointestinal in nature and include watery diarrhea (often accompanied by abdominal cramps), nausea, vomiting, fever, and chills. The illness is largely self-limiting and lasts about 3 days. However, some affected individuals may become dehydrated and require medical attention to treat the dehydration. Much less common, *V. parahaemolyticus* present in warm seawater may cause a skin infection in people when introduced into an open wound. Like *Burkholderia* and *Brucella*, *V. parahaemolyticus* carries two circular DNA chromosomes.

Further Reading

Centers for Disease Control and Prevention. "*Vibrio parahaemolyticus* Infections Associated with Consumption of Raw Shellfish - Three States, 2006." *Morbidity and Mortality Weekly Report* 55 31 (2006): 854-56.

Duncan, Jennifer S., et al. "Contagious Ovine Digital Dermatitis: An Emerging Disease." *Vet J* 201 3 (2014): 265-8.

Krupka, Inke, and Reinhard K. Straubinger. "Lyme Borreliosis in Dogs and Cats: Background, Diagnosis, Treatment and Prevention of Infections with *Borrelia burgdorferi* Sensu Stricto." *Vet Clin North Am Small Anim Pract* 40 6 (2010): 1103-19.

Littman, Meryl P. "Lyme Nephritis." *J Vet Emerg Crit Care (San Antonio)* 23 2 (2013): 163-73.

Wagner, Bettina, et al. "Comparison of Effectiveness of Cefovecin, Doxycycline, and Amoxicillin for the Treatment of Experimentally Induced Early Lyme Borreliosis in Dogs." *BMC Vet Res* 11 (2015): 163.

Chapter 17:

The Anaerobes

Introduction

Obligate anaerobes are unique among bacteria in that they cannot survive in atmospheres containing oxygen. The group contain species with diverse characteristics. They can stain gram-positive or gram-negative. The group can be divided into two main groups depending on whether or not the particular bacterial species can form spores. Another group of anaerobes are termed **facultative anaerobes**. These bacteria are capable of producing energy (i.e., ATP) via aerobic respiration when oxygen is plentiful. When oxygen levels decline or are absent, these organisms can switch to anaerobic fermentation to produce the energy needed to survive and thrive. Examples of these are staphylococci, corynebacteria, *Escherichia coli*, and members of the genus *Listeria*; these genera have been covered in previous chapters and will not be covered here.

Culturing Obligate Anaerobes

Due to their unique gas requirements, it is worthwhile to examine the needs of obligate anaerobes when attempting to culture them in a laboratory. Specimens obtained should be stored at ambient temperatures in air-free containers as the addition of oxygen to specimens can kill the anerobes. For tissue samples, samples of approximately 2 cm^3 or 2 mL can usually provide enough mass to protect the subsurface tissue from coming into contact with lethal oxygen levels. Likewise, residual air should be expelled from syringes containing aspirates. Whenever possible, specimens should be processed within a few hours. In the event that only swabs are available, care should be taken to place the swab immediately into Cary-Blair transport media or other commercially available anaerobic transport system. Culturing anaerobes requires special equipment such as an anaerobic jar or anaerobic chamber (Figure 17.1).

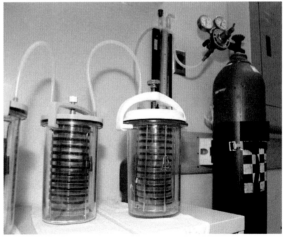

Figure 17.1: A series of anaerobic jars set up in tandem and receiving carbon dioxide (CO$_2$) from a single CO$_2$ tank. Obligate anaerobes cannot live in any amount of oxygen. Therefore, introduction of pure, medical grade CO$_2$ gas from a pressurized tank is necessary.

Spore-forming Anaerobes

Clostridium

Morphology and Staining

Clostridial species are non-motile, spore-forming rod-shaped bacteria. The majority of the species encountered in veterinary medicine stain positive when using the Gram stain; the exception is *Clostridium piliforme*, formerly *Bacillus piliforme*, which stains gram-negative The clostridia also vary in their gaseous requirements. Most *Clostridium* are strict anaerobes. Only *Clostridium perfringens* is relatively aerotolerant.

Sources of Infection

There are two main common sources for clostridial infections. **Exogenous** sources are so-called because they come from outside of the animal's or person's body. In the case of *Clostridium*, the exogenous source is most often the environment (e.g., soil). **Endogenous** sources are those found within or on the animal or person and serve as a reservoir from which to infect individuals in the herd or group. With *Clostridium*, the intestinal tract serves as an endogenous source for infection and disease of other members of the herd. Clostridial species can be described as enterotoxigenic (toxic to the gastrointestinal tract), histotoxic (toxic to various tissues) or neurotoxic (toxic to nervous tissue) depending on the type of disease they cause (Table 17.1).

Table 17. 1: Selected clostridial pathogens important in veterinary medicine and the actions of their toxins.

Species	System Toxin Acts On	Disease Produced
C. botulinum	Nervous	Botulism
C. chauvoei	Muscles	"Blackleg"
C. difficile	Gastrointestinal	Diarrhea Antibiotic-associated diarrhea Colitis
C. tetani	Nervous	Tetanus
C. perfringens Type A	Muscles	Muscle necrosis Gas gangrene
C. perfringens Type D	Gastrointestinal	Enteritis Enterotoxemia
C. piliforme	Heart Gastrointestinal Liver	"Tyzzer's Disease"

Lifecycle

Under optimal environmental conditions, *Clostridium* is present in its vegetative form (Figure 17.2). However, when confronted with conditions of excessive heat or dessication, *Clostridium* forms endospores. These endospores are capable of withstanding these inhospitable conditions for prolonged periods of time (i.e., years). Upon reentering a suitably moist, and slightly cooler environment (e.g., animal host tissues), the endospores germinate and form vegetative bacteria once more. These vegetative bacteria are capable of replicating within the animal host tissues. Once the bacteria are in their vegetative form they are also capable of forming a number of different toxins (see Pathogenesis section, below).

Pathogenesis

Most of the *Clostridium* species produce one or more toxins which perpetrate much of the damage seen in infections. One, an animal or person ingests pre-formed toxin. The second form of intoxication begins when clostridia bacteria are ingested. The *Clostridium* proceed to multiply and increase their numbers inside the body with subsequent production and dissemination of toxin (e.g., infant botulism). The unique aspects of pathogenesis for each pathogen will be handled under their respective sections.

Clostridium tetani

Tetanus, caused by *C. tetani*, is a disease that causes ascending paralysis in affected animals and people. Transmission of *C. tetani* usually occurs subsequent to a wound (e.g., puncture). Environmental spores of *C. tetani* enter the wound and begin to germinate in the anaerobic environment found in the wound. Once in its vegetative form, *C. tetani* produces a neurotoxin. This neurotoxin is taken up by motor nerves and is transported to the spinal nerves (i.e., retrograde) where it inhibits the inhibitory neurotransmitter release within the central nervous system of the host causing the motor neurons to become hyperactive. The increased excitability causes the **rigid** ("spastic") **paralysis** of muscle that is so characteristic of tetanus.

Clinical signs

While any mammals may be affected, the horse is at risk of puncture wounds to the sensitive structures of the hooves. With tetanus, muscle tremors (i.e., "tetanic spasms") are a hallmark of this disease. Due to the increased excitability of the peripheral nerves, affected individuals often have increased or exaggerated responses to stimuli. If the wound and subsequent intoxication is close to the neck or face, paralysis of the horse's muscles of mastication may become paralyzed (i.e., "lock jaw"). Additionally, in the horse, flaring of the nostrils and stiffly erect ears may be seen. A horse's back and tail muscles may become rigid thus leading to the typical "sawhorse stance" (Figure 17.3). If the intoxication is severe and long-standing the ascending paralysis can proceed until it contacts the nerves enervating the respiratory muscles causing respiratory distress.

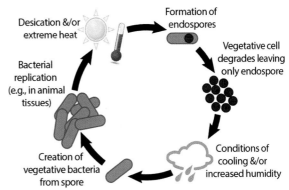

Figure 17.2: Lifecycle of spore-forming bacteria. Under favorable conditions, the bacteria exists in its vegetative form. Under harsh conditions such as extreme heat and desiccation, the vegetative cell forms an endospore.

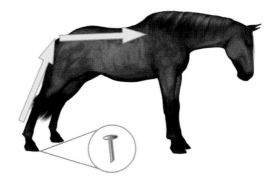

Figure 17.3: Horse exhibiting the "sawhorse" stance that is characteristic of the rigid, ascending paralysis accompanying intoxication with *Clostridium tetani* neurotoxins. Often entry of the clostridial organisms or their toxins is through a wound such as penetration of the soft tissues of the hoof with a nail that has *Clostridium* present on its surface.

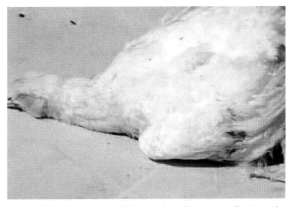

Figure 17.4: "Limberneck" in poultry (lower panel). Note the flaccid paralysis of the neck muscles in both species. Courtesy of The Poultry Site (www.thepoultrysite.com). Used with permission.

151

The respiratory distress can lead to full respiratory paralysis and death.

Clostridium botulinum

Clostridium botulinum causes the disease known as botulism. The disease results from the intoxication of several serologically distinct neurotoxins. There are several forms of botulism, including:

- Foodborne (animal)
- Foodborne (human) – discussed under Human Botulism section
- Wound
- Infant (human)

Foodborne Botulism

In the foodborne (animal) form, a wet, rotting carcass or vegetation are a good environment in which spores of *C. botulinum* can germinate, replicate, and form neurotoxins. When another animal (e.g., dog) comes along and eats the carcass it is also ingesting the preformed toxin. In the case of *C. botulinum*, the neurotoxin produced blocks the release of acetylcholine from the pre-synaptic nerve ending. This results in a failure of the neural signal to propagate across the neural cleft and thus the signal never reaches the muscle. Thus, in contrast to *C. tetani*, intoxication with *C. botulinum* causes **flaccid paralysis**.

A classical presentation of this disease is "**Limberneck**" in waterfowl and poultry (Figure 17.4). Birds that consume *C. botulinum*-contaminated vegetation quickly develop ascending flaccid paralysis. These birds cannot fly nor can they often lift up their heads. Eventually, the birds die due to paralysis of the respiratory muscles.

Wound Botulism

Wound botulism occurs when a wound in the skin is created and contaminated with *Clostridium botulinum* bacteria. The bacteria divide and increase their numbers. All the while they are producing toxin within the wound. Once produced, the actions of the neurotoxin are the same (i.e., flaccid paralysis). Thus, it is not pre-formed toxin, as in the case of foodborne botulism, but post-inoculation toxin formation which causes the clinical signs observed.

Infant Botulism and Shaker Foal Syndrome

In infant botulism, infants ingest either the spores or the vegetative form of *C. botulinum* and not the preformed toxin. While potentially any food could be contaminated with *C. botulinum*, honey has been implicated in multiple cases of infant botulism. The infant is fed a small amount of honey which contains a few viable *C. botulinum* spores. These spores germinate in the infant's gastrointestinal tract and then begin muliplying. Because the infant's gastrointestinal tract has not been fully colonized with healthy gut bacteria, there is more than enough room to support significant colonial expansion of the *C. botulinum*. These vegetative cells then produce the toxin inside the infant's body resulting in the intoxication and subsequent flaccid paralysis. Infants suffering from infant botulism often require respiratory support (e.g., mechanical ventilation) and undergo antitoxin therapy.

As little as 0.25 spores/g of honey can cause disease! It is for this reason that many physicians council parents not to give honey to children under 2 years of age.

While it is not extremely common, a form of infant botulism occurs in foals called "shaker foal syndrome." The source of *C. botulinum* spores is usually the soil. In eating grass or hay placed on the ground, the foal inadvertently also consumes the spores. Thereafter, the pathogenesis of botulism follows the same course as in human infant botulism.

Clostridium perfringens

Clostridium perfringens can produce multiple types of toxins; the damage these toxins produce can be either enterotoxigenic or histotoxic. The diseases caused by *C. perfringens* differ based on the particular toxin produced in a given infection. Infections come from both exogenous (i.e., environmental) as well as endogenous sources.

An example is *Clostridium perfringens* Type D, also known as "overeating disease". This disease is fairly common in suckling lambs. It can also affect calves and kids, though less frequently. The toxin effects the gastrointestinal as well as the central nervous system. The disease is usually preceeded by a sudden change to a very protein-rich diet. This sudden change upsets the normal microflora of the gastrointestinal tract. When a significant amount of this microflora dies, it opens up space for the rapid multiplication of *C. perfringens* within the gut. The production and subsequent uptake of toxin causes rapid CNS damage. The disease can be so acute and severe that individual animals may present as sudden death without any clinical signs.

Diagnostics

Obtaining a thorough history (e.g., recent dietary change) and the observation of compatible clinical signs (e.g., rigid vs. flaccid paralysis) is necessary in order for the veterinary team to correctly diagnose and treat clostridial infections and intoxications. Confirmation of suspected cases will require diagnostics tailored to the clostridial organism(s) which are on the veterinarian's differential diagnosis list.

Culture

Anaerobic culture techniques must be performed on suspected clostridial species (see section "Culturing Anaerobes"). Because environmental *Clostridium* (e.g., *C. perfringens* and *C. septicum*) can rapidly contaminate carcasses, specimens should be taken from recently dead animals. The best specimens are affected tissues (i.e., approximately 4 cm^3) or fluids. Culture is commonly used to detect *C. perfringens* and *C. difficile*, but not recommended for neruotoxic clostridia (*C. botulinum* and *C. tetani*; see "Toxin Detection" and "Animal Testing"). Because they can be normal intestinal inhabitants, enteric isolates of *Clostridium* must be further typed using PCR to determine their pathogenic potential.

Demonstration of Spores

Endospores can be demonstrated through the use of stains like Methylene blue or Malachite green (Figure 17.5).

Fluorescent Antibody Test

Antibodies specific for the histotoxic species of *Clostridia*, conjugated with a fluorescent marker, can be used to detect the organism within tissue. Affected tissues (ex: muscle, liver) are touched to a glass slide which is then treated with the antibodies. Antibodies that bind to the slide preparation are visualized by a fluorescence microscope, and indicate the presence of the particular bacterial species in the original sample. This test is useful for the histotoxic *Clostridia* including *C. chauvoei*, *C. septicum*, *C. novyi* and *C. sordelii*.

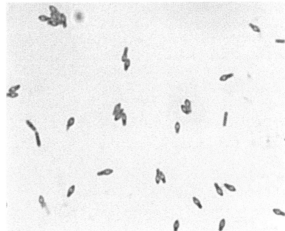

Figure 17.5: Demonstration of endospores in *Clostridium botulinum*. When stained with malachite green, the endospores of clostridial species will stain green while the vegetative bacilli will take on a purple color. Courtesy of the Public Health Image Library, PHIL #1932, Centers for Disease Control and Prevention, Atlanta, 2002.

Toxin Detection

Several tests are available to confirm the presence of clostridial toxin (e.g., ELISA). Ideal samples to submit are contents of the small intestine. Toxins are labile (i.e., prone to breakdown), therefore it is best to obtain the intestinal contents from a recently deceased animal. When submitting samples for toxin detection it is extremely important to inform the reference laboratory which toxins are suspected in each patient. This will aid in the choice of tests used. Call the laboratory prior to sending off the samples as the laboratory may only run the tests on certain days of the week.

Animal Testing

Because of the availability of other methods and animal welfare concerns, animal testing to prove the presence of a *Clostridium* organism (i.e., proving Koch's postulates) is largely no longer necessary. However, the mouse innoculation test is sometimes useful in demonstrating botulism toxin as the mouse bioassay is more sensitive than currently available ELISAs.

Other Clostridial Infections

The toxins of *Clostridium chauvoei* and *Clostridium perfringens* Type A both target muscle tissue resulting in gangrene. In cattle, *C. chauvoei* infections are commonly called "blackleg" due to the accumulation of hydrogen sulfide gas within the muscles and under the skin.

Clostridium piliforme infects a number of hosts including young foals and laboratory animals, such as rodents and rabbits. Called **Tyzzer's disease**, *C. piliforme* causes inflammation of the intestinal tract and associated organs such as the liver.

Treatment of Clostridial Infections

In most clostridial infections, antibiotic therapy is rarely useful. This is because the disease is caused by the toxin and not the organism itself. Treatment is complicated by the fact that the toxins often bind their receptors permanently. In other words, we can't "unbind" a toxin already bound to a receptor. The body has to remove the old, bound receptor and replace it with a new, unbound one. Therefore, antitoxin is only effective against unbound toxin. For this reason, prompt treatment is critical. If, in the case of botulism or tetanus, the respiratory muscles are already affected, respiratory support (e.g., mechanical ventilation) will be necessary. Often, with most of our veterinary patients, this is impractical and euthanasia may be performed.

Prevention: General Strategies

Specific prevention strategies are tailored to each clostridial species. Because it is the toxin which causes the clinical signs, prevention is targeted towards enabling the patient to mount a response against the toxin. To that end, scientists have been able to modify a number of *Clostridium* toxins just enough so that they cannot cause clinical signs yet can be recognized by the immune system, thus producing toxin-neutralizing antibodies. These antibodies will bind any naturally occuring toxin and render the toxin unable to cause the neurologic signs that are so devastating. These altered toxins are packaged in a vaccine called a **toxoid** vaccine.

Tetanus

Vaccination of the mare during gestation with tetanus toxoid helps provide passive immunity to foals through the mare's colostrum. Because wounds, particularly hoof wounds, are common in horses, all adults should be vaccinated with a commercial tetanus toxoid with boosters recommended annually. Additional information about specific vaccination schedules can be found at the American Association of Equine Practitioners website (http://www.aaep.org/info/tetanus).

Botulism

A vaccine against Shaker Foal Syndrome (*C. botulism* type B) is licensed for use within the US. The vaccine is recommended to be given as a series at 2, 4, and 8 weeks of age in endemic areas such as Kentucky and the mid-Atlantic states. Like the tetanus toxoid, mares can also be vaccinated while pregnant to enhance concentrations of toxin-specific antibodies in the colostrum.

Clostridium perfringens Type D

In sheep, ewes are vaccinated before parturition to provide passive immunity to lambs through protective antibodies in their colostrum.

Non-Spore-forming Anaerobes

Dichelobacter nodosus

Dichelobacter nodosus (formerly *Bacteroides nodusus*) is a rod-shaped, gram-negative, oxygen-tolerant anaerobe which initiates the development of foot rot in ruminants, particularly sheep.

Until about the early 2000s, *Fusobacterium necrophorum* (discussed below) was considered the initiator of foot rot, with *D. nodosus* acting only as a secondary, opportunistic infection. However, the weight of scientific evidence, particularly recent molecular pathogenesis studies, has turned this original hypothesis on its head! There is now generally agreement that *D. nodosus* initiates the infection while *F. necrophorum* acts as the opportunistic infection.

Pathogenesis of Foot Rot

D. nodosus can be found on both normal hooves and those exhibiting footroot. Therefore, the simple presence of *D. nodosus* is not enough to cause disease. The creation of foot rot in cattle and sheep requires several things to occur together: a moist/wet environment, low/no oxygen, and the presence of *D. nodosus*. An example of a moist or wet environment is a concrete-floored livestock pen that has not been scraped clean of mud, feces, and urine. Another is a boggy, wet field where livestock continuously stand in deep mud with no access to dry ground.

Constant exposure to wet conditions breaks down the naturally hard, resistant barrier of the hoof wall and, in particular, the softer structures on the underside (i.e., plantar surface) of the hoof. The initial entry of *D. nodosus* into the foot is most often through the soft interdigital space between the two claws. From there it can spread under the sole and the hoof wall. Necrosis of these tissues is very painful and can lead to the complete separation of the hoof wall from the soft, sensitive tissues underneath.

Once *D. nodosus* establishes an active infection, it is not uncommon for *F. necrophorum* (covered in the next section) to enter into the area as an opportunist, thus worsening the clinical disease. Foot rot has a characteristic, fetid "rancid butter" odor, likely caused by the addition of *F. necrophorum*. Once you've smelled it, it is hard to forget!

Clinical Disease of Foot Rot

Partly due to the fact that quadrupeds carry a greater percentage of their body weight on their forelimbs, foot rot and the lameness it found more often in the forelimbs. Because their front feet hurt so badly, they may be observed assuming a kneeling position, sometimes refered to as a "prayer" position (Figure 17.6, top panel) Animals that have foot rot in both hindlimbs will try to shift their weight off of their hindfeet and thus toward their front limbs which causes their head to dip down toward the ground (Figure 17.6, bottom panel).

Diagnostics

In most cases of foot rot, diagnostics are not performed. The observed clinical signs are sufficient to warrant initiation of treatment. Also, remember that *D. nodosus* can be present on clinically normal feet. Therefore, positive culture *by itself* does not

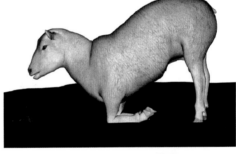

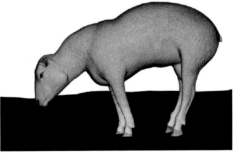

Figure 17.6: Clinical signs associated with foot rot in hoof stock. When the foot rot occurs in one or both front feet, the animal may assume a "prayer" position (**top panel**) in order to take the weight off (and reduce the pain in) the front limbs. Conversely, animals with foot rot in one or both hind feet will shift more weight onto their front limbs causing their head to drop towards the ground (**bottom panel**).

155

mean an animal has foot rot. Culture of the soft affected tissues of the foot might be cultured in the case of treatment failure. This would be to rule-out if the foot rot was caused by another microbe (i.e., independent of *D. nodosus* or *F. necrophorum*)

Treatment

Because both *D. nodosus* and *F. necrophorum* thrive in moist, low-/no-oxygen environments, the first steps in treatment are designed to clean the foot, remove any dead or necrotic material present, and allow oxygen to enter into the tissues. This is done by first washing the gross organic material from the affected feet and then paring out dead and necrotic tissue with a hoof knife. This is followed by topical treatment, such as a 10% zinc sulfate or copper sulfate foot bath. Both of these solutions are drying agents, thus making the environment less hospitable to the agents that contribute to foot rot. During treatment, it is vitally important that the affected hoof is kept clean and dry. Animals should be moved to a clean dry pasture or pen for the duration of treatment.

Prevention

Dry pasture (or pens) and maintaining good hoofcare through regular hoof assessment and trimming are keys to the prevention of foot rot in sheep and cattle. Prompt manure scraping of pens on a regular schedule aids in keeping feet dry as does the practice of periodically rotating animals onto a grassy pasture over packed earth (i.e., not muddy).

Fusobacterium necrophorum

This obligate anaerobe is a cause of liver abcesses in cattle. As it is normally found in the oral cavity and gastrointestinal tract of healthy animals and people, infections are considered to be opportunistic. Additionally, *F. necrophorum* complicates *D. nodosus*-induced foot rot infections.

Morphology and Staining

F. necrophorum is a gram-negative, non-spore-forming fusiform rod. This organism often has a characteristic "rancid butter" odor in culture and clinically.

Pathogenesis

Liver Abcesses

Aggressive grain-feeding results in a lower pH rumen (i.e., more acidic). This acidity is caustic to the epithelial lining of the rumen; the damage renders the rumen susceptible to opportunistic infections, including *F. necrophorum*. When *F. necrophorum* enters the blood stream through the damaged epithelium of the rumen, one of the first organs it colonizes is the liver. These abscesses can be quite large and numerous making the liver unacceptable for human consumption. This can cause economic loss to the farmer.

Foot Rot

F. necrophorum is an opportunistic infection which enters into inflamed hoof structures only after *D. nodosus* has initiated foot rot (see *D. nodosus* section, above). It is thought that the addition of *F. necrophorum* may act synergistically with *D. nodosus* to worsen foot rot when compared to infections consisting only of *D. nodosus*.

Treponemes have been implicated in a newer, somewhat related condition in sheep known as contagious ovine digital dermatitis (CODD). This disease condition is covered briefly in Chapter 16 in the section on *Treponema* species.

Equine Hoof Thrush

Foot rot in horses is termed "**thrush**". Thrush is most often localized to the soft plantar sole of the hoof which usually begins in the area of the frog adjacent to the sulci. The infection and inflamation can spread to other nearby structures including the white line, sole, and other sensitive layers of the foot. Thrush often results in lameness in the affected hoof or hooves. Recently, researchers have proposed that *F. necrophorum*, and not *D. nodosus*, is the likely causative agent of equine thrush. In that study, *F. necrophorum* (and not *D. nodosus*) was present in thrush lesions. However, the authors pointed out that the study did not fullfill all of Koch's postulates. To do that, horses' hooves would need to be experimentally (i.e., purposely) infected with *F. necrophorum* to see if signs of thrush developed. To date, this type of study has not been performed – likely due to both the cost of such a study and ethical concerns. This is an excellent example of how, with some microbes, Koch's postulates have yet to be satisfied – even in this modern era of microbiology!

Treatment and Control

In general, systemic antibiotics are prescribed based on culture and antibiotic susceptibility testing. Additionally, in the case of foot rot, the inflamed hoof tissues are examined. Any abscesses found are lanced and any necrotic tissues are removed. The wound is then usually flushed with antiseptic solution (e.g., copper sulfate) and allowed to drain. To keep the hoof clean and dry, the hoof is bandaged until the wound heals.

A commercial vaccine is available in the US for use in cattle. Cleaning up the environment, preventing cattle from standing in wet conditions, and proper hoof care are all methods used to prevent foot rot. To prevent *F. necrophorum*-induced liver abscesses, farmers should take care not to grain-load their cattle herds.

Bacterioides species

The genus *Bacteroides* contains many species of which *B. fragilis* is the best studied. These bacteria are gram-negative rods that are capable of producing capsule. Members of the genus are common gastro-intestinal commensals and are considered a part of the normal microflora. Infections are largely opportunistic. They usually occur because the bacteria enter into compromised or diseased tissues (e.g., damaged or inflamed intestinal epithelial cells). Calves, lambs, foals, and pigs are susceptible to opportunistic infection. The main result of infection is abscess formation. Selection and handling of samples is the same as for other anaerobes. Many isolates of *B. fragilis* carry β-lactamase enzymes. Therefore use of combination antibiotics like amoxicillin/clavulanic acid are preferred over amoxicillin alone. Because *Bacteroides* spp. are commensals, they may be transmitted to people, especially via dog or cat bites, resulting in local inflammation and abscess formation.

Further Reading

Frosth, Sara, et al. "Characterisation of *Dichelobacter nodosus* and Detection of *Fusobacterium necrophorum* and Treponema Spp. In Sheep with Different Clinical Manifestations of Footrot." *Vet Microbiol* 179 1-2 (2015): 82-90.

Petrov, Kaloyan K., and L. M. Dicks. "*Fusobacterium necrophorum*, and Not *Dichelobacter nodosus*, is Associated with Equine Hoof Thrush." *Vet Microbiol* 161 3-4 (2013): 350-2.

Witcomb, Luci A., et al. "First Study of Pathogen Load and Localisation of Ovine Footrot Using Fluorescence in Situ Hybridisation (Fish)." *Vet Microbiol* 176 3-4 (2015): 321-7.

---. "A Longitudinal Study of the Role of *Dichelobacter nodosus* and *Fusobacterium necrophorum* Load in Initiation and Severity of Footrot in Sheep." *Prev Vet Med* 115 1-2 (2014): 48-55.

Part III:

Veterinary Mycology

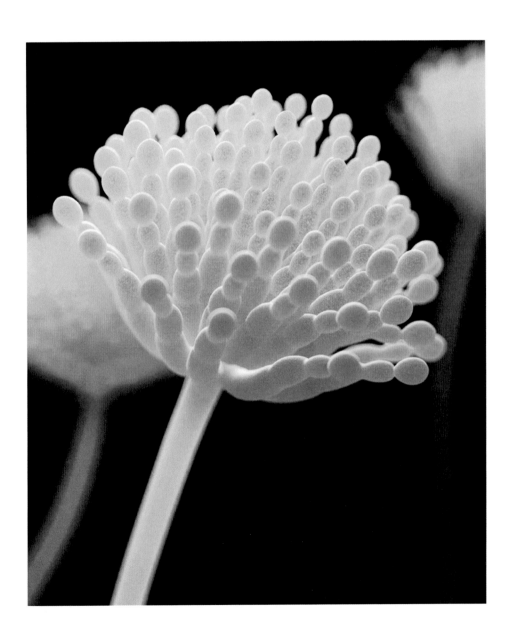

Photo (previous page):

Aspergillus mold. © Can Stock Photos, Image # csp19537542.

Chapter 18:

Mycology: An Introduction

What are Fungi?

The term "fungi"[1] refers to a collection of eukaryotic organisms that possess plant-like cell walls. Depending upon the species of fungus, the cell wall may contain the saccharides cellulose, chitin, glucan, chitosan, or mannan. Fungi may be unicellular or multicellular. Because they are eukaryotic, fungal cells have a nucleus complete with a nuclear membrane that separates the cellular DNA from the cytoplasm. Inside the cytoplasm, fungal organisms contain organelles such as mitochondria, ribosomes, endoplasmic reticulum, lysosomes, secretory vesicles, and the Golgi apparatus. As with other eukaryotes, the cytoplasm contains a network of microtubules; these are part of the cell's cytoskeleton and aid in structural support, especially during cell growth. Unlike plants, fungi are not photosynthetic.

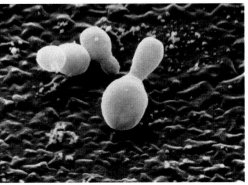

Figure 18.1: Yeast (*Malassezia furfur*) undergoing the process of asexual division (budding), SEM. Courtesy of the Public Health Image Library, PHIL #214, Centers for Disease Control and Prevention, Atlanta, date unknown.

Fungi are strict aerobes. In contrast to most bacteria, fungi are comparatively slow growing and may take a few days up to several weeks before colonies may be seen with the naked eye. Fungi are usually non-motile. Microscopic appearance divides fungi into two main groups: **yeasts** and **molds**. Some fungi are classified as **dimorphic**, and can take on the form of a yeast or mold depending on environmental conditions

Fungal-like agents, although not true fungi, will be discussed later in this chapter as they produce structures that appear very similar to the fungi.

Yeasts

Yeast organisms are oval to spherical single cell fungi that reproduce asexually by budding (Figure 18.1). Asexual reproduction begins with the emergence from the cytoplasm in a process called "budding emergence" (Figure 18.2). DNA replication by mitosis follows. As the bud enlarges, the DNA migrates across the narrow neck into the bud. This is followed by spindle formation. The

---

[1] Pronounced "fun-jeye" – *not* fun-guy.

spindles attach to each chromosome; as they contract toward the poles of the parent and bud, respectively, this allows for chromosomal segregation. Next the cytoplasm at the neck narrows further and eventually the cell walls pinch off in a process called cytokinesis; this leaves a smaller daughter yeast cell and the larger parent cell. The difference in size of the parent and daughter cell is the most visible difference in yeast cell division when compared to bacterial fission. The daughter yeast cell then enters the growth cycle, eventually becoming the same size as the original parent cell. On artificial media, such as agar, most yeast colonies will appear smooth and glistening (Figure 18.3). Examples of yeast include *Candida* and *Malassezia*.

Molds

Molds are multicellular filamentous fungi which consists of masses of threadlike filaments called **hyphae** (Figure 18.4). Hyphae may be separated into chambers by divisions called **septae**. Hyphae grow by elongation of their tips into an intertwining mat called the **mycelium** (Figure 18.5). On artificial media (e.g., agar), most mold colonies will appear "fuzzy" (Figure

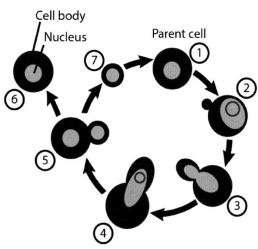

Figure 18.2: Cycle of asexual reproduction in yeast. Steps in the reproductive cycle proceed as follows: (1) the parent cell prepares begin the process; (2) replication of the chromosomal DNA creates 2 duplicate copies while the budding emergence of the cytoplasm begins; (3) budding emergence increases in size; (4) the two chromosomes begin to move to opposite sides of the cell with one located in the bud and one remaining in the parent cell; (5) the nuclei condense and separate as the cytoplasm begins to pinch down and a cross-wall is created to separate the two cells; (6) cross-wall formation is complete thereby releasing the original parent cell to begin another reproductive cycle; (7) the smaller daughter cell is also released and begins to grown in size, soon becoming as large as the original parent cell.

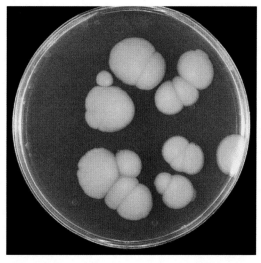

Figure 18.3: *Candida albicans,* a yeast capable of causing disease in multiple species. The colonies appear smooth, white, and glistening. Courtesy of the Public Health Image Library, PHIL #3192, Centers for Disease Control and Prevention, Atlanta, 1969.

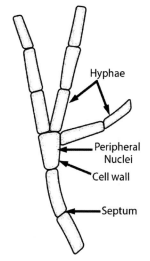

Figure 18.4: Hyphae and other related structures of filamentous fungi. On a microscopic level, molds are made up of filamentous structures called hyphae. Individual fungal cells are separated from one another via a septum.

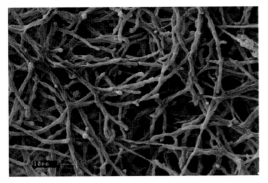

Figure 18.5: Mycelium produced by a fungus, SEM. From: Vadivelan, Ganesan, and Govindarajulu Venkateswaran. "Production and Enhancement of Omega-3 Fatty Acid from *Mortierella Alpina* CFR-GV15: Its Food and Therapeutic Application." *BioMed Research International* 2014 (2014): 657414. *PMC.* Web. Open access.

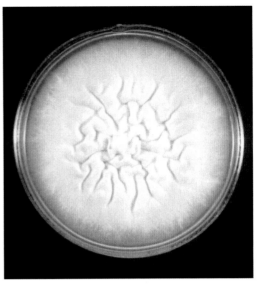

Figure 18.6: Mold (*Trichophyton mentagrophytes*) growing on a Sabouraud's agar plate. Courtesy of the Public Health Image Library, PHIL #14700, Centers for Disease Control and Prevention, Atlanta, 1970, photographer unknown.

18.6). Unlike yeasts, molds can reproduce by either sexual or asexual reproduction. Spores act as the reproductive bodies of fungi. Asexual spores, produced by mitosis, include the sporangiospores and conidia. In those molds that reproduce sexually, spores act as the gametes. For example, zygospores and ascospores are produced by sexual reproduction of *Mucor* and *Aspergillus*, respectively. Most genera of fungi reproduce by a combination of sexual and asexual reproduction; for example, *Rhizopus stolonifer*, known by its common name as black bread mold.

Fungal-like Agents

As the name suggests, fungal-like agents are eukaryotes that are not true fungi. When found in tissues, these species produce elements that resemble fungi. Some fungal-like agents form yeast-like colonies when grown on mycologic media. Genera that are members of this group include *Prototheca*, a type of green algae (Figure 18.7), and *Pythium*, an Oomycete which belong to the same kingdom as diatoms and brown algae.

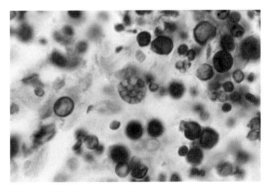

Figure 18.7: *Prototheca*, a fungal-like organism, stained with PAS (Periodic acid-Schiff). Fungal-like organisms share morphologic similarities to fungal organisms. Courtesy of the Public Health Image Library, PHIL #11983, Centers for Disease Control and Prevention, Atlanta, 1971.

Fungal Diseases – General Attributes

Fungal agents can be grouped using two different schema: the ability to cause disease and tissue preference. Like bacteria, fungi can be labeled as pathogenic or opportunistic. Fungal agents may also be grouped by whether they prefer to inhabit one of three locations: superficial (cutaneous), deep (subcutaneous), or systemic tissues (Table 18.1). It is, however, important to remember that a species of fungi may cause a variety of clinical presentations.

Table 18.1: Selected fungal pathogens of interest in veterinary medicine.

Species	Classification	Form	Infection
Dermatophytes (*Microsporum* sp., *Trichophyton* sp.)	Fungi	Mold	Superficial
Aspergillus fumigatus	Fungi	Mold	Systemic (*)
Malassezia pachydermatis	Fungi	Yeast	Superficial
Cryptococcus neoformans	Fungi	Yeast	Systemic (*)
Candida albicans	Fungi	Yeast	Systemic (*)
Sporothrix schenckii	Fungi	Dimorphic	Subcutaneous
Histoplasma capsulatum var. *farciminosum*	Fungi	Dimorphic	Subcutaneous
Histoplasma capsulatum var. *capsulatum*	Fungi	Dimorphic	Systemic
Blastomyces dermatitis	Fungi	Dimorphic	Systemic
Coccidioides immitis	Fungi	Dimorphic	Systemic
Pythium insidiosum	Fungal-like element	N/A	Subcutaneous
Prototheca spp.	Fungal-like element	N/A	Subcutaneous
Rhinosporidium seeberi	Fungal-like element	N/A	Subcutaneous

* May cause superficial or systemic infections.
N/A = not applicable

Diagnostics Used in Mycology

Diagnosis of a fungal infection is largely based on detection of fungal elements in tissues. Whether the fungal elements are observe in tissues or in culture, the single most important information required for species identification is the morphology. In culture, both macroscopic and microscopic morphology are considered for identification. As more is known about genomic differences between species, PCR is gaining importance as a tool for fungal identification. Below is a brief description of methods for diagnosing fungi. A more in-depth discussion of methods can be found in Chapter 23.

Culture

Culturing molds and yeasts requires media specifically formulated to support fungal growth, therefore it is important that fungal culture be specifically requested when a fungal infection is suspected. Sabouraud's and potato dextrose agars are two good general purpose agars capable of supporting the growth of many fungal species, and are routinely used as primary isolation agars. Because fungi often take a much longer time to grow, bacteria contaminating the sample can quickly outgrow any fungi present. For this reason, many fungal culture media contain compounds for the purpose of suppressing the growth of bacteria. In the case of Sabouraud's and potato dextrose agars, the high sugar content and acidic pH of these media inhibit bacterial growth. Adding antibiotics (e.g., chloramphenicol) to fungal media can further inhibit bacterial growth.

Other media are used only with specific types of fungi, such as Dermatophyte Test Medium (DTM) which is used to detect dermatophytes (i.e., a group of fungal agents that target the skin). DTM should not be used to culture non-dermatophytes, deep, or systemic fungi. Thus, it is important to know what fungal organisms the veterinarian suspects when choosing the proper growth media.

Once colonies of fungi become visible, a "tape prep" procedure can be used to mount fungal elements to a slide for examination under the microscope. This is accomplished by touching the sticky side of clear cellophane (e.g., Scotch®) tape to the edge of a colony and then placing the tape on a microscope slide where a drop of lactophenol cotton blue stain has been placed. The combination of macroscopic and microscopic morphology is used to identify the fungal species in question.

Cytology

Aside from fungal culture, examination of skin scrapings and tissue touch preps can be quite useful in the identification of fungal infections. These cytologic specimens contain cellular material that may obscure the technician's ability to correctly identify the fungal agent(s) present. For this reason, potassium hydroxide (KOH) is an important reagent in the veterinary technician's diagnostic tool kit (see Chapter 23). KOH is used in fungal wet mounts as a clearing agent which digests the proteinaceous components of the host cells while leaving the polysaccharide fungal cell wall intact.

Briefly, the sample is applied to a clean glass slide by spreading or touching it to the slide. The sample is then mixed with a drop of KOH. This mixture is allowed to incubate at room temperature for at least 30 minutes. Optimal digestion often can take as long as 4 hours. After the KOH digestion step, examine the slide using the 100x & 400x objectives and look for fungal elements. There are a number of different stains which can be added to the sample preparation to aid in the visualization of the fungal elements. These include: India ink; lactophenol cotton blue; and hematologic stains, such as Giemsa or Romanowsky (Diff-Quik®). Gram stains are generally not used as they can distort fungal morphology making identification extremely difficult.

Further Reading

Larone, Davise Honig. *Medically Important Fungi: A Guide to Identification.* 5th edition. Washington, DC: American Society for Microbiology, 2011.

Chapter 19:

Superficial Fungal Infections

Introduction
Fungi capable of invading the epithelial skin and mucous membranes of animals cause superficial fungal infections. Superficial fungal infections are more common in a clinical setting than subcutaneous or systemic mycoses. Skin and ear infections are the most common manifestations of disease.

The Dermatophytes
A group of superficial fungi that target the skin are known as the **dermatophytes**. These ubiquitous fungi have a world-wide geographic range and are capable of surviving for years in the environment. The two most common genera encountered in veterinary practice are *Microsporum* and *Trichophyton*.

Host and Reservoirs
The dermatophytes are highly infectious and can be passed to other mammals, including humans. Dermatophytes can be subdivided into three groups based on host(s) they are best adapted to and include: **geophilic** (environment), **zoophilic** (animal), and **anthropophilic** (human) dermatophytes. These preferences, however, do not preclude a particular species from infecting hosts other than their preference. For example, zoophilic isolates can infect humans and anthropophilic isolates can infect animals, though this last route is uncommon. Geophilic dermatophytes which live in the soil as saprophytes, can be contracted by exposure to contaminated soil and cause disease in mammals.

Transmission
Risk factors for transmission include crowding, dampness in the environment, and contact with infected animals. Contact with the fungal organisms in the environment or on fomites can also facilitate transmission of disease.

Pathogenesis
Dermatophytes produce conidia (see "Molds", Chapter 18) that are capable of penetrating the top layer of skin (i.e., stratum corneum). They can also invade the hair follicle. While rare, dermatophyte infections do occasionally spontaneously heal. However, most infections become progressively more generalized as autoinfection occurs transferring fungi from one area of skin to another. This usually occurs due to scratching at the lesions and transferring conidia to a separate site, thus making **dermatophytosis** an insidious disease to treat. Dermatophyte infections are very itchy. Secondary bacterial infections are possible (e.g., staphylococci), especially when scratching by the patient is severe and results in damage to the epithelium.

Dermatophyte Species Commonly Seen in Veterinary Medicine
Selected dermatophytes and their reservoir preference are summarized in Table 19.1. Most infections

in veterinary patients are caused by the zoophilic or geophilic dermatophytes; infections by anthropophilic infections are extremely rare.

Table 19.1: Selected dermatophytes, their host preferences and preferred habitat

Dermatophyte	Host species	Classification
Microsporum gypseum	Horses, dogs, rodents	Geophilic
Microsporum nanum	Pigs	Geophilic
Microsporum canis	Cats, dogs	Zoophilic
Microsporum distortum	Dogs, primates	Zoophilic
Trichophyton gallinae	Chickens, turkeys	Zoophilic
Trichophyton equinum	Horses	Zoophilic
Trichophyton verrucosum	Cattle	Zoophilic

Disease

The common name for the disease condition caused by dermatophyte infections is **ringworm**. This name is a misnomer as the infection is caused by a fungus and not a worm. However, the skin lesions often indeed appear ring-like (Figure 19.1). Observations of such lesions on the skin of a human accompanying their pet to see the veterinarian can greatly aid in diagnosing the animal's condition.

Dogs

Dogs are most often infected with either *Microsporum canis* (Figure 19.2 and Figure 19.4) or *Microsporum gypseum*. Lesions will appear scaly with central alopecia and the skin may be thickened. While not the most common cause of ringworm, infection with *Trichophyton mentagrophytes* may cause more extensive scaling, and inflammatory reaction in affected dogs.

Cats

M. canis is the most common species affecting cats (Figure 19.3). However, the infection is often subclinical. Asymptomatic cats can act as mechanical vectors and sources of infection for other animals and people in the household, shelter or cattery. Clinically affected cats present with alopecia surrounding the scaly lesions. In severe cases, infection may to lead the creation of subcutaneous swellings with draining tracts. Lesions may be difficult to observe in long-haired breeds.

Swine

Microsporum nanum infects swine and often

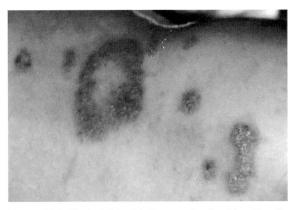

Figure 19.1: Typical "ring" lesions on the shoulder skin of a human patient infected with *Trichophyton verrucosum*, one of several fungal agents responsible for the condition known as ringworm. Courtesy of the Public Health Image Library, PHIL #15436, Centers for Disease Control and Prevention, Atlanta, 1969.

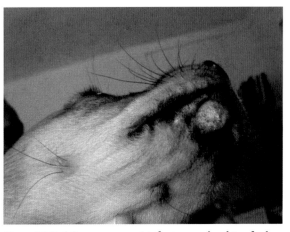

Figure 19.2: *Microsporum canis* infection on the chin of a dog. The lesion is covered with crust. Upon removal of the crust and a skin scraping was taken revealing the *M. canis* organisms. Courtesy of the Veterinary Image Bank, Dr. Giorgio Cancedda, Italy.

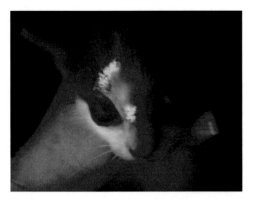

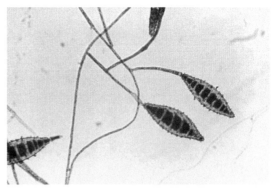

Figure 19.3: Kitten infected with *Microsporum canis* that fluoresces under a Wood's lamp. Only about half of all *Microsporum* isolates, and none of the other dermatophyte species, will fluoresce when placed under the Wood's lamp. Therefore, a negative Wood's lamp test does not mean that an animal is free from dermatophytes. Courtesy of the Veterinary Image Bank, Dr. Galleani Pierantionio.

Figure 19.4: *Microsporum canis,* lactophenol cotton blue. Courtesy of the Public Health Image Library, PHIL #15472, Centers for Disease Control and Prevention, Atlanta, 1964.

presents as brown crusts covering most of the animal's body.

Poultry
Ringworm in fowl, especially chickens and turkeys, is referred to as "favus" or "white comb" and is caused by *Microsporum gallinae*. This is usually a self-limiting condition and involves small to large white patches on the comb. When the fungus spreads to the feathered parts of the bird, emaciation and death may ensue.

Ruminants
Young cattle kept indoors during the winter are at increased risk of developing ringworm lesions. They typically present as alopecic crusts on the face, especially around the eyes, the neck and shoulders.

Horses
Ringworm may be common in large stables, especially when grooming tools, harnesses and blankets are shared. *Trichophyton equinum* is the most likely cause, and outbreaks can be controlled by treating all animals and disinfecting all shared tools and implements.

Rodents
In rodents (e.g., rats, mice, and guinea pigs) and rabbits, the isolate most commonly responsible for ringworm infections is *Trichophyton mentagrophytes* (Figure 19.5).

Diagnostics

Wood's lamp
A Wood's lamp (Figure 19.6) can be a useful first tool in determining if a patient is infected with *Microsporum*. The Wood's lamp may be operated in one of two ways. First, the lamp is turned on and held over any suspected lesions. Alternately, a few hairs from the periphery of

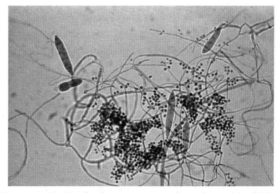

Figure 19.5: *Trichophyton mentagrophytes,* lactophenol blue stain. Courtesy of the Public Health Image Library, PHIL #15105, Centers for Disease Control and Prevention, Atlanta, 1964.

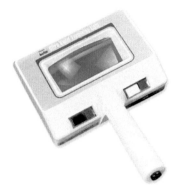

Figure 19.6: Wood's lamp. This piece of equipment is a UV-lamp modified with a viewing window so as to observe for fluorescence of hair shafts infected with dermatophytes. Courtesy of Paragon Medical. Used with permission.

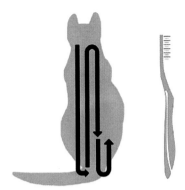

Figure 19.7: Mackenzie brush technique. Typical path used when brushing with a clean toothbrush to ensure systematic coverage all surfaces of the animal during the Mackenzie brush technique. This same pathway can be used for the Wood's lamp examination.

lesions may plucked using forceps or tweezers. These hairs are then examined under the Wood's lamp. About 50 percent of *Microsporum* isolates produce a pigment which fluoresces under a Wood's lamp. However, a Wood's lamp is not useful in determining if *Trichophyton* is present as this species does not fluoresce.

Standard Culture

Obtaining appropriate samples is important for successful isolation of dermatophytes in culture. If an animal is symptomatic, appropriate samples include skin scrapings or hair that is plucked from the periphery of the suspected ringworm lesions. When determining the carrier status of an asymptomatic animal, especially cats, the **Mackenzie brush technique** is recommended. Briefly, a clean unused toothbrush is obtained. The toothbrush is used to brush the entire fur coat of the animal (Figure 19.7). Any loose hyphae or spores should adhere to the bristles of the toothbrush. The toothbrush bristles are gently pressed onto the fungal culture media. The DTM is allowed to incubate at room temperature for up to 14 days.

These fungi are aerobes that grow best at room temperature or slightly warmer (i.e., 25-30°C). The best growth can be seen on Sabouraud's dextrose agar. Due to the slow growth of the dermatophytes, fungal cultures should be incubated for up to 1 month. Once fungal colonies appear, the color and character of the colonies should be noted. Next, small samples can be taken and examined under the microscope in order to identify any macro- or microconidia. Samples should be cleared of host cells using KOH (see previous chapter) before adding a stain. Lactophenol cotton blue is a good stain to aid in identification. The size, shape, and number of compartments of the conidia aid in identification of the dermatophytes present (Table 19.2).

Table 19.2: Comparison of the macro- and microconidia present in *Microsporum and Trichophyton*

	Microsporum sp.	*Trichophyton* sp.
Macroconidia		
Shape	Spindle-shaped	Club-shaped
Wall type	Rough walls	Smooth walls
Chamber number	≥6 chambers	<6 chambers
Microconidia		
Number	Few	Abundant
Shape	Club-shaped	Teardrop-shaped

Dermatophyte Test Medium

A very useful in-house test for the diagnosis of dermatophyte infections is the Dermatophyte Test Medium (DTM). DTM is both a selective and a differential medium (Figure 19.8). It is based on the recipe for Sabouraud's agar. To the basic recipe, an antibiotic (i.e., chloramphenicol) is added to the agar to inhibit a wide range of gram-positive and gram-negative bacteria. Cycloheximide is added to inhibit saprophytic fungi that could potentially contaminate the culture media. Finally, a pH indicator, phenol red, is used to detect the alkaline metabolites produced by dermatophytes. If these alkaline metabolites are produced by the fungi inoculated onto the DTM, then the media will change from its original yellow-orange color to a red color. In addition to recording any color change to the media, record the colony morphology and color. Most dermatophytes produce white colonies. Black, grey, and brown pigmentation is common with saprophytic fungi. To avoid false positive culture interpretations, it is important to observe the media daily to observe simultaneous color change and dermatophyte-like fungal growth.

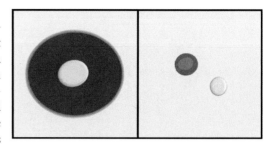

Figure 19.8: Illustration of dermatophyte test medium (DTM) with examples of possible results. Dermatophytes will grow as white colonies and cause the pH indicator (e.g., phenol red) to turn the media red (left). Environmental fungi and other non-dermatophytes will usually grow as pigmented colonies (although there are exceptions) and the media will remain pale yellow (right).

Treatment

There are a variety of options when treating dermatophyte infections. The particular treatment the veterinarian makes is often based on the severity of the infection and ease of client compliance. In cases where there are only a few small lesions, topical antifungal creams, such as miconazole and clotrimazole, may be used. For more generalized disease with lesions extending over a large portion of the skin, medicated baths such as lime sulfur dips may be tried. In both of the above cases, the veterinary technician may be asked to shave the hair from the affected areas. This gives an opportunity for better contact of the medications with the infected skin. The technician should then take care to thoroughly disinfect the clippers and clipper blades directly after use to avoid them from becoming fomites themselves.

Remember this: Sanitize those clippers!
Clippers should be sanitized after using them to shave animals being treated for ringworm. Otherwise **WE** will have created a fomite capable of passing on the infection to our other patients!

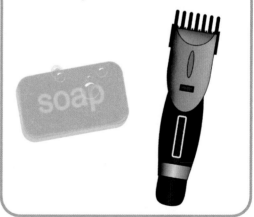

If topical treatments are not an option, or in cases of severe, generalized infections, systemic antifungal drugs (e.g., ketoconazole) may be given by mouth. It is important that clients understand that treatment must continue for the entire time prescribed – even when there are no visible lesions present. If even a small number of conidia are present in the skin, this can cause a recurrence of the dermatophyte infection.

Control

Dermatophytes survive very well in the environment. Luckily, however, they are susceptible to some common disinfectants such as household bleach and iodine. In the case of pets, every surface the pet comes into contact with should be cleaned using a disinfectant. Bedding can be laundered separately from the rest of the household laundry using the hottest water setting available. For livestock, contaminated bedding should be removed and replaced with fresh bedding. Any brushes, halters, clippers, or other fomites should be disinfected thoroughly before using on any other animals. Isolate affected individuals from the rest of the herd until the infection is completely cleared.

Zoonosis

The most common zoonotic dermatophytes are: *M. canis*, *T. mentagrophytes*, and *T. verrucosum*. However, all of the dermatophytes are potential zoonotic fungi. Members of the veterinary team should wear gloves when handling infected or suspect animals. Practicing good hygiene (e.g., hand washing) is essential to preventing occupationally-acquired infections.

Anthroponosis

The dermatophytes are highly contagious. While rare, it is possible for humans to transfer a dermatophyte infection to the animals, such as pets or livestock that they handle. Furthermore, there are dermatophytes that are host-adapted specifically to people (e.g., *M. audouini* and *T. rubrum*). Therefore, members of the veterinary team should be cautious before blaming an animal, particularly one that has no visible lesions (e.g., the family cat) if an owner reports that a family member is suspected of having a ringworm infection. Cultures should be taken from asymptomatic animals in order to attempt to establish whether or not they may be harboring a dermatophyte, although a causal relationship between the cat's dermatophyte infection and the human infection is difficult to prove (See also: "Mackenzie Brush Technique", above).

Malassezia

An oval-shaped budding yeast, *Malassezia* prefers an aerobic or microaerophilic environment (Figure 19.9). Its reservoir is the skin (i.e., stratum corneum) of healthy animals and is rarely found in the environment. Thus, *Malassezia* is an opportunist pathogen with infections usually originating from endogenous sources. There are several species of *Malassezia*, but *Malassezia pachydermatis* is most commonly associated with disease in animals.

Pathogenesis

Because *Malassezia* is a member of the normal skin flora of most animals, in order for it to cause disease there must be either an alteration of the normal skin flora or the skin surface must be compromised in some way, such as by trauma. Areas of the skin that are warm and moist support the growth – and overgrowth – of *Malassezia*. Animal species or breeds that have long external ear canals (e.g., Cocker Spaniel) or excessive skin folds (e.g., Chinese Shar-Pei) are at higher risk for clinical infections due to the overgrowth of *Malassezia*. Another factor which predisposes animals to *Malassezia* infections is immune system malfunction as is the case with allergies (e.g., canine atopy) and immunocompromised states.

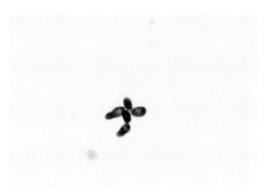

Figure 19.9: *Malassezia pachydermatis*, Gram stain. Courtesy of the Public Health Image Library, PHIL #268, Centers for Disease Control and Prevention, Atlanta, date unknown.

Disease conditions

Otitis externa is a common clinical manifestation of *Malassezia* overgrowth in dogs and has also been reported in llamas. *Malassezia* causes dermatitis in horses, dogs and cats.

Diagnostics

Cytology

Swabs of the external ear or skin lesions can be rolled gently on clean glass slides to make cytologic preparations for examination with a light microscope. Similarly, cellophane tape can be touched to a lesion and then placed on a clean glass slide. Slides may be stained with Gram stain or Diff-Quik®, though budding yeast are often visible even without the use of a cytological stain. The budding yeast have been described as having the shape of a "footprint", "peanut", or "bottle". Cytology is often a more sensitive method for identification than histopathology.

Culture

Malassezia can grow on regular blood agar used for bacterial isolation, but is easily overgrown by bacteria. Therefore it is best grown on solid fungal media (agar) containing antibiotics to inhibit bacterial overgrowth. Plates should be incubated at 32-37°C for up to one week.

Treatment and Prevention

Treatment of infections uses a two pronged approach. Topical antifungal treatments can be used effectively to kill the *Malassezia*. However, as this is most often an opportunistic infection, treatment must also be aimed at the predisposing factors involved (e.g., atopy and/or anatomic conformation). Owners should institute regular ear or skin fold cleaning to ensure the removal of debris and thorough drying of these areas that are prone to overgrowth and clinical disease.

Zoonotic potential

While zoonotic infections of *Malassezia* are thought to be rare, there is one report of dog-to-human-to-human transmission involving a neonatal intensive care unit (NICU) nurse living in the same household as an infected dog. The nurse is thought to have passed the infection onto a child in the NICU.

Further Reading

Bond, Ross. "Superficial Veterinary Mycoses." *Clin Dermatol* 28 2 (2010): 226-36.

Cafarchia, Claudia, Luciana A. Figueredo, and Domenico Otranto. "Fungal Diseases of Horses." *Vet Microbiol* 167 1-2 (2013): 215-34.

Frymus, Tadeusz, et al. "Dermatophytosis in Cats: ABCD Guidelines on Prevention and Management." *J Feline Med Surg* 15 7 (2013): 598-604.

Chapter 20:

The Subcutaneous Mycoses

Introduction
Fungi found in this group infect and cause damage to the skin, the subcutaneous skin tissue, and the associated local lymphatics. While the infections due to these fungi are most often limited to the aforementioned tissues, infection can spread systemically, especially in susceptible species or those individuals that are immunocompromised.

Sporothrix schenckii
While not the only member of the genus, *Sporothrix schenckii* is the most common causative species of sporotrichosis in our domestic animal species. The organism is a saprophyte, preferring soil rich in decaying matter. A dimorphic fungus, *S. schenckii* is found in its filamentous form with hyphae at room temperature (25°C) and its yeast form when *in vivo* or cultured at 37°C.

Distribution of *Sporothrix schenckii* is worldwide, but is most abundantly found in tropical and semi-tropical climes. *S. schenckii* can survive in the soil, especially where sphagnum moss grows or in decaying organic material.

Disease
A number of species can act as host to *Sporothrix schenckii* including cats, dogs, horses, parrots, rodents and humans. However, the cat is particularly sensitive to infection. Disease in animals tends to be sporadic, but outbreaks have been reported (e.g., Brazil, 1998-2004).

Infection is most commonly contracted when the mold form gains access to a host via traumatic inoculation. Exudate from lesions may be infectious, especially if it is a cat, as their exudate has a large quantity of organisms. Inhalation of spores has resulted in infection, but is quite an uncommon route.

Clinical presentations of sporotrichosis can be described as cutaneous, cutaneolymphatic or disseminated. In immunocompetent patients, infections are most commonly cutaneous or cutaneolymphatic. Immunosuppression can predispose the patient to the

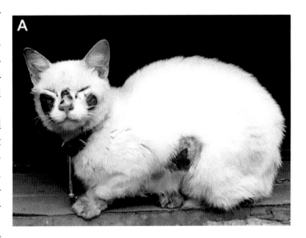

Figure 20.1: Clinical signs of sporotrichosis in a cat. Note the wet, ulcerated skin lesions. From: Montenegro, H., et al. Montenegro, Hildebrando, et al. "Feline Sporotrichosis Due to *Sporothrix brasiliensis*: An Emerging Animal Infection in São Paulo, Brazil." *BMC Vet Res* 10 (2014): 269. Open access.

disseminated form. The exception is the cat. Immunocompetent felines will develop cutaneolymphatic or disseminated disease.

Lesions most often appear on the lower half of the limbs. In some small animal cases, the head or tail base may also be affected (Figure 20.1). At first, the lesions look much like any other draining abscess, but later develop into ulcerated, cutaneous nodules. Large crusts may be present in ulcerated areas. Not surprisingly, because *Sporothrix* is a fungus, the infection shows incomplete response to antibiotic therapy. Infection may follow the lymphatics, resulting in thickened lymphatic vessels and new nodules appearing along the lymph pathway. This is referred to as the **cutaneolymphatic** form. The disseminated form is very rare, except in cats, and can involve multiple sites in the body including viscera, joints, bones and the central nervous system.

In a retrospective study of 337 cats, about 3% were asymptomatic carriers with another 27% of cats transiently but asymptomatically infected. The remaining cats (approximately 60%) exhibited clinical disease ranging from cutaneous to systemic illness.

Diagnostics
Sample choice will depend on the clinical signs and extent of the disease. *S. schenckii* organisms can be demonstrated in exudate (i.e., pus), biopsies submitted for histopathology, or blood (i.e., systemic infections).

Cytology
Sporothrix schenckii is usually readily visible in cytologic specimens of exudate from infected cats or other immunocompromised hosts (Figure 20.2). They are not as readily visible in the wounds of horses or dogs. Because of the scarcity of the organism found in infections within these species, it is imperative to use KOH to clear host debris before attempting to view samples under the microscope and look for the yeast cells. The organism's yeast form can appear round- to cigar-shaped. If only the round form is present, it can be difficult to distinguish from other fungal pathogens.

Histopathology
The tissue processing required for histopathologic examination can result in altered morphology of the organism and misidentification. Therefore, immunofluorescent labeling which specifically targets the organism of interest can be helpful in making a correct diagnosis. It is wise to contact the reference laboratory prior to collecting and sending tissues as the lab may require that special procedures be followed. Not following these procedures may result in samples that are not diagnostic.

Culture
The organism grows readily on standard fungal media. Definitive identification requires growth in both the mold and yeast forms. At 25°C most colonies of *S. schenckii* appear in 5-7 days, and are initially moist, white to creamy and become fuzzy and pigmented (i.e., brown to black) after several days of incubation. However, a small subset of isolates may produce pigmented colonies almost immediately. *Sporothrix* produces colonies that are flat, not fluffy, when grown on agar. The yeast form of *S. schenckii* can be induced between 35 to 37°C on blood agar. Yeast colonies are smooth and white and appear within a few days. Culture can be a risk to laboratory personnel so precautions should be taken (e.g. wearing proper PPE) to avoid laboratory-acquired infections.

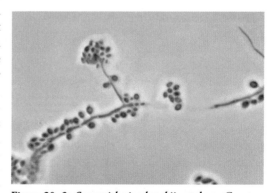

Figure 20. 2: *Sporotrichosis schenckii,* cytology. Courtesy of the Public Health Image Library, PHIL #4208, Centers for Disease Control and Prevention, Atlanta, 1972.

Other Tests

Serologic tests are available, but infrequently used for testing animals. PCR tests available from some academic or commercial reference labs are useful for direct identification of the organism in clinical samples, and also for identification of culture isolates. Contact the reference laboratory prior to collecting and shipping samples.

Treatment

A variety of antifungal drugs are effective against sporotrichosis. Itraconazole is often the veterinarian's first choice of treatment.

Zoonosis

People working, handling, or living with cats infected with *S. schenckii* are at risk of the disease. These individuals should wear latex or nitrile gloves when handling infected cats. Asymptomatic animals may also be a source of infection. Disease manifestation in people is similar to animals and can present as cutaneous, subcutaneous, or systemic.

It is important to note that people, particularly those who garden, are at risk of acquiring the disease independent of handling animals. This disease in humans is often referred to as "rose gardener's disease." Sphagnum moss has been identified as a source of environmentally acquired human infections. Thus, human sporotrichosis is not necessarily due to contact with animals. The veterinarian will be able to advise clients with sporotrichosis on options to try and identify if an animal was involved in the transmission of the disease to a person(s).

Control

Because of the ubiquitous nature of *Sporothrix schenckii*, it is impossible to completely eliminate the organism from the environment. However, animals should be kept away from Sphagnum moss and decaying organic material. Intact toms are more likely to fight other males for breeding access to receptive females. As *Sporothrix* is often transmitted via trauma, clients should be advised to spay and neuter their cats to decrease aggressive behaviors.

Histoplasma capsulatum var. *farciminosum*

This variety of *H. capsulatum* causes epizootic lymphangitis, also known as pseudoglanders. It does not cause disseminated disease, known as histoplasmosis, which is discussed in Chapter 21. Like *Sporothrix* sp., *H. capsulatum* is a dimorphic fungus, taking on the mold form at room temperature (25°C) and the yeast form at body temperature (37°C). The saprophytic (mold) form is most at home in nitrogen-rich soils. Endemic areas include some Mediterranean countries, and parts of Africa and Asia, including India, Pakistan and Japan.

Disease

Epizootic lymphangitis most commonly infects horses, donkeys and mules, but has been reported in other species. The first sign of infection is a skin nodule. That innocent looking nodule will develop into an abscess that ruptures, leaving behind an ulcerated lesion. The typical course of disease involves failure of complete healing, recurrence and spread of nodules. Lesions are most commonly noted on the head, neck and limbs. Cases of pneumonia and ulcerative conjunctivitis have also been attributed to *H. capsulatum* var. *farciminosum*.

Diagnostics

A diagnosis can be reached by examination of stained exudates or by isolation of the organism on standard fungal media. Macroscopic and microscopic morphology can allow differentiation of *H. capsulatum* var. *farciminosum* from other *H. capsulatum* varieties.

Treatment

A variety of antifungal drugs have been effective in treating epizootic lymphangitis. However, in non-endemic regions, destruction of the infected animal is recommended, and often required.

Fungal-like agent: *Pythium insidiosum*

Formerly classified as a fungus, *Pythium* is now considered an oomycete, belonging to the same kingdom as diatoms and brown algae. *P. insidiosum* causes disease in animals, including horses, cattle, dogs and cats. Because of the association with stagnant ponds, the disease is commonly referred to as "swamp cancer."

Disease

In cases of cutaneous pythiosis, lesions appear ulcerative, granulomatous and may contain fistulous. Lesions are most often found on the limbs and ventrum, which are the areas of the body most likely to contact the standing water where the organism resides. The organism gains entry through skin lesions, even small scratches. Dogs, however, are more likely to present with gastrointestinal disease, and transmission is thought to occur via drinking contaminated water.

Diagnostics

Many diagnostic tests are available. Direct cytology of clinical specimen may reveal fungal like elements that closely mimic hyphae. PCR and serology tests are available. The organism will grow on standard fungal media, and identification of motile zoospores confirms the diagnosis.

Treatment

Surgical debridement of lesions and treatment with a systemic antifungal, such as amphotericin B, are appropriate treatments.

Control

Keep animals away from stagnant ponds. Prevention of pythiosis is only one of many reasons to avoid stagnant water.

Further Reading

Barros, Monica B., Rodrigo de Almeida Paes, and Armando O. Schubach. "Sporothrix Schenckii and Sporotrichosis." *Clin Microbiol Rev* 24 4 (2011): 633-54.

Lloret, Albert, et al. "Sporotrichosis in Cats: Abcd Guidelines on Prevention and Management." *J Feline Med Surg* 15 7 (2013): 619-23.

Schubach, Armando, Monica B. Barros, and Bodo Wanke. "Epidemic Sporotrichosis." *Curr Opin Infect Dis* 21 2 (2008): 129-33.

Schubach, Tania M., et al. "Evaluation of an Epidemic of Sporotrichosis in Cats: 347 Cases (1998-2001)." *J Am Vet Med Assoc* 224 10 (2004): 1623-9.

Spickler, Anna Rovid. "Fact Sheet: Epizootic Lymphangitis." Center for Public Health and Food Safety, 2009. Web. At http://www.cfsph.iastate.edu/Factsheets/pdfs/epizootic_lymphangitis.pdf.

Chapter 21:

The Systemic Mycoses

Introduction

While the fungi targeting the superficial and subcutaneous tissues can cause substantial damage to their respective host tissues, by far the most serious fungal infections are the systemic (or "deep") mycoses. Because these fungi possess the capability to invade deeper host tissues and target multiple organ systems, they are the most dangerous in terms of morbidity and mortality. Thus, the veterinarian must make a prompt and accurate diagnosis and members of the veterinary team must be vigilant in their continuing assessment and care of these patients.

The four most common systemic fungi will be discussed in this chapter: *Blastomyces, Histoplasma, Coccidioides*, and *Cryptococcus*. The first three are dimorphic fungi, existing in the mold form in nature or when cultured at room temperature (25°C), and in the yeast form in host tissue or in culture at 37°C. Due to the potential hazard of live cultures, it is recommended that samples be submitted to reference laboratories and not cultured in-house. Treatment of systemic fungal infections requires a long course of therapy.

Blastomyces dermatitidis

Blastomyces dermatitidis represents the species of most significance in veterinary medicine within this genus.

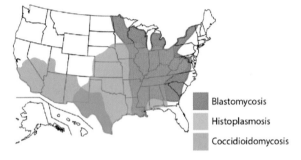

Figure 21.1: Current distribution of common fungal diseases occurring in the United States. Illustration created by the authors using aggregate data from the Centers for Disease Control.

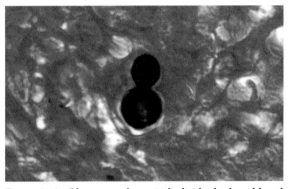

Figure 21.2: *Blastomyces dermatitidis* **divides by broad-based budding.** Courtesy of the Public Health Image Library, PHIL #2889, Centers for Disease Control and Prevention, Atlanta, 1978.

Reservoir and Geographic Distribution

Blastomyces dermatitis inhabits the soil preferring the sandy, acid soils found near bodies of water. The geographic distribution of most reported clinical cases is found around the Mississippi and the St.

Laurence rivers (Figure 21.1). *Blastomyces* produces spores capable of surviving for long periods, especially when soil is enriched with rotting vegetation. *Blastomyces* divides by broad-based budding (Figure 21.2).

Hosts and Transmission

Inhalation of spores constitutes the primary method of transmitting *B. dermatitidis* between individuals (Figure 21.3). The spores germinate once inside the body and quickly transition from the mycelial to yeast phase in the lung. Occasionally, the fungus can enter the body via wound contamination with the yeast phase of *B. dermatitidis* (e.g., dog bite or other accidental contamination). Hosts can include dogs, humans, cats, horses, ferrets and wildlife.

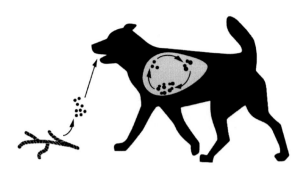

Figure 21.3: **Typical transmission and pathogenesis of infections caused by** *Blastomyces dermatitidis.* Animals typically acquire infections via inhalation of spores from fungal elements. Once in the lung, the fungus transitions from the mycelial phase to the yeast phase quickly asexually reproducing and creating more yeasts.

Risk Factors

Drought, dust, excavation activity, and living near water are all considered risk factors for becoming infected with *Blastomyces*. While infections in strictly indoor animals have occurred, animals with outdoor activity or those that live exclusively outdoors are at highest risk for infection. There is a seasonal influence as well with the spring usually being too wet to sustain the infections. Infections are usually seen from summer-winter. Dogs are very sensitive to infection and are considered the species at greatest risk. Sporting and large breeds, intact males, and dogs between the ages of 1-5 years are at highest risk among all dogs. *What do these groups have in common?* The answer: *an increased tendency toward roaming.*

Compared to dogs, humans and cats are considered intermediately sensitive. Horses can be infected but are considered to be relatively resistant when compared to the other species mentioned.

Clinical Disease

Asymptomatic infections do occur. Clinical infections may remain localized in the pulmonary system causing pneumonia and clinical signs such as dyspnea. Often dissemination occurs via the vascular and lymphatic systems. Clinical signs depend on tissue(s) affected. Preferred sites of dissemination include: skin, bone, eye, lymph node, testes, brain, subcutaneous tissue, and the external nares. However the organism can settle in just about any location in the body.

Diagnostics

Exudates and tissues are appropriate samples. Contact the reference laboratory for detailed instructions.

Culture

For reasons of occupational safety, samples should be submitted to a reference laboratory for culture. These laboratories have additional safety features allowing them to culture the fungi with minimal risk to the laboratorians.

Other Methods

Serology is useful for looking for antibodies produced against *B. dermatitidis*, however antibodies may remain at detectable levels even after the patient has cleared the infection. Molecular methods, such as PCR, are also diagnostic options. The veterinarian will be able to decide what option is the safest and most reliable method for a particular patient.

Treatment

Because blastomycosis is a deep, systemic fungus, systemic antifungals must be used. The drug of choice is itraconazole, but amphotericin B and ketoconazole, alone or in combination, are also effective. Topical drugs will not be useful.

Human infections

Transmission from animals to humans is rare, however caution must be taken when handling infected animals or their tissues. Transmission to humans via dog bites has been reported, though is rare. More commonly, individuals with blastomycosis acquired the agent from the environment.

Client Education

Due to the tenacious nature of the fungus, clients should be advised that treatment may take several months. Some infections have taken over a year to resolve; luckily this is rare. In any case, relapses may occur. The client should be informed of these possibilities so as not to have unrealistic expectations of a very quick cure.

Histoplasma capsulatum var. *capsulatum*

Histoplasmosis is caused by two varieties: *H. capsulatum* var. *capsulatum* (worldwide distribution) and *H. capsulatum* var. *duboisii* (Africa). The third variety, *H. capsulatum* var. *farciminosum*, causes epizootic lymphangitis and was discussed in Chapter 20.

Reservoir

Histoplasma capsulatum var. *capsulatum* tends to inhabit sandy, acidic soil found near bodies of water, a feature is shares with *Blastomyces*. The geographic distribution of *Histoplasma* infections, though wider than that of *Blastomyces*, still centers on the Mississippi River, Ohio River and their tributaries (Figure 21.1). Sporadic cases occur worldwide. The fungal spores of *Histoplasma* are capable of surviving in the environment for long periods of time.

Host preference

Dogs and cats are the primary domestic species that act as hosts for *Histoplasma* infections. Disease due to any species of *Histoplasma* in ruminants, swine, and poultry is rare.

Transmission

Individuals become infected by inhaling microconidia or hyphal fragments. Much less common routes of transmission include ingestion and wound inoculation. Transmission has been reported in people involved in excavation activities and other activities that involve increased soil turnover and dust. Animals subjected to similar circumstances, by living in areas where these activities are occurring, are presumably also at risk for infection.

Pathogenesis

Once inhaled, *Histoplasma capsulatum* converts to the yeast phase in the lung (37°C). The organism is capable of surviving and reproducing within macrophages. These same macrophages inadvertently aid the yeast in its dissemination.

Risk factors

Risk factors for histoplasmosis are the same as those for blastomycosis.

Disease

Dogs and cats infected with *H. capsulatum* var. *capsulatum* may experience one of two main forms of the disease. The disease may be restricted to the pulmonary system; this occurs most frequently with dogs. Infections in both dogs and cats may progress to disseminated disease. This form is progressive and debilitating. Multiple tissues are affected in the disseminated form (e.g., liver, spleen, central nervous system, eyes, and bone marrow).

Diagnostics

Tissues and blood may be appropriate samples. Contact the reference laboratory for detailed instructions.

Microscopic Examination

Both cytology and histology are useful diagnostics. Macrophages with intracellular yeast forms are easily demonstrated with cytology (Figure 21.4). The yeast cells have a "teardrop" or an "eggplant" appearance to them. Histologic preparations usually require special stains to appropriately contrast the yeast organisms with the host tissue. Be sure to call the laboratory ahead of sample collection to optimize sample selection and handling.

Culture

Submit samples to a reference laboratory for culture. Round microconidia and nodular macroconidia are characteristic features of the mycelium. Yeast cells have a relatively thin cell wall and no capsule is present.

Treatment

Treatment is very similar to blastomycosis.

Human infections

Exercise caution when handling open wounds as there is potential for zoonotic transmission, though most human infections are acquired from the environment. Both the respiratory and systemic forms may occur in people. The disease is also referred to as "Ohio River Valley fever". Persons with pre-existing lung disease (e.g., emphysema) and those that are immunocompromised are at greatest risk of infection as well as more severe disease manifestations.

Coccidioides immitis

Coccidioides immitis is considered to be the most virulent fungal pathogen of all those that infect humans and other domestic animals. Because of this, *C. immitis* has been classified as a potential bioterrorist organism by the US government.

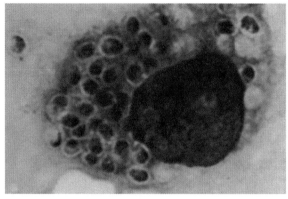

Figure 21.4: *Histoplasma capsulatum* var. *capsulatum* within the cytoplasm of a macrophage. Courtesy of the Public Health Image Library, PHIL #14423, Centers for Disease Control and Prevention, Atlanta, date unknown.

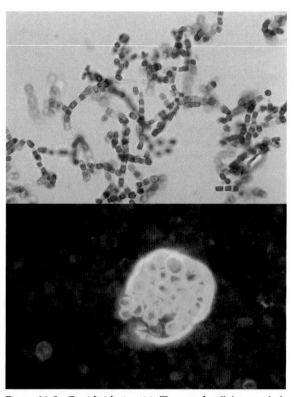

Figure 21.5: *Coccidioides immitis*. Top panel: cellular morphology consists of thick-walled hyphae containing bridge-like structures (cytology, lactophenol blue). Bottom panel: Endospores are contained within a structure called a spherule (calcofluor stain). Courtesy of the Public Health Image Library, PHIL #12196 and #481, Centers for Disease Control and Prevention, Atlanta.

The fungal morphology consists of hyphae with thick-walled or barrel-shaped arthroconidia alternating with bridge-like structures (Figure 21.5, top panel). The asexual endospores are enclosed in a structure called a **spherule** (Figure 21.5, bottom panel).

Reservoir

Coccidioides persists in the sandy, alkaline soil found in the Southwestern United States (Figure 21.1). This contrasts to the preference for acidic soil by both *Blastomyces* and *Histoplasma*. Soil disturbances increase exposure to the fungal arthroconidia. Increased release of arthroconidia also occurs after a heavy rainfall due to mechanical disturbance.

Pathogenesis

Infection begins when the host inhales or ingests the mold arthrospores (Figure 21.6). Once within the host, the fungus changes into the yeast phase within a spherule. Spherules contain endospores which divide by binary fission. Once there is no more room for the dividing endospores, the spherule ruptures, releasing endospores to infect adjacent tissues. In this way, the infection spreads within the host.

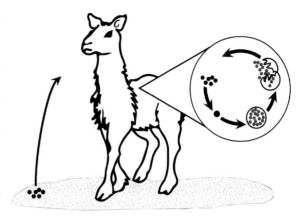

Figure 21.6: Transmission and pathogenesis of *Coccidioides immitis*. Once an animal inhales the arthrospores, typically from the soil, *Coccidioides* changes from the mold to the yeast form. The yeast produces endospores surrounded by a spherule. High production of endospores within the spherule cause the spherule to rupture thus releasing the endospores and aiding in systemic spread of the disease.

Hosts

Dogs, horses, llamas, and humans may all serve as hosts to infection. Llamas appear to be highly susceptible; disease in this species also tends to be more severe.

Clinical Disease

Most infections, approximately 80%, are confined to the lung with the remaining 20% of cases becoming systemic (Figure 21.7). Llamas, however, appear more likely to become ill with the disseminated form. Hosts with inadequate cell-mediated immunity may experience disseminated disease, occurring most commonly in the bone and skin, but potentially occurring in almost any body location.

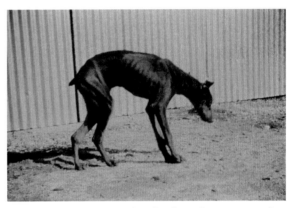

Figure 21.7: Systemic *Coccidioides* infection in a dog. Courtesy of Public Health Image Library, PHIL #15739, Centers for Disease Control and Prevention, Atlanta.

Diagnostics

Microscopic examination

Appropriate samples to examine for the presence of spherules include: sputum samples, transtracheal washes, tissues and fine needle aspirates (e.g., lymph node). Samples can be examined in wet mounts containing KOH or in fixed smears prepared with a fungal stain. Histopathology can identify both the agent and the characteristic lesions using standard cytological and/or fungal stains.

Culture

Submit samples to a reference laboratory for culture. Conversion between the mold form (arthroconidia) and the yeast form (sporangia) requires a special medium and culture conditions.

Other methods
Serology is useful for demonstrating the presence of anti-*Coccidioides* antibodies. PCR can be used to detect the agent in clinical samples.

Treatment
Systemic antifungals (amphotericin B in humans and fluconazole in small animals) have been effective in treating *Coccidioides* infections.

Prevention
Avoid bringing animals into endemic areas when possible. Avoid activities that increase exposure to dust, especially in these endemic areas.

Human infections
Humans become infected from exposure to the environment, just like veterinary species, therefore this is not considered to be a zoonotic infection. However, it is prudent to exercise caution when handling infected animals just to be on the safe side.

Cryptococcus neoformans
Cryptococcus exists as a yeast both in the environment and the tissues, making it a monomorphic yeast. The species of most concern is *Cryptococcus neoformans*. *C. neoformans* is the only encapsulated systemic mycoses infecting animals and humans. Encapsulation aids the yeast in avoiding killing by host macrophages.

Reservoirs
The two most important reservoirs of this yeast is the soil and bird (especially, pigeon) excreta. The pigeon is the major urban reservoir of this disease. The pathogen has a worldwide distribution.

Pathogenesis
Animals acquire the infection solely from the environment (Figure 21.8). No animal-to-animal transmission has been reported. This is known as a "dead-end" lifecycle. The yeast is inhaled, and due to its small size, it can travel all the way down to the alveoli of the lung. It has also been reported to enter a host via skin wounds and, in the bovine, teat mucosa. Its thick capsule helps it avoid being phagocytosed by macrophages. If, however, it finds itself within a macrophage's phagolysosome, the organism employs other mechanisms to avoid destruction. Infections can be subclinical, or involved the skin, lungs and nervous tissues. The organism has a tropism for the central nervous system due to the plentiful supply of nitrogen-containing substances that it can metabolize.

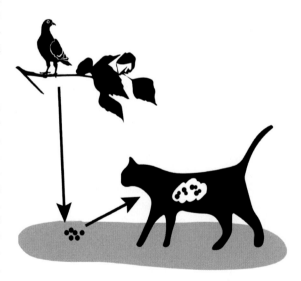

Figure 21.8: *Cryptococcus* lifecycle. Animals inhale the yeast either from the soil or bird (e.g., pigeon) droppings. Once inhaled, the yeast travels down into the lungs where it can undergo asexual reproduction. The yeast can migrate to the brain and cause meningitis. Cryptococcal organisms escape destruction by the host immune system by survival within the macrophage phagolysosome.

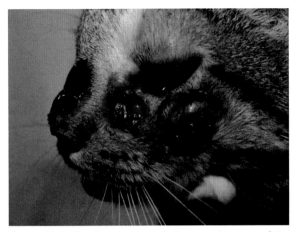

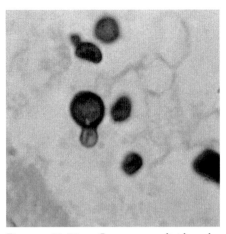

Figure 21.9: Nasal cryptococcosis in a cat. Courtesy of Dr. J. Noxon, Iowa State University, College of Veterinary Medi-cine, Department of Veterinary Clinical Sciences and the Cen-ter for Food Security and Public Health (CFSPH). Used with permission.

Figure 21.10: *Cryptococcus* divides by **narrow-based budding.** Courtesy of Public Health Image Library, PHIL #9857, Centers for Disease Control and Prevention, Atlanta, 1969.

Clinical Disease

Cats

Most often, *Cryptococcus neoformans* infection results in a fungal rhinitis. Owners may report that their cat is sneezing and has nasal discharge. If the infection invades the facial bones, distortion of the nasal cavity may result (Figure 21.9). In some cases, the infection penetrates the bony border between the nasal cavity and the brain (i.e., cribriform plate) invading the olfactory bulbs and causing meningitis.

Dogs

Cryptococcal infections are much less common in dogs than in cats. In dogs, the disease affects the respiratory tract with rhinitis that may occasionally progress to pneumonia. Infections of the skin (i.e., cutaneous *Cryptococcus*) may also occur via hematogenous spread.

Cattle

Cows acquire infection iatrogenically through contaminated intramammary treatments. While the infection seldom travels past the regional lymph nodes, irreversible damage to the mammary glands can result.

Diagnostics

Microscopic examination

Impression smears of lesions and the collection of body fluids, like nasal discharge or cerebrospinal fluid, make good samples for cytology. Slides stained with Romanowsky-type stains (Wright's and Giemsa) allow visualization of a pale or clear capsule surrounding the darker staining yeast. Sample sediment can be mixed with India ink to enhanced visualization of the thick capsule. Additionally, cryptococcal organisms divide using **narrow-based budding** (Figure 21.10). This contrasts to fungi like *Blastomyces* which divide using broad-based budding. If the slide contains budding yeast, this can be very helpful in correct species identification. Similarly, in histopathology preparations the capsule will appear as a clear zone surrounding the yeast.

Culture

Fungal culture is best performed using Sabouraud's Dextrose Agar, incubated at 25°C, and blood agar, incubated at 30°C. Microscopy and biochemical tests are used to confirm the identity of yeast colonies. Because some normal dogs and cats harbor *C. neoformans* in their nasal cavities, culture results should be interpreted in light of direct smears and/or detection of antigen in serum.

Other Methods
Serology, to identify capsular antigens of *Cryptococcus*, is also very helpful. Both serum and CSF are useful sample types. Even clinically normal dogs who harbor the organism in their nasal cavity will be negative for capsular antigen in their serum and CSF.

Treatment
Systemic antifungals, such as fluconazole and itraconazole, are the preferred treatment. In some cases, surgery to remove pockets of infection and debris may be required. Clients should be forewarned about the long treatment regimen. It is not unusual for treatment to continue for 1-2 months *past the resolution of clinical signs* so as to insure a complete cure. It is advisable to confirm that antigen is no longer present in serum and CSF before discontinuing treatment.

Prevention
Lime sulfur fungicide solutions and powders can be used to disinfect contaminated surfaces such as attics and pigeon lofts. It is critical that masks be worn by the individual performing this task to avoid infection.

Candida albicans
Candida albicans is found on the mucous membranes of most mammals and birds, and can cause disease when the host's immune system is compromised. Factors that predispose a host to candidiasis include stress or prolonged use of antibiotics, steroids or hormonal therapy.

Disease
Candidiasis is usually an infection of squamous epithelium, but occasionally can cause disseminated disease involving the respiratory system or intestinal tract. Birds experience thrush (crop mycosis) which is often fatal. Swine and foals present with ulcerative lesions in the gastrointestinal tract. Horses also can have candidiasis of reproductive organs affecting their ability to conceive and give birth to live young. Calves receiving intensive antibiotic treatment can develop disseminated candidiasis. Bovine mastitis due to *C. albicans* is usually self-limiting. Cats and dogs present with ulcerative mucosal lesions in the mouth, upper respiratory tract, gastrointestinal tract, genitals or urinary tract.

Diagnostics
C. albicans grows well on standard culture media, both those intended for bacterial and fungal organisms. Colonies are whitish and shiny, resembling bacterial colonies. Microscopically, budding yeasts can be appreciated. Because *C. albicans* inhabits clinically normal hosts, it's important to correlate culture results with disease. Better yet, visualization of *C. albicans* in direct smears from lesions can support this organism as a player in the disease process.

Treatment
Systemic antifungals (fluconazole or flucytosine) are used in cases of disseminated disease. Local infections may be successfully treated with topical antifungals. Attempts should be made to correct the underlying cause of immune disturbance; for example, stopping antibiotic treatment and reestablishing normal flora.

Aspergillus fumigatus
Aspergillus spp. are ubiquitous in nature. This mold can be found in soil, vegetation, feed, water and even the air. They are hard to avoid. *Aspergillus fumigatus* is the species most often associated with disease in animals and humans.

Disease

Because it is ubiquitous in nature, *A. fumigatus* is easily acquired by inhalation or ingestion. Luckily, some breech in the host's immune system is required for disease to develop; this is often combined with a heavy dose of exposure. Additionally, this fungus can gain entry into the bovine mammary gland via intramammary inoculation. Once the organism are present in the host tissues, the immune system quickly recognizes them as invaders and mounts an inflammatory immune response. The release of inflammatory compounds results in damage to host tissues while the fungus hides within macrophages, avoiding destruction.

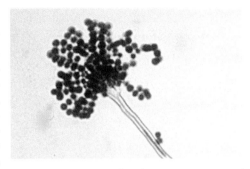

Figure 21.11: *Aspergillus fumigatus.* Courtesy of Public Health Image Library, PHIL #300, Centers for Disease Control and Prevention, Atlanta, date unknown.

Most animal species can develop pulmonary and disseminated disease, often involving the kidneys and central nervous system. Avian aspergillosis is primarily respiratory and usually associated with stress and heavy exposure. The most common presentations of bovine aspergillosis are abortion and mastitis. Dogs can be affected with aspergillosis in their nasal sinuses, so it is a differential in cases of epistaxis, especially in dolichocephalic (long nose) breeds.

Diagnostics

Microscopically, *Aspergillus* can be recognized directly in stained preparations of clinical specimens (Figure 21.11). The organism grows readily on standard fungal media, but care should be taken to obtain samples from lesions (e.g., sinus plaques). Because *Aspergillus* is ubiquitous in nature, a positive culture is not definitive of a causal relationship, and clinical signs must be correlated with culture results. For example, culturing *A. fumigatus* from a nasal swab is of little value in reaching a diagnosis.

Treatment

Systemic antifungal drugs are used to treat disseminated aspergillosis. Canine nasal aspergillosis is treated with nasal infusions while the patient is under sedation. Bovine mastitis caused by *A. fumigatus* may be treated with both intramammary and intra-arterial miconazole.

Control

Avoiding exposure altogether is simply impossible, but removal of moldy feed and bedding can prevent concentrated, high-dose exposure.

Fungal-like sytemic infection: *Prototheca*

Prototheca is a type of green algae that does not contain chlorophyll, thus it is not green in color. Protothecosis has been reported in domestic and wild animals. Ubiquitous in nature, a host may acquire *Prototheca* via ingestion, through skin wounds, or in the case of dairy cows, inoculation can occur directly into the mammary gland. (For cytology photo of *Prototheca*, see Chapter 18, Figure 18.7)

Disease

Dogs most commonly experience disseminated disease in the form of hemorrhagic diarrhea and lesions of the eyes and central nervous system. In contrast, feline and human disease is limited to the skin. Bovine mastitis due to *Prototheca* is chronic and progressive.

Diagnostics

Prototheca grows on standard fungal media as cream-colored yeast-like colonies and can be identified by microscopic and biochemical means. Direct microscopy of clinical specimen may be adequate to demonstrate the presence of the organism.

Treatment

Treatment is usually not effective in animals. Systemic anti-fungal drugs are used in human patients. Cows with mastitis due to *Prototheca* should be culled or, at the very least, milked last.

Control

Keep animals away from areas of standing water. However, because of its ubiquitous nature, infections may occur in areas with no obvious standing water.

Further Reading

Brömel, Catharina, and Jane E. Sykes. "Epidemiology, Diagnosis, and Treatment of Blastomycosis in Dogs and Cats." *Clin Tech Small Anim Pract* 20 4 (2005): 233-9.

---. "Histoplasmosis in Dogs and Cats." *Clin Tech Small Anim Pract* 20 4 (2005): 227-32.

Lloret, Albert, et al. "Rare Systemic Mycoses in Cats: Blastomycosis, Histoplasmosis and Coccidioidomycosis: ABCD Guidelines on Prevention and Management." *J Feline Med Surg* 15 7 (2013): 624-7.

Pennisi, Maria G., et al. "Cryptococcosis in Cats: ABCD Guidelines on Prevention and Management." *J Feline Med Surg* 15 7 (2013): 611-8.

Shubitz, Lisa F. "Comparative Aspects of Coccidioidomycosis in Animals and Humans." *Ann N Y Acad Sci* 1111 (2007): 395-403

.

Part IV:

Laboratory Procedures

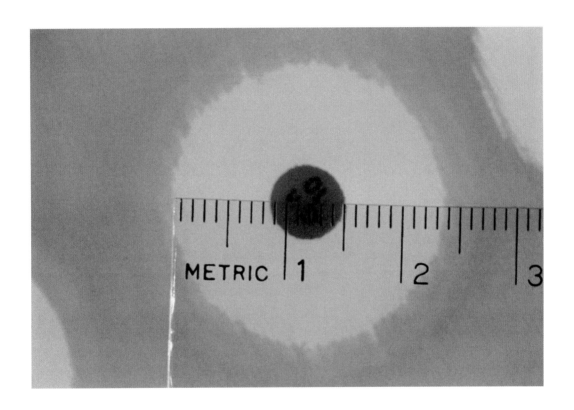

Photo (previous page):

Zone of inhibition observed during an antibiotic sensitivity test. Light micrograph. Courtesy of the Public Health Image Library, PHIL #15145, Centers for Disease Control and Prevention, Atlanta, 1972.

Chapter 22:

Bacteriological Laboratory Procedures

"Chance favors the prepared mind."

— *Louis Pasteur, 1881*

Introduction

While most veterinary clinics do not have a full service in-house microbiology laboratory, familiarity with the principles of proper sample collection and basic microbiological procedures is desirable. At first glance, the sheer number and variety of microbiological testing techniques may appear overwhelming. The purpose of this chapter, as well as the one immediately following it, will be to acquaint you with the most common techniques that the veterinary technician should at least be familiar with. Most of the following chapters will deal with techniques that can successfully be applied in most veterinary settings, be they clinical, hospital, or field. The cultivation and identification of some pathogens, however, can be potentially dangerous if done in a typical hospital or clinical setting. When a technique is best done in a specialized laboratory using special equipment or enhanced safety procedures, special mention will be made.

Sample Collection

General Principles

The importance of proper sample collection and handling cannot be overemphasized. Poor sampling technique renders culture results useless: "Garbage In equals Garbage Out". The following must be avoided: desiccation, extreme temperatures, and delays between sampling and culturing. Desiccation can be avoided by collecting an adequate amount of sample, or if a swab must be used, ensuring that it is properly placed in a moistened environment (see "Collection Devices", below). Samples should be stored only briefly in the refrigerator (~4°C) and shipped to a reference lab on an ice pack. If culturing will be performed in-house, cultures should be sent the same day as samples are collected whenever possible. It is important not to leave a sample in the refrigerator more than a few days. If, for example, a sample will be stored more than 2 or 3 days due to other lab results pending, or approval from an owner, or there is a shipping delay due to a holiday, it is best to store the sample in the freezer (i.e., approximately -20°C) instead of the refrigerator (~4°C) to avoid overgrowth of bacteria. The goal is not for bacteria in the sample to grow during transport to the lab, but rather that they maintain their numbers. This way, upon arrival in the laboratory, the sample represents its state at the time of collection.

Collection Devices

There are many options of commercially available swabs and tubes for samples destined for bacterial culture. Generally speaking, the sample needs to be placed into a sterile container with no additives. Appropriate containers include red top tubes, usually used for blood collection for blood chemistries, and sterile sample bags such as Whirl-Pak® bags (Nasco). A liquid sample or tissue sample of at least 0.5 mL or 0.5 cm³ usually does not desiccate. However, achieving a sample size of at least 2 mL or 2 cm³ is desirable and will preserve anaerobes, should anaerobic culture be required. If a tissue sample is very small, as is often the case with biopsies, they can be placed in a red top tube with 0.5 to 1 mL of sterile saline. When appropriate, a swab may be used to collect material for culture. Such is the case when a piece of tissue or fluid itself is not available. For example, appropriate scenarios for use of a swab include culturing conjunctiva of a bovine patient for pinkeye, intra-operative peritoneal swabs (though, if there is free fluid in the abdomen, gathering 2 mL in a red top tube is preferred), and obtaining deep swabs of a wound or draining tract. A swab may also be useful for submitting a sample collected by fine-needle aspirate (FNA) which often is quite small. Commercial culturettes may be used, which include a sleeve with a moistened material at the end to prevent desiccation during transportation of the swab to a bacteriology laboratory. Alternately, a sterile wooden cotton-tipped swab may be used to collect the sample and then placed in a red top tube with 0.5 mL of sterile saline.

Two special situation of note include swabs for anaerobic culture and blood cultures. As mentioned above, having sufficient volume of tissue or liquid ensures survival of anaerobes. But what if only a swab sample is available and anaerobic culture is required? In those cases, special transport tubes containing a solid transport media are recommended such as Port-A-Cul™ tubes (Becton Dickinson). Blood cultures must be collected in yellow top tubes (Table 22.1) or in blood culture bottles. Contact your reference lab for their recommended method. Standard blood tubes such as red top tubes and lavender top tubes are not appropriate for blood culture. Furthermore, purple top tubes are never appropriate for samples to be cultured because these tubes contain EDTA which kills microbes.

Table 22.1: Common sample collection tubes and their uses in bacteriology

Tube top color	Additive	Primary clinical use	Use in bacteriology
Red	Coagulant	Collection of serum; serum biochemistry	Useful for biopsy collection *Not useful for blood culture*
Yellow	Sodium polyanethol sulfonate	Blood culture	Blood culture
Green	Sodium heparin anticoagulant	Collection of plasma; plasma biochemistry	*Not appropriate for use due to bactericidal effect*
Purple/lavender	EDTA anticoagulant	Collection of plasma; hematology	*Not appropriate for use due to bactericidal effect*

Media for the Culturing of Bacteria

It is perhaps only a slight exaggeration to say that there are as many types of media for culturing bacteria as there are, well, *bacteria!* It is, therefore, important to have a working knowledge of the most common types of bacterial media. **Bacterial media** is nothing more than a substrate allowing for the growth and cultivation of bacteria either on or in it. Media may be of two basic types: solid or liquid. Media consists of a special "recipe" of nutrients mixed into solution. The ingredients in a particular medium are optimized to provide the correct formulation of these nutrients to ensure the optimal growth of a particular group of bacteria. Media can be liquid or, when agar is added at varying concentrations, semi-solid or solid. Liquid and semi-solid media are generally found in tubes, while solid media can be in a tube, usually as a slant, or in a plate.

Selective, Differential, and Enrichment Media

To isolate and identify particular microorganisms, especially those from animals with infectious diseases, selective, differential, or enrichment media are often used. Such special media are an essential part of modern diagnostic microbiology, with one type of media often fitting more than one definition.

Selective Media

A **selective medium** is one that encourages the growth of some organisms but suppresses the growth of others. For example, Mannitol salt agar or MSA contains a high concentration (~7.5%- 10%) of salt (NaCl), making it selective for staphylococci (and *Micrococcaceae*) since this level of NaCl is inhibitory to most other bacteria. Another example, to identify *Clostridium botulinum* in food samples suspected of being agents of food poisoning, the antibiotics sulfadiazine and polymyxin sulfate (SPS) are added to anaerobic cultures of *Clostridium* species. This culture medium is called SPS agar. It allows growth of *C. botulinum* while inhibiting growth of most other *Clostridium* species.

Differential Media

A **differential medium** has a constituent that causes an observable change (usually a color change) in the medium when a particular biochemical reaction occurs. This change allows microbiologists to distinguish a certain type of colony from others growing on the same plate. MSA and SPS agar also serve as a differential medium (MSA contains mannitol and the indicator phenol red). Mannitol-fermenting staphylococci produce yellow colonies with yellow zones, whereas those that do not ferment mannitol produce small pink or red colonies with no color change to the medium. Colonies of *C. botulinum* formed on SPS medium are black because of hydrogen sulfide made by the organisms from the sulfur-containing additives.

Enrichment Media

An **enrichment medium** contains special nutrients that allow growth of a particular organism that might not otherwise be present in sufficient numbers to allow it to be isolated and identified. Unlike a selective medium, an enrichment medium does not suppress other microbes. For example, because *Salmonella typhi* organisms may not be sufficiently numerous in a fecal sample to allow positive identification, they are cultured on a medium containing the trace element selenium, which supports growth of the organism. After incubation in the enrichment medium, the greater numbers of the organisms increase the likelihood of a positive identification.

Bacteriological Media: Common Types

The most common types of media are discussed below. Some media are commercially available in combination plates (bi-plates) which may be convenient in private veterinary practice. For a comprehensive listing and description of the types of media and their uses, it is a good idea to consult manufactures of microbiological media, such as the Difco™ and BBL™ Manual, 2nd edition. The manual may be found online at: http://www.bd.com/ds/technicalCenter/misc/difcobblmanual_2nded_lowres.pdf. Other manufactures will have similar catalogs.

Table 22.2: Hemolytic patterns found on blood agar plates

Hemolysis pattern	Changes to media	Examples
Alpha (α) hemolysis	Partial lysis of red blood cells with reduction of hemoglobin to methemoglobin result in greenish discoloration of medium	*Enterococcus faecalis*
Beta (β) hemolysis	Complete lysis of red blood cells; complete breakdown of hemoglobin and used by the microorganism; the area appears lightened (yellow) and transparent	*Streptococcus canis* *Streptococcus equi ssp. equi* *Staphylococcus aureus* *Streptococcus pseudintermedius*
Gamma (γ) hemolysis	No lysis no change in the media	*Pasteurella multocida*

Blood Agar

Due to the rich nutrients most bacteria can extract from red blood cells, serum, and plasma proteins, blood agar is a good all-purpose enriched media. Blood agar is also useful in differentiating organisms that can cause the hemolysis, or breakdown, of red blood cells. Sheep's blood is used because its hemolysis is more clearly defined than other blood from different species when used in the agar medium. Hemolytic patterns are detailed in Table 22.2 and may be visualized in Figure 22.1. Pathogenic bacteria are generally β-hemolytic.

MacConkey Agar (MAC)

MacConkey Agar (MAC) is a combination agar in that it is both selective and differential. MAC is available with many different formulations that have slightly different ingredients. Therefore it is critical that the veterinary technician be aware of what specific MAC formulation is needed for a given sample. The basic formulation of MAC contains Crystal Violet, bile salts, and Neutral Red. Crystal Violet and bile salts inhibit growth of gram-positive bacteria while allowing growth of gram-negative bacteria. MacConkey agar also contains the sugar lactose plus a pH indicator (i.e., Neutral Red) that turns colonies of lactose fermenters red and leaves colonies of non-fermenters colorless and translucent. Although there are some exceptions, most organisms that are normally found in the human intestines ferment lactose, whereas most pathogens (disease-causing microorganisms) do not. For example, *Salmonella* sp. are non-lactose fermenters (colorless colonies) and *E. coli* ferment lactose (pink colonies).

Mannitol Salt Agar (MSA)

MSA is both a selective and differential media as discussed above in the section "Selective, Differential, and Enrichment Media".

Tryptic Soy Agar (TSA)

Tryptic Soy Agar (TSA) is a general-purpose agar used most commonly to prepare an inoculum for antimicrobial susceptibility testing by the Kirby Bauer disk diffusion method. See "Antibiotic Susceptibility Testing" section later in this chapter.

Mueller Hinton Agar

Mueller Hinton Agar is used mainly to prepare an inoculum for antibiotic susceptibility testing by

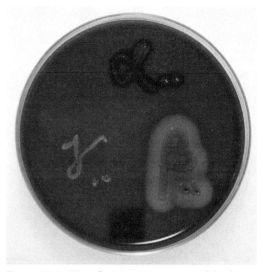

Figure 22.1: Hemolysis patterns seen on blood agar media. Clockwise from top: alpha hemolysis (green discoloration of agar), beta hemolysis (complete lysis of RBCs and clearing of agar), and gamma "hemolysis" (non-hemolytic). For a more detailed explanation of how hemolysis patterns are formed, see chapter text.

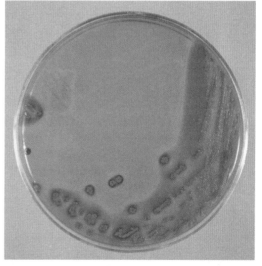

Figure 22.2: MacConkey (MAC) agar. MAC contains Crystal violet and bile salts that inhibit the growth of gram-positive organisms, thus selecting for gram-negative bacteria. In addition, phenol red is an indicator used to determine if the organism is a lactose-fermenter (pink colonies) or non-fermenter (colorless colonies).

the broth microdilution method. For fastidious organisms, 5% sheep's blood may be added to the formulation.

Selective and Differential Media for *Salmonella*

Xylose-Lysine-Desoxycholate Agar (XLD) Agar
Desoxycholate inhibits gram-positive organisms. Phenol red is the pH indicator, and colonies appear yellow to yellow-red when the media is acidic. *Salmonella* revert the pH to an alkaline state, resulting in transparent or red colonies. *Salmonella* colonies also have a black center due to H_2S production, detectable in this media due to the indicator (ferric ammonium citrate) and sulfur source (sodium thiosulfate). A variation of this formula is xylose-lysine-tergitol 4 (XLT4) agar, which has been shown to be superior for recovery of non-typhi *Salmonella* from chicken and poultry farm environmental samples.

Desoxycholate Inhibits Gram-Positive Organisms.
Phenol red is the pH indicator in this media, and colonies appear yellow to yellow-red when the media is acidic. *Salmonella* revert the pH to an alkaline state, resulting in transparent or red colonies. *Salmonella* colonies also have a black center due to H_2S production, detectable in this media due to the indicator (ferric ammonium citrate) and sulfur source (sodium thiosulfate). A variation of this formula is xylose-lysine-tergitol 4 (XLT4) agar, which has been shown to be superior for recovery of non-typhi *Salmonella* from chicken and poultry farm environmental samples.

Brilliant Green (BG) agar
A high concentration of brilliant green dye selects against most gram-positive and gram-negative bacteria. Phenol red is the pH indicator which results in yellow-green colonies of sucrose and lactose fermenters, and white to reddish pink colonies with a surrounding red zone for non-fermenters such as *Salmonella*. *Salmonella* serovar Typhi is inhibited by brilliant green dye so BG agar cannot be used for its isolation.

Selective Broths
Selective enrichment broths can be a helpful first step when attempting to isolate *Salmonella* from fecal or intestinal samples. In tetrathionate broth, bile salts select against gram-positive organisms and tetrathionate inhibits normal intestinal flora. In selenite broth, selenite inhibits coliforms and enterococci, and cystine enhances the growth of *Salmonella* spp.

Anaerobes: Special Considerations
As mentioned previously, anaerobes can be maintained in a sample if there is enough quantity of the sample or if the

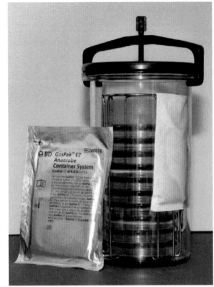

Figure 22.3: An anaerobe jar: chemical induction method. The container of the jar has a screw top lid and O-ring allowing it to be completely sealed from outside air. Air in the chamber is removed using a chemical reaction in which hydrogen gas is produced (GasPak™, Becton Dickinson). The hydrogen combines with the available oxygen and generates water, thus effectively removing free oxygen from the chamber.

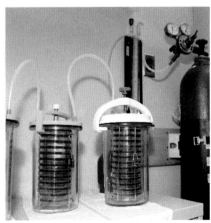

Figure 22.4: Multiple anaerobic jars set up in a reference laboratory. Here, instead of relying on a chemical method to remove available oxygen, the jars are connected to a continuous source of pressurized gaseous carbon dioxide in the form of a CO_2 tank. Photo taken with permission of the Animal Disease Diagnostic Laboratory (ADDL), Purdue University, West Lafayette, IN.

sample is placed in a transport container designed to preserve anaerobes. Once in the diagnostic laboratory, samples are applied to appropriate media which is incubated under anaerobic conditions. A common non-selective enriched media for anaerobes is Brucella agar, a blood agar supplemented with vitamin K and hemin. Selective and differential media are available for specific anaerobes such as cycloserine cefoxitin fructose agar (CCFA) plates for *Clostridium difficile* and Bacteroides bile esculin (BBE) plates for *Bacteroides fragilis*. Media must be pre-reduced (i.e., have excess oxygen removed), by reducing agents or by storing under anaerobic conditions. Anaerobic conditions can be created in multiple ways: anaerobic chamber, jars or pouches. An anaerobic chamber offers incubator space and bench space such that subcultures and identification can be performed under anaerobic conditions. Pouches and jars can be made anaerobic by use of sachets or connection to gas tanks containing an anaerobic mix. Historically, anaerobic conditions were created in candle jars which involved sealing a jar with a lit candle inside along with the culture plates. The candle would burn out once the flame had consumed most of the oxygen in the jar. The candle jar method has been largely supplanted by chambers as well as modern jars (Figures 22.3 and 22.4) and pouches; however, it remains an effective method for creating anaerobic conditions.

Inoculating Solid Media

A routine setup may include a blood agar plate to support general growth and a MacConkey plate for selection and differentiation of gram-negative organisms. If the sample is from a normally sterile site, then an enrichment broth such as thioglycolate may also be inoculated. If *Salmonella* is the species of interest, tetrathionate broth should be inoculated in addition to selective and differential plates such as XLT4 and brilliant green. Other bacteria require special conditions and will not grow on blood or MacConkey agars or in thioglycolate broth. These organisms include *Campylobacter* sp., *Chlamydia* sp., *Mycoplasma* sp., *Anaplasma* sp. and anaerobes.

Isolating Single Colonies of Bacteria on Agar Plates

A pure culture of a bacterial species is necessary for identification purposes. Theoretically one bacterial cell will form one bacterial colony, so a mixed bacterial population is "streaked out" on a solid agar medium in order to separate and spread out the bacterial cells. From each viable cell, one bacterial colony will develop after incubation. The most popular method is the **quadrant streak method** (Figure 22.5). Briefly the following procedure is followed.

1. The first quadrant of the agar plate is inoculated by a loop that has just been dipped in broth or liquid sample, or has touched to surface of a colony. The loop is gently brought into contact with the agar surface of quadrant ① and streaked back and forth. (Alternately, quadrant ① can be inoculated by directly touching the cut surface of a tissue sample to

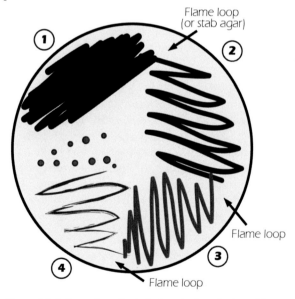

Figure 22.5: Procedure for isolating single colonies of bacteria on solid agar media. The method relies on using an inoculation loop to which some bacteria are adhered. Each time the loop touches the surface of the agar, bacteria adhere to the agar. Each pass of the loop across the agar surface helps to dilute out the density of bacteria, making isolation of single colonies possible. The procedure is also sometimes referred to as "streaking for isolated colonies". For a detailed description, see chapter text.

the agar.)

2. Flame the loop and cool. Note: If using pre-sterilized plastic loops, stab agar between streaking of each quadrant. Do not flame the loop as this will cause it to melt. When streaking is complete in all four quadrants, safely dispose of the contaminated plastic loop in a biohazard container.

3. Streak once or twice into quadrant ① to pick up the organism, then draw the loop into quadrant ② and streak back and forth several times.

4. Flame the loop and cool.

5. Repeat step 3 twice more (quadrants ③ and ④) to carry fewer organisms into the subsequent quadrants. Keep streak lines close together and cover rest of plate, taking care not to return to a previous quadrant. Isolated colonies are expected in quadrant ④.

A pure culture on an agar plate must be judged visually. If you see a colony on the plate which differs from the majority, it may be a mutant of the same species or it may be a contaminant. If you suspect a contaminant, determine whether it likely came from the source culture or whether it simply contaminated your agar plate (e.g., from the environment). If it is on a streak line, the contaminant may be throughout your culture. If the colony is not on a streak line, then it is probably a surface contaminant, and the rest of the source from which this streak was obtained is probably okay. To confirm the purity of the culture, a Gram stain is performed on a typical isolated colony. The pure culture can be used to inoculate other media and tests to identify the organism.

Inoculating Liquid Media

Once a pure culture is obtained using agar plates, differential and selective media in tubes are often used for the determination of biochemical properties, motility, etc. Liquid media can be inoculated from a solid or liquid culture source. Use a sterile needle to touch the top of a well-isolated colony from solid media, or a loop to obtain a loopful of liquid culture and inoculate the surface of the liquid media. Always sterilize the transfer apparatus (loop or needle) before and after transferring.

> In order to inoculate solid media in a tube, the following steps are used:
>
> 1. Heat-sterilize a wire needle or use the needle end of a disposable plastic apparatus.
> 2. Touch the top of a well-isolated colony on an agar plate.
> 3. Open tube and stab the needle straight down to the bottom of the tube.
> 4. Withdraw the needle as straight as possible.
> 5. If the tube you are using has a slant surface, you may streak the slant surface in a zig-zag motion after you have done the stab.
> 6. Loosely cap the tube and incubate as desired.
> 7. Heat sterilize wire needle or disinfect plastic needle.

Biochemical Tests

Catalase Test

Catalase is the enzyme that breaks down hydrogen peroxide (H_2O_2) into water (H_2O) and oxygen (O_2). Using an inoculating loop, a small amount of culture (1-2 small colonies) is mixed into a drop of H_2O_2 on a clean microscope slide. If a bacteria produces the catalase enzyme, the enzyme will begin to break down the hydrogen peroxide almost immediately resulting in the release of oxygen, evidenced by the generation of bubbles. In bacteria that do not carry the catalase enzyme, there will be no bubbles released or, rarely, only a few scattered bubbles. Catalase testing is done mainly on gram-positive cocci to differentiate between *Staphylococcus* (catalase positive) and *Streptococcus* (catalase negative) species. Caution: be careful to not pick up blood agar along with the colonies as this can result in a false positive result.

Coagulase Test

The coagulase test identifies whether an organism produces the enzyme coagulase, which causes the fibrin of blood plasma to clot. Organisms that produce coagulase can trigger blood plasma clotting and form protective barriers of fibrin around themselves, making the bacteria highly resistant to phagocytosis, other immune responses, and some other antimicrobial agents. Coagulase exists in two forms: bound coagulase (also called "clumping factor"), which is bound to the cell wall, and "free coagulase", which is liberated by the cell wall. Bound coagulase is detected by the slide coagulase test, whereas both bound and free coagulase are detected by the tube coagulase test. The coagulase test is usually performed to differentiate between coagulase-positive and coagulase-negative *Staphylococci*. Most pathogenic *Staphylococcus* species are coagulase-positive, however there are exceptions. *S. aureus* produces coagulase (i.e., coagulase-positive) whereas *S. epidermidis* does not (i.e., coagulase-negative).

Oxidase Test

The oxidase test is a test used in microbiology to determine if a bacterium produces certain cytochrome C oxidases. Oxidase enzymes play a vital role in the operation of the electron transport system during aerobic respiration. Cytochrome oxidase catalyzes the transport of electrons from donor compounds (NADH) to electron acceptors (oxygen). In the oxidase test, an artificial final electron acceptor N,N,N',N'-tetramethyl phenylenediamine dihydrochloride (TMPD) is used in the place of oxygen. This acceptor is a chemical that changes color to a dark blue/purple when it takes the electron from cytochrome oxidase in the electron transport chain. The oxidase test aids in differentiation among members of the genera *Pasteurella* and *Pseudomonas*, which are oxidase-positive, and Enterobacteriaceae (e.g., *E. coli* and *Salmonella*), which are oxidase-negative. Commercial products such as swabs or plastic slides are also available that contain oxidase reagent and will turn pink to dark purple when a heavy inoculum of an oxidase-positive organism adheres to the product.

Urease Test

The urease test determines the ability of microorganisms to degrade urea by means of the enzyme urease. Urease is a hydrolytic enzyme that attacks urea and forms the alkaline end product ammonia, which can be detected in the media by pH indicator phenol red. The presence of ammonia created alkaline environment that causes phenol red to turn to a hot pink color. This is a positive reaction for the presence of urease. Failure of a hot pink color to develop is evidence of a negative reaction.

Indole Test

The indole test determines if an organism is able to produce indole from deamination of tryptophan by tryptophanase. This test can be performed in a tube or on a piece of filter paper. The tube test uses either Ehrlich reagent or Kovac's indole reagent, and a positive test is evidenced by a red ring forming at the interface of medium and reagent phase or at the surface of the medium, respectively. The spot indole test is performed by applying a colony to a piece of filter paper moistened with the test reagent, and a positive result appears as blue to blue-green color development.

Methods of Performing Multiple Biochemical Tests

Many diagnostic laboratories use identification systems that contain a panel of biochemical tests, such as the Enterotube™ test (Benton Dickinson BBL™) or the Analytical Profile Index (API)® (bioMérieux). These systems allow simultaneous determination of an organism's reaction to a variety of carefully chosen diagnostic tests from a single inoculation. The advantages of these systems are that they use small quantities of media, occupy little space in an incubator, and provide an efficient and reliable means of making positive identification of infectious organisms.

Analytical Profile Index (API)

The API consists of a plastic tray with 20 microtubes called cupules, each containing a different kind of dehydrated substrate for the demonstration of enzymatic activity and carbohydrate fermentation (Figure 22.6). Each cupule medium is rehydrated and inoculated with a suspension of bacteria from an isolated colony. The tray is incubated; the metabolic end products are detected by indicator systems or the addition of reagents. Carbohydrate fermentation is detected by color change in the pH indicator, test results are determined, and a set of values (i.e., 1, 2, and 4) are determined and summed for seven test sets. There are three tests per test set. The seven-digit profile number identifies the organism. An example of the API system is the API-20E test. This test kit is useful for identifying bacterium usually found in the gastrointestinal system (i.e., the enterics) such as *Escherichia coli* and *Salmonella* species.

Automated Biochemical Testing

Platforms also exist for performing multiple biochemical tests with automated reading and interpretation such as the Vitek® (bioMérieux) and Omnilog® (Biolog) systems. After testing is complete, a printout is available detailing the reaction of each biochemical test and an identification of the organism with a level of confidence. The confidence in the identification is based on how well the biochemical profiles match that of the species in the software database.

Other Test Methods

MALDI-TOF MS

Matrix Assisted Laser Desorption Ionization – Time of Flight Mass Spectrometry (MALDI-TOF MS) is a method, currently only available in reference laboratories, for identifying bacteria based on

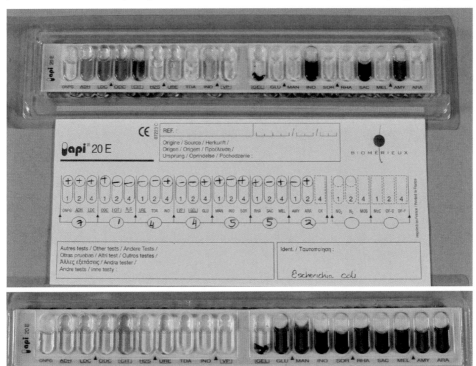

Figure 22.6: Analytical Profile Index (API) test. This system tests for up to 20 different biochemical tests from the same bacterial isolate. The test uses color indicators to indicate a positive or negative test result. **Top Panel:** API20E results for an isolate identified as *Escherichia coli*. Included is the worksheet for figuring out the seven-digit profile number. **Bottom panel:** shows the API20E as it appears when all of the individual tests are negative. For a more detailed explanation of the test, see chapter text.

their protein profiles and not on biochemical tests. A single colony is applied to a metal target (plate) and overlaid with a matrix that positively charges the proteins. As the laser blasts the bacteria on the target, proteins are released from the target and travel through a vacuum tube to a detector which senses the positive charges. The results are represented as a mass spectrum made up of multiple peaks of different intensity and size – determined by the time it took each protein to travel from the target to the detector (time of flight). Each spectrum is mapped to a database and an identification is made along with a confidence score. This entire process is complete in minutes, instead of the hours (often overnight) required for traditional biochemical tests.

Polymerase Chain Reaction (PCR)

PCR is a useful tool in microbiology laboratories for rapid detection of organisms from animal samples. PCR methods are carefully designed to detect a specific piece of DNA that is only found in the organism of interest. For example, a fecal sample can be submitted for PCR to test for a specific pathogen or panel of pathogens, such as *Salmonella*, but not to check for all bacteria present in the sample. PCR can also be used to further characterize isolates from the bacteriology lab based on the presence of certain toxin genes, for example. The identification of toxin genes in intestinal isolates of *E. coli* and *Clostridium perfringens* supports their contribution to clinical signs, whereas without this evidence they may be considered normal intestinal flora.

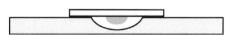

Figure 22.7: Motility tube test. The three test tubes show results of the motility tube test (from left to right): stab line (just inoculated); a non-motile organism (24 hours growth) with growth only just along the stab line; a motile organism (24 hours) with growth far from the stab line indicating motility.

Other Specialized Tests

Motility Tests

Many of the bacteria discussed in this book are motile, such as *Escherichia coli* and *Salmonella*. The two most common tests used to determine if a bacteria is motile are the motility tube test and the hanging drop method.

Motility Tube Test

Motility test medium is a semisolid agar that supports the growth of most non-fastidious organisms and permits the movement of motile bacteria (like *Listeria*). An inoculum of the bacterium is stabbed into the agar using an inoculating needle or loop. As the cells use up the nutrients in the area of the initial stab line, they must either cease growth (non-motile) or move to areas of the medium that still contain nutrients (motile) (Figure 22.7)

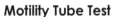

Figure 22.8: Hanging drop method for determining motility. This method requires a glass slide with a concave depression. A drop of liquid culture that has been incubated for 2-4 hours is placed on a glass cover slip. The cover slip is then inverted onto the glass slide.

Hanging Drop Method

The hanging drop method is useful when examining motility of bacteria inoculated into liquid media. A drop of liquid culture that has been incubated for 2-4 hours is placed on a glass cover slip. The cover slip is then inverted onto a glass slide that has plastic ring "spacer" attached to it or that has a concave depression (Figure 22.8). The slide is then ready at 400X using a light microscope. Motile bacteria move purposefully through the media. Brownian motion, a slight "jiggling" of the bacterium back-and-forth with no specific trajectory, is not motility.

CAMP Test

The CAMP test is based on interacting hemolysins and whether they enhance or inhibit one another. It is named after its creators: Christie, Atkins, Munch-Petersen. It is commonly used to confirm identification of *Streptococcus agalactiae* (not strongly beta-hemolytic on its own). *S. agalactiae* produces CAMP factor which enhances the β-hemolysis of *S. aureus* by binding to already damaged red blood cells. The two bacteria are streaked perpendicular to one another on blood agar without touching. An isolate is considered CAMP-positive if enhanced hemolysis, seen as an arrowhead of increased hemolysis (Figure 22.9), is produced between the two streaks. Other organisms that have a positive CAMP reaction with *S. aureus* include: *Rhodococcus equi*, *Corynebacterium renale*, and *Listeria monocytogenes* (weakly CAMP-positive).

Reverse CAMP Test

A modification of the CAMP test, the Reverse CAMP test is commonly used to identify *Corynebacterium pseudotuberculosis*. *S. aureus* is streaked perpendicular to *C. pseudotuberculosis* in the same manner as the CAMP test (see above). *C. pseudotuberculosis* exports substances into the media that inhibit the effect of the staphylococcal hemolysins (Figure 22.10). In contrast, *C. pseudotuberculosis* has a positive CAMP reac-

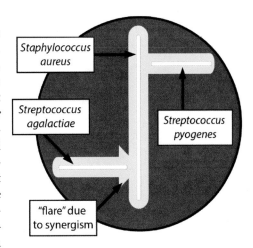

Figure 22.9: The CAMP test. The test is used to identify those bacteria that produce CAMP-factor, a substance that when contacting the red blood cells already damaged by B-hemolysis and actually enhances the β-hemolysis creating a hemolytic "flare" or arrowhead. In this illustration, *S. pyogenes* is β-hemolytic, but CAMP-negative. *S. agalactiae* is both β-hemolytic and carries the CAMP factor, thus the flare is seen at the intersection of *S. agalactiae* and *S. aureus*. *S. pyogenes* is included as a negative-CAMP isolate (negative control)

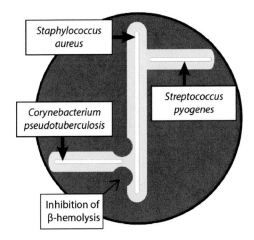

Figure 22.10: The Reverse CAMP test. This test is used primarily to identify *Corynebacterium pseudotuberculosis*. *Corynebacterium* exports a substance into the blood agar that inhibits the β-hemolysis produced by S. aureus, thus creating a "notching" effect (thin arrow). S. pyogenes is included as a positive control for β-hemolysis.

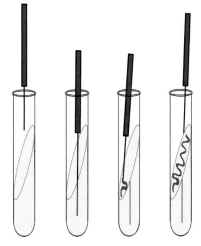

Figure 22.11: Procedure for setting up a TSI slant (Left to right): The stab stick is introduced into the agar slant tube taking care not to touch the mouth or sides of the tube. Next, the agar is stabbed using a perpendicularly. Upon withdrawing the needle of the stab stick, the needle is drawn back and forth over the agar slant surface, inoculating the surface.

tion with *Rhodococcus equi*. Often *C. pseudotuberculosis* suspects are streaked perpendicular to both *S. aureus* and *R. equi* for identification.

Triple Sugar Iron (TSI)

All enterobacteria are capable of fermenting glucose, and the small amount (0.1%) will be attacked preferentially and rapidly. At this early stage both butt and slant will be yellow due to acid production. Phenol red, the pH indicator in the media, turns yellow under acidic conditions and red under alkaline conditions. After glucose utilization, however, under aerobic conditions, the slant will revert to the red alkaline condition if the organism cannot ferment lactose or sucrose. This is because of the oxidative breakdown of proteinaceous substrates leading to alkaline pH (e.g. deamination). The relatively anaerobic butt will remain yellow (i.e., acidic). To allow this oxidative deamination reaction to occur, the TSI medium must always be used in loosely-capped tubes. To illustrate this, *Salmonella* has a red over yellow TSI reaction and produces H_2S which appears as a black precipitate in the bottom of the agar.

If the organism can ferment lactose and/or sucrose in addition to glucose, the lactose and/or sucrose will now be attacked resulting in acid production, and the medium will be acidic (yellow) throughout. Lactose and sucrose are present in 1% quantities so there is sufficient quantity to maintain acid conditions in the slant, which will remain yellow. For example, *E. coli* has a yellow over yellow TSI reaction.

Gas production is evidence by lifting of the butt of the tube, with or without obvious gas bubbles. Organisms that typically produce gas include *Salmonella*, *E. coli*, *Enterobacter*, *Citrobacter* and *Klebsiella*, for example.

RODAC Plates

Replicate Organism Detection and Counting (RODAC) plates are solid agar microbial media plates used for the detection and enumeration of aerobic bacteria present on a surface (e.g., surgery table). RODAC plates are most often used to assess the efficacy of a sanitization program (e.g., within a clinic, hospital, or laboratory).

An example of a proper sanitation procedure is as follows: First, the room and all surfaces are cleaned to remove any organic material (e.g., dirt, blood, pus) that may be present. Use soap and water. Once the surface has dried, an appropriate disinfectant is applied to the clean surfaces and allowed to sit for a designated amount of time. *The time needed to properly disinfect a given surface is dependent upon the particular disinfectant used and which microbial agent(s) you are trying to kill or inactivate.* Once the disinfected surface has dried, the veterinary technician may validate the efficacy

---

How to Use a RODAC Plate:

1. Remove the lid of the RODAC plate.

2. Gently touch the surface of the recently sanitized surface. This should be done within 1-2 hours of the sanitization process. Waiting longer could allow the surface to be colonized by environmental contaminants and would not accurately reflect the quality of the recent cleaning and disinfection.

3. Quickly replace the lid. This is to avoid undue contamination of the agar by environmental contaminants (e.g., from the air) not associated with the cleaned surface.

4. Incubate the plate upside down in an incubator at 37°C for 48 hours.

5. Plates are checked at 24 and 48 hours of incubation. Any bacterial colonies are noted and counted.

A 5-log reduction in organisms normally present on surfaces is considered a high-level of disinfection.

of the sanitation method through the use of a RODAC plate as follows:

ATPase Bioluminescence
Covered in Chapter 4.

Antibiotic Susceptibility Testing

Microorganisms vary in their susceptibility to different chemotherapeutic agents, and susceptibilities can change over time. Ideally, the appropriate antibiotic to treat any particular infection should be determined before any antibiotics are given. In the case of predictably susceptible bacteria, an appropriate agent can be prescribed as soon as the causative organism is identified from a laboratory culture. More often, tests are needed to show which antibiotics inhibit the organism. Several methods like disk diffusion, dilution, and automated methods are available to do this. Interpretive standards for both the disk diffusion and broth microdilution methods are established by the Clinical Laboratory Standards Institute (CLSI).

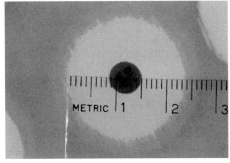

Figure 22.12: Measuring the zone of inhibition. Kirby-Bauer disk diffusion method of antimicrobial susceptibility testing. Courtesy of Public Health Image Library, PHIL #10787, Centers for Disease Control and Prevention, Atlanta, 1972.

Disk Diffusion Method (i.e., Kirby-Bauer)

In the disk diffusion method, or Kirby-Bauer method, a suspension of standard density of the causative organism is uniformly spread over an agar plate. Several filter paper disks impregnated with specific concentrations of selected chemotherapeutic agents are then placed on the agar surface, and the plate is incubated. During incubation, each chemotherapeutic agent diffuses radially from the disk. Agents with lower molecular weights diffuse faster than those with higher molecular weights.

Following the appropriate incubation times, areas around the disks where bacteria have failed to grow are called **zones of inhibition** (Figure 22.12). The size of a zone of inhibition is not necessarily a measure of the degree of inhibition because of differences in the diffusion rates of chemotherapeutic agents. An agent of large molecular size might be a powerful inhibitor even though it might diffuse only a small distance and produce a small zone of inhibition. Thus, zones of inhibition cannot be compared between agents, but instead should be compared to CLSI standards to determine the final interpretation.

Dilution Method (Minimum Inhibitory Concentration or MIC)

The dilution method of testing antibiotic sensitivity was first performed in tubes of culture broth; it is now performed in shallow wells on standardized plates. In this method a suspension of standard density of the organism to be tested is introduced into a series of broth cultures containing decreasing concentrations of a chemotherapeutic agent. Due to the conical shape of each well and the force of gravity, bacteria growing in the suspension will move to the bottom center of the well. Growth can be visualized as a whitish dot in the bottom of a well, commonly referred to as the "button". After an appropriate incubation time (usually 16 to 20 hours) the tubes or wells are examined for the lowest concentration of the agent that prevents visible growth. This concentration is the **minimum inhibitory concentration (MIC)** for a particular agent acting on a specific microorganism. This test is commercially available in 96-well plates pre-coated with antibiotic such that after adding the correct volume of the appropriate bacterial suspension, each well has a known concentration of antibiotic. This test is usually performed in reference labs using software to interpret the MIC values in light of CLSI standards to designate the tested bacterium as being sensitive, intermediate, or resistant to a particular agent.

E-Test (Formerly Known as the Epsilometer test)

Several antibiotics are available in the E-Test format (Figure 22.13). In a similar fashion to setting up a Kirby-Bauer test, a plate is inoculated and then an E-Test, a strip impregnated with a range of concentrations of an antibiotic is placed on the surface of the agar. After the appropriate incubation time, the point at which the zone of clearing crosses the strip is the MIC. Interpretive criteria is available in the product insert.

Interpretation

Zones of inhibition for the disk diffusion and E-test methods and the MIC for the broth microdilution method must be carefully interpreted. CLSI standards for disk diffusion and broth microdilution methods and product inserts for E-tests are available. Appropriate interpretation is critical since treatment decisions are often based on these results. Furthermore, it is important to recognize that these tests are based on expected serum concentrations and may not be necessary or informative if only topical therapy is being considered. Susceptibility testing results should be used as a tool to aid in developing the treatment plan for the patient, and must be interpreted in light of the patient's clinical status. If a drug with a "susceptible" interpretation is being used, but the patient is getting worse, another drug choice should be considered. If a drug with a "resistant" interpretation was chosen empirically, and the patient is getting better by the time MIC results are available, there may be no need to change the treatment plan. The diagnostic lab providing antimicrobial susceptibility testing and results should have a consulting microbiologist available to answer any questions.

Cytologic Stains Used in Bacteriology

Direct stains are a valuable tool in veterinary practice because they can provide quick information that guides the formulation of a treatment plan. This section describes the most common stains utilized in the identification of bacterial species. The basic underlying mechanics of how each stain works, general recommendations for their use, and expected results are discussed here.

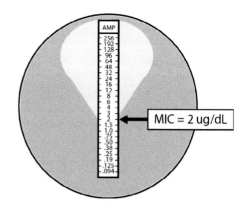

Figure 22.13: The E-test. This test is used to test the antibiotic susceptibility of bacterial isolates taken from clinical samples, similar to the Kirby-Bauer method.

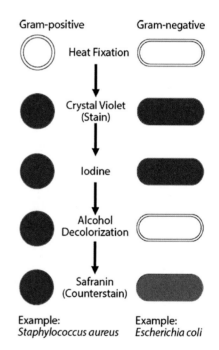

Figure 22.14: The Gram Stain, the most common cytologic stain used in bacteriology. See text for a detailed explanation of the procedure.

Stains, Decolorizers, and Counterstains

Cytologic stains greatly aid in our ability to identify specific features about bacteria. Most staining procedures consist of up to three components: the primary stain, decolorizer, and counterstain. Not all staining procedures have all three components. Some simple stains consist only of the primary stain. The **stain** is a dye that attaches to some part of the bacterium, usually irreversibly, and gives it a contrasting color to that of the general background, thus allowing for better visualization. A **decolorizer**, such as ethyl alcohol, is used to remove any unbound stain. Thus, any unbound stain present in the background is washed away leaving the remaining stain that is bound to the bacterium. At this point, some staining protocols call for the addition of a counterstain. The **counterstain** contains a pigment of a different color and targets a different structure than the main stain. The use of a counterstain is especially helpful in **differential stains**, or those staining protocols designed to differentiate between two different types of bacteria. The Gram stain and the acid-fast stain are both examples of differential stains.

Specific Stains Used in Bacteriology

Gram Stain

The most common cytologic stain used in bacteriology is, by far, the Gram stain. This relatively simple stain can be performed in clinical locations including mobile veterinary services. The simple knowledge of a sample's Gram reaction helps the veterinarian make an educated decision as to which antibiotics to prescribe. This is especially important in critically ill patients who cannot wait for culture results prior to beginning treatment.

The amount of peptidoglycan is the major determinant whether the cell will stain gram-positive or gram-negative. The staining procedure (Figure 22.14 and callout box, right) is done on a sample of bacteria that has been heat fixed to a glass microscope slide. The more peptidoglycan a bacterium possesses in its cell wall, the harder it is for the alcohol to remove the Crystal Violet. Gram-positive bacteria, with their thick peptidoglycan layer, retain Crystal Violet after the treatment with alcohol and thus appears purple when viewed under the microscope. Gram-negative bacteria, which have a thinner peptidoglycan layer, are easily decolorized and appear the color of the counterstain (pink).

The Gram Stain Procedure

Briefly, the Gram staining procedure is as follows:

1. Apply Crystal Violet (primary stain) to the sample for 1 minute.
2. Rinse with water.
3. Apply Gram's iodine solution (mordent). Wait 1 minute.
4. Rinse with water.
5. Rinse with 95% ethyl alcohol (decolorizer) until the alcohol runs clear (0-20 seconds).
6. Rinse with water.
7. Apply Safranin (counterstain). Wait 30-60 seconds.
8. Rinse with water.
9. Air dry or blot slide carefully and examine under the microscope.

Acid-Fast Stain

The cell wall of some bacteria do not Gram stain well. This is the case for bacteria of the genus *Mycobacterium*. Their lipid-rich cell wall contains mycolic acids that do not readily take up and retain the Gram stain. These bacteria are more readily stained using an acid-fast stain. The acid-fast stain is performed by serially applying carbol fuchsin (the primary stain), an acid-alcohol decolorizer, and methylene blue (the counterstain). Bacteria that are acid-fast stain red due to the retention of carbol fuchsin; essentially, these bacteria hold fast to the primary stain in the face of acid alcohol. Non-acid-fast bacteria and eukaryotic cells, such as inflammatory or skin cells, stain blue because the acid alcohol readily removes (decolorizes) the carbol fuchsin and the blue counterstain is taken up.

Methylene Blue Stain

Methylene blue is a non-specific dye. It stains most bacteria a uniform deep blue color. Therefore, it is useful in determining the presence and morphology of bacteria that may be present in a sample. However, it does not differentiate between the different genera of bacteria. Therefore, methylene blue is classified as a **simple stain**.

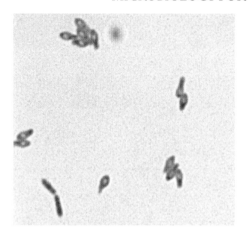

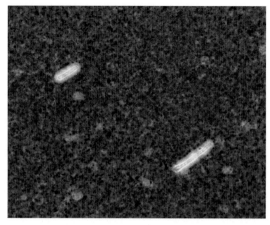

Figure 22.15: Malachite green endospore stain used to visualize the endospores of *Clostridium difficile*. Courtesy of Public Health Image Library, PHIL #1932, Centers for Disease Control and Prevention, Atlanta, 2002.

Figure 22.16: India ink stain used to observe the capsule of *Bacillus anthracis*. The background fluid and the vegetative cell pick up some of the ink stain. However, the capsule remains a transparent "halo" surrounding the vegetative cell body. Courtesy of Public Health Image Library, PHIL #1882, Centers for Disease Control and Prevention, Atlanta, 2001.

Giemsa & Wrights Stains

The Romanowsky-Giemsa and Wrights stains are used most commonly in cytology, but are also used for aiding in the identification of bacteria. Some intracellular bacteria, such as *Anaplasma* sp. in bovine blood smears and *Chlamydia* sp. in feline conjunctival scrapings, will appear blue with these stains.

Endospore Stain

Bacteria such as *Bacillus* and *Clostridium* are capable of forming endospores under harsh environmental conditions. The Dorner Method and the Schaeffer-Fulton Method are two specific endospore stains. Because the endospore is quite a hardy structure, both methods require that the stains be applied under heated conditions so as to "drive" the stain into the endospore. The Dorner Method uses carbolfuchsin and nigrosine solution in this staining procedure. The vegetative bacterium remains colorless while the endospore stains black. In the Schaeffer-Fulton Method, malachite green is the stain and safranin the counterstain. Thus the vegetative bacterium stains red while the endospore stains green (Figure 22.15).

Capsule Stain

Visualizing the capsule may be achieved via several capsule stains. Anthony's capsule stain, the Maneval method, and India ink method are some of the methods used. Unlike endospores, capsule is quite fragile. Therefore, the bacterial smear is air-dried, but not heat-fixed. Heat-fixing may distort or destroy the capsule making identification difficult to impossible. Using India ink, the ink stains the vegetative cell and the background fluid medium (Figure 22.16). By contrast, the capsule remains transparent.

Further Reading

Markey, B. K. *Clinical veterinary microbiology*. 2nd ed. Edinburgh: Elsevier, 2013. Print.

Chapter 23:

Fungal Laboratory Procedures

"To raise new questions, new possibilities, to regard old problems from a new angle, requires creative imagination and marks real advance in science."

— *Albert Einstein*

Introduction
Fungi are ubiquitous in nature. Most of the time, as members of the veterinary team, we spend most of our time trying to keep contaminating fungi out of our diagnostic cultures (e.g., bacterial or cell cultures). In this chapter, however, we will discuss methods for how to successfully isolate and identify clinical fungal specimens that cause disease in our veterinary patients.

Histopathology
Examination of an infectious agent in tissues exhibiting pathologic changes is often diagnostic. Special stains such as Gomori methenamine silver (GMS) aid in the visualization of fungi in tissues.

Molecular Diagnostics
PCR is available for certain fungal agents, and results are available usually within 24 hours in contrast to the weeks that culture may take. Caution must be used in interpreting the results of PCR alone, as many fungi are common in the environment. A positive PCR result does not necessarily indicate that the agent is the cause of clinical disease.

Culture
Fungal culture must be specifically requested when samples are submitted to a diagnostic laboratory. Simply indicating that you want a culture with no further explanation may lead to only a bacterial culture being performed. Most fungal cultures should be incubated at room temperature (25°C), but a few require incubation at body temperature (37°C).

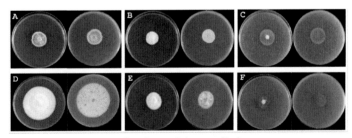

Figure 23.1: Fungi inoculated onto Sabouraud's dextrose agar, a common fungal media. From: Oh, Taek J., et al. "NMR and GC-MS Based Metabolic Profiling and Free-Radical Scavenging Activities of *Cordyceps pruinosa* Mycelia Cultivated under Different Media and Light Conditions." *PLoS One* 9 6 (2014): e90823. Open access.

Thus, it is important to include a list of the veterinarian's top differential diagnoses on the laboratory submission form. With the exception of dermatophyte culture, fungal cultures are best sent to reference laboratories with highly trained personnel and high level safety features. Dermatophyte cultures may be grown safely and successfully in-house.

Sample Collection

Specific sampling recommendations will depend on the clinical presentation. Generally, samples should be taken from a sterile site (e.g., blood, tissue, urine collected by cystocentesis) or directly from a lesion (e.g., fungal plaque in canine nasal sinus or equine guttural pouch). Some fungi are ubiquitous in the environment and are common culture contaminants, therefore typically "dirty" or contaminated samples such as nasal or skin swabs should be avoided.

Culture Media

While nutrient agars used for bacterial culture (blood agar, for example) will support fungal growth, fungi are often outcompeted by bacteria which generally grow much more quickly. Overgrowth of bacteria on a plate makes isolation and identification of fungal organisms challenging to outright impossible. To solve this problem, fungal media was designed to support the growth of fungi, while inhibiting bacteria. Fungal media may or may not include antibiotics to specifically inhibit bacteria and/or an antifungal agent to inhibit the growth of rapidly growing molds that are unlikely to be pathogens. Common fungal media include Sabouraud's dextrose agar (SDA, Figure 23.1), potato dextrose agar (PDA), brain-heart infusion (BHI), and when dermatophytes are suspected, dermatophyte test media (DTM). DTM has an additional diagnostic feature in that the agar changes color from yellow to red when a dermatophyte grows, aiding diagnosis.

Gross Examination of Fungal Cultures

Careful examination of colony characteristics on solid media is critical for proper identification. Colonies should be examined on the **obverse side** of the plate (i.e., the side that was inoculated) as well as the **reverse side** (i.e., looking through the bottom of the petri dish). Color (e.g., white, brown, yellow) and consistency (e.g., fluffy, powdery) are key features to note. Table 23.1 shows the importance of careful examination of fungal growth and its power to aid identification. It is best to check dermatophyte cultures daily so that the color change in the DTM can be correlated with growth of the dermatophyte, as any fungal growth may eventually turn the media to red.

Table 23.1: Gross examination of dermatophytes on solid DTM

Organism	Colony Color and Texture		Media color
	Obverse	Reverse	
Microsporum canis	White with yellow/orange periphery; fluffy	Yellow/orange	Bright Red
Trichophyton mentagrophytes	White-to-cream-colored; powdery	Brownish tan, colorless, red or yellow	Bright Red
Non-dermatophyte fungi (e.g., saprophytes)	Black, green or grey; various	Black, green, or grey	No Change*

* Color change must be noted on the same day that fungal growth appears.

Microscopic Examination

Microscopy is critical for examining direct preparation of clinical material and for examining growth in culture. Microscopic examination allows identification of fruiting heads and spores, which are often unique enough to allow genus or species level identification. Clinical material can be used to prepare a smear or touch prep on a glass slide. Culture material that appears fuzzy (mold-like), should be transferred to a slide using clear tape or tweezers. These methods are known as tape preps (see "A Step-by-Step Guide to Performing a Tape Prep", below) or tease preps and allow aerial hyphae to be

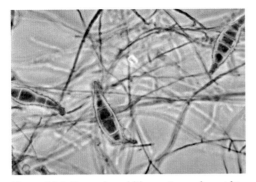

Figure 23.2: Lactophenol blue stain used to aid in the identification of fungal elements, in this case, the macroconidia of *Microsporum distortum.* Courtesy of Public Health Image Library, PHIL #4325, Centers for Disease Control and Prevention, Atlanta, 1970.

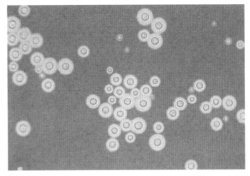

Figure 23.3: India ink preparation of cerebrospinal fluid from a patient with cryptococcal meningitis showing the budding yeast cells of *C. neoformans* surrounded by a characteristic wide gelatinous capsule. From: Kushawaha, Anurag, et al. "*Cryptococcus neoformans* Meningitis in a Diabetic Patient--The Perils of an Overzealous Immune Response: A Case Report." *Cases J* 2 (2009): 209. Open access.

gently transferred from the culture to the slide. Yeast can be transferred to a glass slide using an inoculating loop or needle, just as bacteria would be handled. Several staining techniques are useful for aiding microscopic examination of fungi.

Lactophenol Cotton Blue

Lactophenol cotton blue contains three ingredients: phenol, to kill any live organisms; lactic acid to preserves fungal structures; and cotton blue which stains the chitin present in fungal cell walls. The Lactophenol cotton blue staining technique described below can be used to examine dermatophytes as well as other non-dermatophyte fungi (Figure 23.2).

A Step-by-Step Guide to Performing a Tape Prep

1. Obtain a clean glass slide and apply a drop of Lactophenol cotton blue dye.
2. Take a small piece of cellophane ("Scotch") tape.
3. Lightly touch the tape (sticky side down) to the fungal colony you wish to examine.
4. Place the tape on the glass slide (sticky side down) and examine the specimen under the microscope.

India Ink

India ink is used mainly to visualize *Cryptococcus neoformans* and other encapsulated yeasts (Figure 23.3). India ink is unable to penetrate the capsule, so the technician will observe a dark background and unstained yeast cells.

Gram Staining

It is not recommended to Gram stain any samples to be examined for fungi or fungal elements. Gram and similar stains tend to distort the fungal morphology making successful identification difficult, if not impossible. The exception is some yeast, such as *Candida* and *Malassezia*, whose morphology can be appreciated in a Gram stained preparation. This comes in handy when Gram staining ear smears from dogs and cats, as the technician can identify both bacteria and yeast with one slide preparation.

The section below is dedicated to diagnosing a dermatophyte infection.

Culturing Dermatophytes

Dermatophytes grow best on Sabouraud's dextrose agar. This agar has peptone & glucose that the fungi can use for nutrients. It also has an acidic pH (5.6) & contains other inhibitors to inhibit bacterial growth. Dermatophytes are aerobes which grow best at 25-30°C. For this reason, you can easily culture fungi at room temperature in the clinic or hospital. Most dermatophytes take 7-10 days to grow; some take slightly longer. Therefore, *do not throw out cultures before 14 days of incubation.*

Systematic Examination

To ensure that a diagnostic sample is obtained, it is best to take a very systematic approach to collecting samples. Remember that some animals may carry dermatophytes and never show any clinical signs. Yet, these animals can be a source of infection within the household or the herd. Successful identification of dermatophytes can be achieved through a multi-step process (see sidebar).

Systematic Examination of Patients Suspected of Having a Dermatophyte Infection

1. Wood's lamp
2. Mapping suspected lesions
3. Sampling of suspected lesions
    a. Hair plucking
    b. Mackenzie brush technique
4. Growth on agar
    a. Sabouraud's Agar
    b. Dermatophyte Test Media (DTM)
    c. Other specialized agars, as needed
5. Microscopic examination of fungal morphology (e.g., Lactophenol cotton blue mount)

Remember to always wear gloves when performing diagnostic tests if a dermatophyte inspection is suspected. Dermatophytes are zoonotic organisms.

Wood's Lamp

A Wood's lamp is a hand-held device that emits long-wave ultraviolet light. Certain genera of bacteria and fungi will fluoresce under the UV light. A Wood's lamp is particularly useful in identifying dermatophyte infections. However, remember that only 50 percent of *Microsporum* spp. will fluoresce under UV light, emitting a bright green color. Areas that do not fluoresce will be cast in a blue light. Other genera within the dermatophytes (e.g., *Trichophyton, Epidermophyton*) will not fluoresce.

To use the Wood's lamp, turn on the light and angle the light so that it shines on the animal's fur and skin. Make slow sweeping motions over the length of the animal covering all surfaces of the animal. Include the face and tail, taking care to protect the animal's eyes. While using a Wood's lamp, be careful not to shine the light into anyone's (including the animal's) eyes as UV light can cause retinal damage. In areas that fluoresce, choose samples from these areas by either hair plucking or the Mackenzie brush technique (covered below).

Mapping Lesion

Because fungal infections take a fairly long time to heal, it is important to know how the infection is proceeding. *Are the lesions getting smaller? Are they getting bigger? Are their more lesions than there were at the previous exam?* For this reason, it is a good idea to "map" the lesions using a picture (Figure 23.4). Separate maps are used to record the occurrence, distribution, and extent of lesions on the dorsum and ventrum, respectively.

Hair Plucking

For visible lesions, pick an area on the edge of the ringworm lesion. This is the spot most likely to contain active fungal organisms. Easily epilated (removed) hair is likely damaged from the fungus inhabiting the hair follicle and makes an excellent sample. The hairless center of the lesion is the *least*

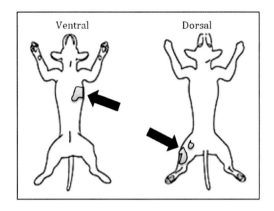

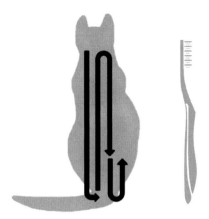

Figure 23.4: Mapping lesions. A typical map of a canine patient showing both the ventral and dorsal surfaces of the animal. Lesions are shown on both surfaces (arrows) as an example.

Figure 23.5: Typical path used to ensure systematic coverage all surfaces of the animal during the Mackenzie brush technique. This same pathway can be used for the Wood's lamp examination.

likely area to find actively growing fungi. Use a pair of clean hemostats or tweezers to pluck the hairs and transfer the hairs and inoculate fungal media (see "Dermatophyte Test Media", below).

If no areas fluoresce, yet dermatophyte infection is still suspected, proceed to performing the Mackenzie brush technique.

Mackenzie Brush Technique

This technique (Figure 23.5) is particularly useful when a patient is not showing clinical signs (i.e., no obvious lesions present) yet the animal is suspected of carrying a dermatophyte and possibly infecting others in the household or herd.

Take a clean, unused toothbrush out of its packaging. Proceed to brush the animal's entire coat using the toothbrush. Take care to cover any areas with suspected lesions. It is okay if hair sticks to the toothbrush. Use the toothbrush to inoculate fungal media.

Do not touch the toothbrush bristles with your hands. If you do, two things may happen. One, environmental fungus that are hanging out on the skin may contaminate the culture complicating the results. Two, you might infect yourself with ringworm!

Dermatophyte Test Media (DTM)

The most common media used for testing animals suspected of having ringworm is **Dermatophyte Test Media (DTM)** (Figure 23.6). DTM contains Sabouraud's dextrose agar with cycloheximide, gentamicin, and chlortetracycline as antifungal and antibacterial agents to retard the growth of contaminant organisms. It also contains a pH indicator, phenol red. The inclusion of phenol red makes DTM a differential media. There are two main ways to obtain a sample for the DTM. If a patient has obvious ringworm lesions, pluck the hairs on the periphery of the lesion as noted previously (see "Hair Plucking", above). If there are no lesions, then the Mackenzie brush technique should be used.

In this method, the sample is placed gently on

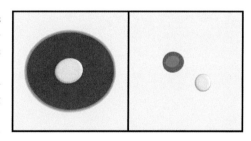

Figure 23.6: Illustration of dermatophyte test medium (DTM) with examples of possible results. Dermatophytes will grow as white colonies and cause the pH indicator (e.g., phenol red) to turn the media red (left). Environmental fungi and other non-dermatophytes will usually grow as pigmented colonies, although there are exceptions, and the media will remain pale yellow (right).

209

the surface of the media. It is okay if hair from the patient sticks to the DTM surface. The DTM is allowed to incubate at room temperature (i.e., 25-30°C) for a minimum of 10-14 days. A sample of possible results are detailed in Table 23.1.

Microscopic Examination of Pure Fungal Cultures

Once fungal colonies have grown on the fungal media of your choice, you can take a sample to examine under the microscope. One of the most useful stains for the microscopic examination of fungi is lactophenol cotton blue.

Further Reading

Larone, Davise Honig. *Medically Important Fungi: A Guide to Identification.* 5 ed. Washington, DC: American Society for Microbiology, 2011.

Part IV:

Appendices

Appendix A:

Reportable (Bacterial) Diseases

This is a list of bacterial diseases that the veterinarian is required, by law, to report to the USDA. There are currently no fungal organisms that are reportable. A variety of viruses, parasites, and prion diseases are also reportable but will not be covered here.

Bacterial Agent	Species*	Common Disease Term
Anaplasma marginale, A. centrale	B	Anaplasmosis
Babesia bovis, B. bigemina	B	Babesiosis
Bacillus anthracis	B, C, O, E, P	Anthrax
Brucella spp.	B, C, O, P	Brucellosis, Bang's Disease
Campylobacter fetus subsp. *venerealis*	B	Genital/Venereal Campylobacteriosis
Chlamydia psittaci	C,O	Enzootic Abortion Of Ewes
	A	Avian Psittacosis/Ornithosis
Cowdria ruminantium	B, C, O	Heartwater Disease
Coxiella burnetii	B	Q-Fever
Francisella tularensis	C, O, P	Tularemia
Leptospira spp.	B, C, O, E, P	Leptospirosis
Mycobacterium avium subsp. *paratuberculosis*	B, C, O	Johne's Disease
Mycobacterium bovis	B, C, O	Bovine Tuberculosis (Tb)
Mycoplasma spp.	B	Contagious Bovine Pleuropneumonia
	C	Contagious Caprine Pleuropneumonia
	O	Contagious Agalactia
Mycoplasma gallisepticum, M. synoviae	A	Mycoplasmosis
Pasteurella multocida, serotypes B/Asian or E/African	B	Hemorrhagic Septicemia
Pasteurella multocida	A	Fowl cholera
Salmonella abortus subsp. *ovis*	C, O	Salmonellosis
Salmonella gallinarum	A	Fowl typhoid
Salmonella pullorum	A	Pullorum disease
Taylorella equigenitalis	E	Contagious equine metritis

Table adapted from: Animal and Plant Health Inspection Service. "National Animal Health Reporting System (NAHRS) reportable disease list." United States Department of Agriculture, 2011. 4. Web. https://www.aphis.usda.gov/animal_health/nahrs/downloads/2011_nahrs_dz_list.pdf. Accessed on November 18, 2015.

*Species Key
A=avian (poultry)
B=bovine (cattle)
C=caprine (goats)
O=ovine (sheep)
P=porcine (pigs)

Appendix B:

Glossary of Terms

A

Adaptive immune system – a subsystem of the body's immune response composed of highly specialized system cells and processes designed to eliminate and/or prevent pathogen growth and reproduction; also referred to as the acquired immune system

Adhesins – special molecules on the surface of pathogens enabling the recognition and binding to particular host cell receptors; also known as ligands

Aerobes – those microbes that grow only in the presence of free oxygen

Agglutination – clumping (especially of red blood cells) due to crosslinking of antibodies to the surface of the cells

Alpha hemolysis – a process that occurs when a bacterial species (e.g., streptococci) contains an enzyme enabling it to reduce the hemoglobin within the erythrocytes immediately adjacent and touching the bacteria to methemoglobin; methemoglobin imparts a greenish cast on the agar; the colony appears to be surrounded by a "halo" of green

Amphitrichous – a bacterium possessing two flagella, one on each pole (end) of the bacterium

Anaerobes – those microbes that only grow in the absence of oxygen

Animalcules – the name Anton van Leeuwenhoek called the single-celled organisms we now refer to as microbes

Antagonism – drugs that when used in combination are less effective than when each is used alone

Anthroponosis – a disease where humans are the natural host and which is capable of being transmitted to animals

Anthropophilic – a microorganism (e.g., fungal organism) that is adapted to colonizing humans

Antibiotic – a drug which targets bacteria to either kill it or inhibit its growth

Antibiotic resistance – the ability of bacteria to acquire mechanisms allowing them to survive in the presence of antibiotics

Antifungal – a drug which targets fungi to either kill it or inhibit its growth

Antigen-presenting cell (APC) – a cell in the immune system which engulfs, processes, and presents foreign antigens to T-cells; cells with this function include dendritic cells, macrophages, and B-cells

Antimicrobial drug – a drug which kills a microorganism or inhibits its growth

Antimicrobial peptides – short chain amino acids that are produced by some cells of the body (e.g., skin) which are capable of killing or slowing the growth of many bacteria, viruses, and fungi

Antimicrobial resistance – the ability of microbes to acquire mechanisms allowing them to survive in the presence of antimicrobials

Antiphagocytic – the property of a component of bacteria (e.g., capsule) whereupon macrophages and other immune cells that would normally engulf (eat) the bacterium cannot do so.

Antiseptic – a chemical agent that can safely be used externally on living tissue to destroy microorganisms or to inhibit their growth

APC – see Antigen-presenting cell

Acquired immune system – see Adaptive immune system

Atopy - a condition where individuals are predisposed to develop allergic reactions to allergens that are inhaled or contact the skin. Atopy is thought to be an underlying factor in a number of skin infections

Autoclave – a chamber using high pressure saturated steam used for sterilization of equipment and supplies

Autoclave indicator tape – adhesive tape which is applied to the outside of equipment or materials (e.g., spay pack) to undergo autoclave sterilization; the achievement of a minimally effective temperature is usually shown by the tape undergoing a color change (e.g., clear to black)

Avirulent – nonpathogenic; a microbe that is incapable of causing disease in a host

B

Bacterial media – a substrate allowing for the growth and cultivation of bacteria either on or in it; it may be either liquid or solid

Bactericide – an agent that kills vegetative (actively growing) bacteria; most such agents do not kill spores

Bacterin – a vaccine made from killed or attenuated (i.e., weakened) bacteria

Bacteriocidal – a drugs capable of killing the pathogen directly

Bacteriophage – a virus capable of infecting a bacterial cell; see also Transduction

Bacteriostatic – a drug that inhibits the growth of the pathogen allowing the host immune response time to eliminate the pathogen

Bacteriostatic agent – an agent that inhibits the growth of bacteria

Beta hemolysis – complete lysis of the erythrocytes in the blood agar plate by a bacterium harboring beta hemolysins; this causes the affected blood agar to appear clear and translucent

Binary fission – process of asexual reproduction utilized by many microorganisms where the parent cell divides and produces two genetically identical daughter cells

Biofilm - a grouping of bacteria of a single species with a distinct architectural structure that can adhere to a surface and be subjected to heavy shear stress (e.g., high water velocity) without being dislodged from the surface; biofilms are made up of two main parts: a core of bacteria and an outer layer of extracellular polysaccharides

Biological indicators – a non-pathogenic microbe spore-former (e.g., *Bacillus subtilis*), used to validate that the sterilization method was adequate to kill spores, the most resistant form of microbes

Biosecurity – a set of operations or procedures designed to decrease the likelihood of a disease entering an area or facility

B-lymphocyte – a specific type of white blood cells produced in the bone marrow (or Bursa of Fabricius in birds) that is part of the humoral arm of the adaptive immune response

Botryomycosis - the chronic granulomatous reaction consisting of neutrophils and activated macrophages, present as multinucleated giant cells that surround the infection, especially in staphylococci infections

Broad-based budding – a form of asexual reproduction of some fungi (e.g., cryptococci) where the parent and daughter cells are attached by a thick neck

Broad spectrum – an antimicrobial capable of targeting a wide range of pathogens

Bumblefoot – laymen's term for chronic pododermatitis; see also Pododermatitis

C

Capnophilic – those microbes requiring 3-10% carbon dioxide in the environment to initiate growth

Capsule – an outer protective layer made up of polysaccharides produced by some bacteria

Caseous lymphadenitis – caseous necrosis of the lymph nodes; name for the condition caused by *Corynebacterium pseudotuberculosis* in sheep

Caseous necrosis – necrotic tissue that grossly appears cheese-like

Catalase – an enzyme that can break hydrogen peroxide down into oxygen and water

Cell membrane – a structural component of a bacterium consisting of a double layer of phospholipid sheets interspersed with proteins

Cell wall – made up of polysaccharides, the cell wall holds all of the constituents of the cell's cytoplasm. The bacterial cell wall acts as a protective barrier for the bacterium.

Chemoattractants – chemical compounds released from damaged or dying cells which immune cells, such as phagocytes, can sense and will migrate towards

Chromosome – a highly folded circular, double-stranded piece of DNA containing the genetic sequences encoding all of the structural and functional components of a cell. The genes that are necessary to sustain life are contained in the chromosome.

Clonal expansion – the process where one parent cell divides into two genetically identical daughter cells, which each divide into two additional daughter cells, thus causing the microbial population to double at the end of each round of binary fission

Clone – see Daughter Cells

Coccobacillus –very short bacterial rods that can be mistaken for cocci during microscopic examination

Colony – a small circular patch of clonally expanded bacteria growing on an agar plate descended from a single progenitor (parent) cell

Commensals – bacteria which live on or within the body of normal, healthy individuals; also called normal flora

Complement system – a part of the innate immune system consisting of a large number of plasma proteins that possess the ability to attach and break down pathogen cell walls, attract phagocytes, and stimulate inflammation

Conjugation – the process by which the bacterial DNA of one cell is copied and the copy is transferred to another bacterial cell using a hollow bridge-like structure known as a sex pilus; see sex pilus

Counterstain – cytologic dye that contains a pigment of a different color and targets a different structure than the main stain

Cross-wall – a new cell wall that is formed by an invagination of the growing cell wall and that then separates the growing cell into two daughter cells during binary fission.

Cystitis – inflammation of the urinary bladder

Cytokines – small proteins that are important in cell signaling, particularly in signaling and coordinating the host immune response

Cytologic stain – a dye, that when applied to cells, aids in visualization of the cell and/or cell structures

D

Dark field microscope – type of microscope which relies on oblique illumination of the subject in order to enhance visualization; typically used for very small or thin microbes, such as spirochetes; the microorganism is visualized as a bright structure on a dark background; see also Light microscope

Daughter cells – the product of a parent cell following binary fission. The daughter cells are genetically identical to the parent cell. These daughter cells may also referred to as a clone of the parent cell.

Death phase – period of time where the microbial death rate significantly outpaces the growth rate due to a severe depletion of available nutrients along with a significant increase in toxic waste products; the total number of live organisms in a culture decreases sharply

Decolorizer – substance that is used to remove any unbound stain (e.g., ethyl alcohol)

Denaturation – the process of permanently altering the three-dimensional structure of a protein, thus inactivating the protein's activity; compounds capable of causing denaturation include strong acids or bases, organic solvents, and quaternary ammonias

Dermatophyte – a superficial fungus that targets and colonizes the skin

Differential media – artificial media containing a constituent that causes an observable change (usually a color change) in the medium when a particular biochemical reaction occurs

Differential stain – a staining protocol designed to differentiate between two different types of bacteria

Dimorphic – those fungi that can take on the form of a yeast or mold depending on environmental conditions

Diptheroidal – having a shape like a club

Disinfectant – a chemical agent used on inanimate objects to destroy microorganisms

Disinfection – the reduction of the number of pathogenic microorganisms to the point where they pose no danger of disease

Disseminated intravascular coagulopathy (DIC) – a rare but often fatal condition characterized by the overwhelming systemic activation of blood clotting that results in clots lodging in multiple organs and subsequent severe organ dysfunction; after a time, clotting factors are used up and uncontrolled hemorrhaging results

Dry (oven) heat – a method of sterilization utilizing heat devoid of humidity to sterilize objects that would degrade if water vapor were added (e.g., powders)

E

Efflux pump – a channel present within the cell wall of a microbe that is capable of actively exporting antimicrobials and other compounds out of the cell

Electron microscope – type of microscope that creates an image of the sample by first bombarding it with electrons; electron microscopy allows for the visualization of objects that are as small as or smaller than 1 nanometer (nm); abbreviated EM

EM – see Electron microscope

Empiric treatment – the practice of choosing an antimicrobial based on a practitioner's "best guess" as to the identity of the pathogen; usually done while culture and antimicrobial susceptibility testing results are still pending

Endogenous infection – an infection originating from within the individual or the herd

Endospore – a small, tough, non-replicating structure produced by some bacteria in order to survive stressful environmental conditions

Endotoxic shock – host circulatory system collapse due to the actions of endotoxins, such as lipo-polysaccharide (LPS) of gram-negative bacteria

Endotoxins – poisonous parts of the microbe that can cause serious, adverse physiological effects in the host, such as fever and shock; e.g., LPS of gram-negative bacteria

Enrichment media – media that contains special nutrients that allow the growth of a particular organism that might not otherwise be present in sufficient numbers to allow it to be isolated and identified

Exogenous infection - an infection originating from within the individual or the herd

Exotoxins – poisonous proteins secreted by a variety of pathogens

F

Facultative anaerobes – those microbes that grow in either the absence or presence of free oxygen, but must obtain oxygen from oxygen-containing compounds (e.g., inorganic sulfates)

Facultative intracellular pathogens – a pathogen capable of surviving in the environment in addition to thriving within a host cell.

Filtration – physical method of removing microbes from liquids where the liquid is passed through a filter with small pores (e.g., 0.2 μm filter) and any microbes are trapped on the filter paper while the liquid portion freely passes through the filter into a sterile container below

Fimbriae – tiny, bristle-like structures distributed evenly over the entire surface of the bacterial cell

Fine needle aspirate (FNA) – a biopsy technique using a syringe and small needle

Flagella – structure of motile microbes consisting of three or more thread-like proteins, called flagellins, that are twisted upon each other like a rope; flagella are capable of spiraling and twisting (e.g., like the propeller on a motor boat) and thus capable of both powering and steering the microbe to its destination

Fomite – an inanimate object that can harbor and transmit microbial infections

Frank pathogen – see Obligate pathogen

Fungicide – an agent that kills fungi

G

Gamma hemolysis – non-hemolytic bacteria

Gangrene – is a type of necrosis due to a lack of blood supply to the tissues

Generation time – the time it takes for the process of binary fission to proceed from one parent cell to the creation of two daughter cells

Geophilic – a microorganism (e.g., fungal organism) that is adapted to living in the environment

Germ theory – Louis Pasteur's ground-breaking theory that microorganisms are the cause of many diseases

Germicide – an agent capable of killing microbes rapidly; some such agents effectively kill certain microorganisms but only inhibit the growth of others

Gram stain – the most common differential stain used by microbiologists. Invented by Hans Christian Gram in 1884, the Gram stain relies on differences in cell wall structure, especially the amount of peptidoglycan, between bacteria in order to distinguish between them. Bacterial cells are classified as either gram-positive or gram-negative.

H

Helper T-cell – lymphocyte of thymus origin (i.e., T-lymphocyte) that is involved in the adaptive immune response, particularly cell-mediated immunity

Host-agent-environment triad – the interaction of host, microbial agent, and environmental factors which, when taken together, determine if a given microbe will cause disease in a particular patient

Humoral immunity – portion of the immune system responsible for the production of antibodies, the regulation of the complement system, and the activities of antimicrobial peptides

Hyphae – threadlike filaments that make up the structure of molds

I

IgA – a secretory immunoglobulin produced by B-lymphocytes and then transported to the mucosal surfaces of the body where they prevent microbial pathogens and toxins from traversing the epithelium by a series of actions that result in the entrapment and clearance of these entities from the body; also called Secretory Immunoglobulin A

Innate immune system – a relatively non-specific secondary line of defense composed of many factors, including phagocytes, extracellular killing mechanisms, the inflammatory response, and the complement system

Intracellular pathogen – disease-causing microbe capable of surviving and replicating inside a host cell; see also Obligate intracellular pathogen

Ionizing radiation – a particle carrying enough energy to ionize or remove electrons from an atom; e.g., "x-rays"

Isolate – a pure culture derived from a single colony that arose from a single microbial organism

J

Jumping gene – common name for a transposon; see Transposon

L

Lag phase – period of time where the microbe is adjusting to its new environment and thus is not expending much energy in dividing; the number of bacteria in this phase remains relatively constant

Lancefield grouping system – a method of classifying streptococci based on the different surface antigens present among different species

Ligands – see Adhesins

Light field microscope – see Light microscope

Light microscope – an instrument using light in conjunction with optical lenses to magnify objects rendering them visible to the human eye; the most common type of microscope found in microbiology laboratories; also called light field microscope

Lipopolysaccharide (LPS) – also known as LPS. LPS is a cellular structure made up of three subunits: lipid A, core oligosaccharide and O-antigen and can produce endotoxic shock in people and animals.

Log phase – period of maximum growth rate of a microbe due to the maximum rate of binary fission taking place; also known as the logarithmic phase

Logarithmic phase – see log phase

Lophotrichous – a bacterium possessing multiple flagella located at only one pole of the bacterium

LPS – see lipopolysaccharide

Lysosome – a membrane-bound organelle located within the cytoplasm of eukaryotic cells containing degradative enzymes, such as lysozyme

Lysozyme – an enzyme produced by many host cells (e.g., epithelium, macrophages) capable of destroying bacteria through the enzyme's ability to disrupt the bacterial cell wall polysaccharides

M

MAC – see Membrane attack complex

Mackenzie brush technique – method of sampling for dermatophytes in a potential asymptomatic carrier

Macroconidia – large asexual spores (i.e., conidia) of certain fungi

Macrophage – a specific type of white blood cell capable of phagocytosing foreign material, such as microorganisms; macrophages are also antigen-presenting cells; see also Antigen-presenting cell

Magnification – how enlarged an object appears (i.e., the image size) when compared to the actual size of the object being observed

Mastitis – inflammation of the udder

Membrane attack complex – the last step in the complement system resulting in the creation and insertion of a pore into the cell wall of a bacterium resulting in its rupture and death; also referred to as MAC

Memory cell – a specific type of B-cell that is formed in lymph nodes following an initial infection and that are important in generating an accelerated, more robust antibody-mediated response in cases of subsequent reinfection with the same pathogen

Mesophiles – microbes that grow best at temperatures between 20-40 °C

Microaerophilic – those microbes that grow best in oxygen levels less than those present in ambient air

Microbes – microscopic organisms, such as bacteria, viruses, and certain fungi and parasitic organisms

Microbiology – a branch of biology that deals with microorganisms (such as bacteria, viruses, and certain fungi and parasitic organisms) and their effects on other living organisms

Microconidia – small asexual spores (i.e., conidia) of certain fungi

Minimum inhibitory concentration – the lowest concentration of an antimicrobial drug that prevents visible growth of the bacteria; also referred to as MIC

Moist heat – a method of sterilization used by most autoclaves; sterility using this method requires a minimum time, temperature, and pressure to ensure the entire object(s) placed in the autoclave is sterilized

Mold – multicellular filamentous fungi consisting of masses of threadlike filaments (i.e., hyphae)

Morbidity – a diseased condition or state

Mortality – a diseased condition or state resulting in the death of the individual; being subject to death

Monotrichous – a bacterium possessing only one polar flagella

Mucin - a group of mucoproteins released from the apical membrane of epithelial cells and that forms a protective barrier which limits the exposure to commensal bacteria and prevents adhesion of pathogenic organisms; mucins may be found in various substances of the body such as saliva, gastric juices, and other mucous secretions

Mycelium – in fungi, an intertwining mat of hyphae

N

Narrow-based budding – a form of asexual reproduction of some fungi (e.g., cryptococci) where the parent and daughter cells are attached only by a very narrow neck

Narrow spectrum – an antimicrobial that targets a limited range of microorganisms

Neutrophil – one of the most abundant white blood cells in mammals and which is one of the key cell types involved in the innate immune response; neutrophils contain special granules capable of damaging pathogens when the granules are released into the extracellular environment

Niche – a particular location or environment that a given pathogen is particularly adapted to

Non-ionizing radiation –a particle of electromagnetic radiation that does not carry enough energy to ionize or remove electrons from an atom; e.g., microwave and infrared radiation

Normal flora – see Commensals

Nosocomial infection – an infection acquired from a hospital setting

O

Obligate intracellular pathogens – a disease-causing microorganism which must live and replicate within a host cell; it cannot survive in the extracellular environment

Obligate pathogen – a disease-causing microorganism which does not survive outside of the host

Obverse side – the side of the agar plate upon which the bacteria or fungi are inoculated

Opportunistic pathogen – a microorganism which causes disease only under certain conditions, such as when the host is immunocompromised

Organic material – carbon atom-based materials (e.g., soil, dust, blood, pus) of plant- or animal-origin which can interfere in the actions of disinfectants

P

PAMPs – see Pathogen-associated molecular patterns

Parent cell – the original cell from which, during binary fission, two genetically identical daughter cells are produced; see also Daughter cells and Binary fission

Pasteurization – the process of super-heating liquids, such as milk or apple cider, to kill any viable microorganisms present

Pathogen – a disease-causing microorganism

Pathogen-associated molecular patterns – molecules of pathogens associated with cell structures such as the peptidoglycan or lipoteichoic acids within the cell wall which the host immune system recognizes as foreign or "non-self"; also referred to as PAMPs

Pathogenesis – the disease process caused by infection by a pathogen

Pathogenic – microbes capable of causing disease

Peptidoglycan – a structural polymer consisting of polysaccharide and peptide chains. The two most common components of the peptidoglycan layer are teichoic acid and lipoteichoic acid

Peritrichous – a bacterium possessing numerous flagella that are interspersed over the bacterium's entire surface

Phagocytes – immune cells that can engulf ("eat") microorganisms, e.g., macrophages

Phagolysosome fusion – the act of joining the phagosome and lysosome into one combined organelle containing the contents of both organelles: the phagocytosed material (e.g., pathogen) and the lysosomal enzymes, respectively; see also Phagosome and Lysosome

Phagosome – a membrane-bound organelle formed by the invagination of the cell membrane around a substance that the cell is engulfing ("eating")

Pili – long, thick hair-like structures made of polymerized protein molecules, called pilin

Plasma cell – antibody-producing B-cell

Plasmid – a piece of circular, double-stranded DNA capable of replicating on its own and independent from the chromosome. Helpful, but not absolutely necessary genes, are often found on plasmids (e.g., antimicrobial resistance genes). Plasmids can be exchanged between bacterial cells.

Pleomorphic – having more than one shape

Pododermatitis – inflammation of the skin, and sometimes underlying structure, of the foot

Potency – refers to the level of effectiveness of a substance, e.g., a chemical antimicrobial agent

Primary pathogen – see Obligate pathogen

Primary stain – see Stain

Prodromal period – during the development of disease, the period of time consisting of early, usually non-specific, signs of a disease that occur just before the more characteristic signs of the disease appear

Psychrophiles – microbes that grow best at temperatures between 0-30°C

Pyelonephritis – inflammation of the kidneys

Pyoderma – pus in the skin; microscopically, the predominant leukocyte is neutrophils

Q

Quadrant streak method – a method used to separate and spread out bacterial cells so as to get isolated colonies, especially for use in further diagnostic tests

Quorum sensing – the regulation of gene expression within the population of bacteria in response to the density of the cell population

R

Resolution – the shortest distance between two points on a specimen that can be distinguished visually by the observer

Reticle – an ocular ruler built-in to some light microscopes that helps to calibrate and estimate the size of objects seen through the microscope

Reverse side – looking through the bottom of the agar plate to examine that side of the bacterial or fungal culture

Ringworm – common term for a dermatophyte infection

RODAC plates – Replicate Organism Detection and Counting plates are solid agar microbial media plates used for the detection and enumeration of aerobic (i.e., oxygen-loving) bacteria present on a surface (e.g., surgery table)

S

Sanitizer – a chemical agent typically used on food-handling equipment and eating utensils to reduce bacterial numbers so as to meet public health standards. Sanitization may simply refer to thorough washing with only soap or detergent.

Saprophyte – a microorganism that lives in and derives its nutrition from dead or decaying organic material

Scanning electron microscope – a type of electron microscope used to visualize the surface of cells

Secretory Immunoglobulin A – see IgA

Selective media – artificial media that encourages the growth of some organisms but suppresses the growth of others

Selective pressure – a concept first developed by Charles Darwin, in which genetic traits that confer an advantage to an organism's reproduction and survival (or can mitigate a threat to its survival) are retained within the population

Selective toxicity – a drug which causes more harm to the pathogen than to the host; usually this is due to the ability of the antimicrobial drug to recognize structures or processes of the pathogen, but not the host

Septae – in fungi, a thin partition forming separate chambers within the hyphae

Septicemia – an infection in the blood

Sex pilus – a hollow bridge-like structure that forms between two cells for the purpose of transferring genetic material between the two cells in a process known as conjugation; see also Conjugation

Simple stain – a staining procedure consisting of only a primary stain

Sonication – a physical method of cleaning by removing organic material from a surface (e.g., surgical instruments, tooth surface) via the use of ultrasonic vibrations

SOP/SOPs – see Standard Operating Procedures

Spectrum of activity - the range of microorganisms that an antimicrobial drug can kill or inhibit

Spherule – structure of certain yeasts that encloses the asexual spores of those yeasts

Sporicide – an agent that kills bacterial endospores or fungal spores

Stage micrometer slide – a device used to calibrate the ocular reticle present in some models of light microscopes

Stain – a dye that attaches to some part of the bacterium, usually irreversibly, and gives it a contrasting color to that of the general back-ground, thus allowing for better visualization

Standard Operating Procedures – a set of written instructions that ensure uniformity and compliance with common practices and procedures of an institutions (including veterinary hospitals and clinics); e.g., how to correctly set up and run the autoclave to sterilize surgical packs; also referred to as SOPs

Stationary phase – period of time where the number of replicating microbes equals those that are dying, thus the total number of organisms in a culture appears static

Sterility – having no living organisms in or on a material

Sterilization – the killing or removal of all microorganisms in a material or on an object

Strain – a group of isolates that are indistinguishable from each other yet can be differentiated from a completely different group of isolates

Strangles – the common name for the disease caused by *Streptococcus equi* ssp. *equi*

Synergism – administration of two drugs together exerts an additive effect (i.e., a better outcome than if each antibiotic were given singly)

T

Therapeutic index – a mathematical formula used to estimate the ratio of the drug's effectiveness versus it's toxicity to the host; calculated by dividing the maximum tolerated dose of the drug by the minimum therapeutic dose; a drug with a higher therapeutic index is more effective and less toxic than one which has a lower therapeutic index

Thermophiles – microbes that grow best at temperatures between 40-80 °C

T-lymphocyte – a white blood cell originating from the thymus that is directly involved in cell-mediated immunity

Transduction – a process whereby bacterial DNA is transferred from one bacterium to another inside a virus capable of infecting bacteria (i.e., bacteriophage); see bacteriophage

Transformation – a process by which bacteria can scavenge naked DNA floating in the extracellular environment, internalize it, and incorporate it into their own DNA

Transposon – a DNA genetic element which possess the necessary machinery which allows them to not only replicate but also to "cut-out" a copy of themselves and pass that copy onto another species of bacteria

U

Ultraviolet (UV) light radiation – radiation from the short-wavelength "ultraviolet spectrum" (~280-360 nm); used as a germicidal method to kill or inactivate microorganisms by destroying or severely damaging their DNA leaving the microbes unable to replicate or perform many important cellular functions

Urolithiasis – urinary bladder stones

V

Vegetative – an actively growing and developing microbial cell

Virulence factors – attributes that enable pathogens to attach to the host, escape destruction by the immune system, and cause disease

Virulent – a highly pathogenic microbe; a microbe capable of causing significant disease and/or incapacitation of a host

Y

Yeast –oval to spherical single-celled fungi that reproduce asexually by budding

Z

Zones of inhibition – areas around the antibiotic disks where bacteria have failed to grow, such as in the Kirby-Bauer method of antimicrobial susceptibility testing

Zoonoses – a disease where animals are the natural host and which is capable of being transmitted to humans

Zoophilic – a microorganism (e.g., fungal organism) that is adapted to colonizing animals

Zoospores – motile asexual spores of some algae and lower fungi (e.g., the genus *Dermatophilus*)

Index

f=figure
t=table, sidebar, or callout box

Made in the USA
Monee, IL
22 December 2019

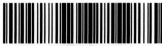